Artificial Intelligence in Medicine and Dentistry

Lobat Tayebi · Sachin Shetty · Seyedmisagh Imani

Artificial Intelligence in Medicine and Dentistry

Advancing Science, Education, and Clinical Practice

Springer

Lobat Tayebi
Department of Electrical and Computer Engineering/Institute for Engineering in Medicine, Health, and Human Performance (EnMed)
Old Dominion University
Norfolk, VA, USA

Seyedmisagh Imani
Department of Electrical and Computer Engineering/Institute for Engineering in Medicine, Health, and Human Performance (EnMed)
Old Dominion University
Norfolk, VA, USA

Sachin Shetty
Department of Electrical and Computer Engineering/Office of Enterprise Research and Innovation/Institute for Engineering in Medicine, Health, and Human Performance (EnMed)
Old Dominion University
Norfolk, VA, USA

ISBN 978-3-032-15976-2 ISBN 978-3-032-15977-9 (eBook)
https://doi.org/10.1007/978-3-032-15977-9

This Springer imprint is published by the registered company Springer Nature Switzerland AG
The registered company address is: Gewerbestrasse 11, 6330 Cham, Switzerland

Acknowledgement The authors acknowledge the use of AI-based tools for proof-reading, basic grammar and spelling checks, and improving overall readability. All content, including the attribution of ideas, is original and properly cited.

Competing Interests The authors have no competing interests to declare that are relevant to the content of this manuscript.

Introduction

Artificial Intelligence (AI) is no longer a distant promise in medicine and dentistry; it is here, shaping how we diagnose, treat, learn, and manage care. From reading complex medical images in seconds to guiding surgical decisions, from monitoring patients at home to supporting administrators behind the scenes, AI is steadily moving into the everyday fabric of health systems. What makes this moment important is not only what AI can already do, but how quickly its capabilities are expanding and how deeply they are beginning to touch both medicine and dentistry. This book was written to make that fast-moving landscape understandable, practical, and useful. It brings together the "why," the "what," and the "how" of AI across diagnosis, treatment, education, and management, so clinicians, students, researchers, and leaders can move forward with clarity and confidence.

At the heart of AI's value is its ability to see patterns in data such as images, signals, text, and longitudinal records, that are too large, too complex, or too subtle for human eyes and memory alone. In health care, that means earlier detection of disease, decision support that reduces variation, more personalized therapies, and better use of scarce resources. In dentistry, it means more consistent image analysis, earlier recognition of caries and periodontal disease, better planning of orthodontic movement and implants, and smarter chairside tools that free clinicians to focus on the patient. Equally important, AI is a team sport: computer scientists and engineers work alongside clinicians, educators, and administrators to embed tools into real workflows where accuracy, safety, equity, and trust truly matter. This book recognizes that collaboration and aims to be a shared reference, which is technical enough to be credible and plain-spoken enough to be used.

The book is organized into seven chapters, each building on the last.

Chapter 1 introduces core AI ideas in the context of health care. It defines the scope of AI and walks through key methods such as Machine Learning, Deep Learning, Natural Language Processing, Computer Vision, Robotics, and Knowledge Representation and Reasoning. It also covers performance metrics and model evaluation, sketches the chronological evolution from rule-based systems to today's data-driven approaches, and highlights current trends and future outlook. The goal is to give readers a common language and a realistic sense of what AI can and cannot do.

Chapter 2 focuses on AI in medical diagnostics. It explains how modern algorithms support radiology and imaging tasks such as detection, segmentation, and pattern recognition across X-ray, CT, and MRI and then explores early disease detection through predictive analytics, genomics, and large-scale screening programs. The chapter closes with digital pathology, where AI assists slide interpretation, tumor grading, and even molecular prediction. Throughout, the emphasis is on accuracy, workflow, and the way decision support can make diagnoses both more reliable and more timely.

Chapter 3 turns to treatment and patient care. It shows how AI helps personalize therapy using genomic and clinical data, supports chronic disease management with continuous monitoring and proactive interventions, and strengthens surgical planning and risk assessment. It also looks at robot-assisted surgery and telemedicine, where AI-enabled triage and remote monitoring extend high-quality care beyond the hospital walls. The message is simple: diagnosis is just the beginning. AI can also help select, deliver, and evaluate care.

Chapter 4 examines AI in medical education and healthcare management. On the education side, it covers intelligent learning platforms, adaptive tutoring, simulation-based training with virtual patients, and AI-supported assessment and curriculum design. On the management side, it reviews AI for hospital administration, resource allocation, governance, policy, and regulatory compliance. Together, these sections show how AI improves both how professionals learn and how institutions run, linking the classroom, the ward, and the boardroom.

Chapter 5 brings the lens to dental diagnostics. It outlines the foundations of AI in dental imaging, including enhancement, segmentation, landmark detection, and 3D reconstruction. It then reviews AI for disease detection, from caries and periodontal disease to endodontic lesions and oral cancers, and discusses clinical decision support in dentistry, commercial software solutions, and the challenges and opportunities ahead. The focus is on earlier, more consistent, and more equitable diagnostic decisions.

Chapter 6 addresses AI in dental treatment. It discusses personalized treatment planning, improvements in restorative and prosthetic workflows, orthodontic planning and prediction, AI support in endodontics, and computer-guided and robotic assistance in implantology and oral surgery. Periodontal and soft tissue therapies, as well as post-treatment monitoring and patient engagement, round out the chapter. The throughline is precision and predictability, using AI to plan better, execute safer, and follow up smarter.

Chapter 7 looks at AI in dental education and practice management. It covers how AI enhances preclinical and clinical training, supports adaptive curricula, and powers practical tools for patient scheduling, workflow, communication, and secure data management. This chapter emphasizes that modern dentistry is not only clinical; it is operational, and AI can help practices and academic clinics work more efficiently and communicate more effectively with patients.

Why does this book matter now? Because adoption is accelerating, expectations are rising, and the cost of misunderstanding AI, whether through hype or hesitation, is high. Clinicians need clear explanations and practical examples. Students need a foundation that will remain useful as tools change. Administrators need a balanced view of value, risk, and implementation. Dental professionals need resources that treat dentistry as more than a footnote to medicine. And all stakeholders need a shared, human-centered perspective that keeps patients first, while welcoming innovation.

This book aims to meet those needs. It offers a structured overview across domains, written in simple, direct language, grounded in the workflows where care is delivered and learned. It highlights both promise and limitations, so readers can make responsible decisions. Most of all, it connects the dots: between algorithms and outcomes, between diagnostics and treatment, between the simulation lab and the clinic, and between individual encounters and system-level performance.

AI will not replace the clinician, the educator, or the manager. But those who understand and thoughtfully use AI will likely set new standards for accuracy, safety, efficiency, and access. If this book helps you see what is possible, avoid common pitfalls, and design better ways to deliver dental and medical care, then it will have done its job.

Contents

Abbreviations

2D	Two-Dimensional
3D	Three-Dimensional
3D-DCGAN	3D-Deep Convolutional Generative Adversarial Network
A2C	Advantage Actor-Critic
AAE	American Association of Endodontists
Adam	Adaptive Moment Estimation
ADR	Adenoma Detection Rates
AGI	Artificial General Intelligence
AI	Artificial Intelligence
ANN	Artificial Neural Network
API	Application Programming Interface
AQS	Adaptive Quizzing System
AR	Augmented Reality
ASA	American Society of Anesthesiologists
AUC	Area Under a Curve
AUC-ROC	Area Under the Receiver Operating Characteristic Curve
AutoML	Automated Machine Learning
CAD	Computer-Aided Design
CAM	Computer-Aided Manufacturing
CBCT	3D Cone-Beam Computed Tomography
CDSS	Clinical Decision Support System
cGAN	Conditional Generative Adversarial Network
CGM	Continuous Glucose Monitor
CLO	Course Learning Outcome
CMS	Centers for Medicare & Medicaid Services
CNN	Convolutional Neural Network
COPD	Chronic Obstructive Pulmonary Disease
CPT	Current Procedural Terminology
CPU	Central Processing Unit
CRF	Conditional Random Field
CV	Computer Vision

DBSCAN	Density-Based Spatial Clustering of Applications with Noise
DCIS	Ductal Carcinoma in Situ
DDPG	Deep Deterministic Policy Gradient
DETR	DEtection TRansformer
DL	Deep Learning
DM	Dental Monitoring
DNN	Deep Neural Network
DT	Decision Tree
ECG	Electrocardiogram
ED	Emergency Department
EDR	Electronic Dental Record
EEG	Electroencephalogram
EHR	Electronic Health Record
ER	Estrogen Receptor
FAIR	Facebook AI Research
FDA	U.S. Food and Drug Administration
FID	Frechet Inception Distance
FKGL	Flesch–Kincaid Grade Level
FL	Federated Learning
FNN	Feedforward Neural Network
FP-Growth	Frequent Pattern Growth
GAN	Generative Adversarial Network
GBM	Gradient Boosted Machine
GDPR	General Data Protection Regulation
GLCM	Gray-Level Co-occurrence Matrix
GPT	Generative Pre-trained Transformer
GPU	Graphics Processing Unit
Grad-CAM	Gradient-weighted Class Activation Mapping
GRU	Gated Recurrent Unit
H&E	Hematoxylin and Eosin
HER2	Human Epidermal Growth Factor Receptor 2
HESI	Health Education Systems, Inc.
HIPAA	Health Insurance Portability and Accountability Act
HMD	Head-Mounted Display
HMM	Hidden Markov Model
IoT	Internet of Things
IoU	Intersection-over-Union
IPGx	Interprofessional Pharmacogenomics
K-NN	K-Nearest Neighbor
KR&R	Knowledge Representation and Reasoning
LA-PSO	Linearly Adaptive Particle Swarm Optimization
LASR	Levels of Autonomy in Surgical Robotics
LF-CNN	Late Fusion Convolutional Neural Network
LinReg	Linear Regression
LLM	Large Language Model

LMS	Learning Management System
LogReg	Logistic Regression
LSA	Latent Semantic Analysis
DT	Decision Tree
ECG	Electrocardiogram
ED	Emergency Department
EDR	Electronic Dental Record
EEG	Electroencephalogram
EHR	Electronic Health Record
ER	Estrogen Receptor
FAIR	Facebook AI Research
FDA	U.S. Food and Drug Administration
FID	Frechet Inception Distance
FKGL	Flesch–Kincaid Grade Level
FL	Federated Learning
FNN	Feedforward Neural Network
FP-Growth	Frequent Pattern Growth
GAN	Generative Adversarial Network
GBM	Gradient Boosted Machine
GDPR	General Data Protection Regulation
GLCM	Gray-Level Co-occurrence Matrix
GPT	Generative Pre-trained Transformer
GPU	Graphics Processing Unit
Grad-CAM	Gradient-weighted Class Activation Mapping
GRU	Gated Recurrent Unit
H&E	Hematoxylin and Eosin
HER2	Human Epidermal Growth Factor Receptor 2
HESI	Health Education Systems, Inc.
HIPAA	Health Insurance Portability and Accountability Act
HMD	Head-Mounted Display
HMM	Hidden Markov Model
IoT	Internet of Things
IoU	Intersection-over-Union
IPGx	Interprofessional Pharmacogenomics
K-NN	K-Nearest Neighbor
KR&R	Knowledge Representation and Reasoning
LA-PSO	Linearly Adaptive Particle Swarm Optimization
LASR	Levels of Autonomy in Surgical Robotics
LF-CNN	Late Fusion Convolutional Neural Network
LinReg	Linear Regression
LLM	Large Language Model
LMS	Learning Management System
LogReg	Logistic Regression
LSA	Latent Semantic Analysis
LSTM	Long Short-Term Memory

LUAD	Lung Adenocarcinoma
LUSC	Lung Squamous Cell Carcinoma
MaxEnt	Maximum Entropy
MDP	Markov Decision Process
MIDAS	Meaningful Integration of Data Analytics and Services
MIRS	Master Interview Rating Scale
ML	Machine Learning
MLP	Multi-Layer Perceptron
MPCA	Morphological Principal Component Analysis
MR	Mixed Reality
MSE	Mean Square Error
NLG	Natural Language Generation
NLP	Natural Language Processing
NLU	Natural Language Understanding
NN	Neural Network
NPV	Negative Predictive Value
OMFS	Oral and Maxillofacial Surgery
OPMD	Oral Potentially Malignant Disorder
OR	Operating Room
OSCC	Oral Squamous Cell Carcinoma
OSCE	Objective Structured Clinical Examination
PACS	Picture Archiving and Communication Systems
PALM	Perceptual and Adaptive Learning Module
PAR	Peer Assessment Rating
PBL	Problem-Based Learning
PCA	Principal Component Analysis
PDC	Partial Dental Crown
PDR	Polyp Detection Rate
PII	Personally Identifiable Information
PLO	Program Learning Outcome
PMS	Practice Management System
PPO	Proximal Policy Optimization
PPV	Positive Predictive Value
PR	Progesterone Receptor
PRS	Polygenic Risk Score
RBF	Radial Basis Function
R-CNN	Region-based Convolutional Neural Network
RF	Random Forest
RL	Reinforcement Learning
RNN	Recurrent Neural Network
ROC	Receiver Operating Characteristic
RPD	Removable Partial Denture
RPM	Remote Patient Monitoring
RR	Relative Risk
SaMD	Software as a Medical Device

SAS	Surgical Apgar Score
SGD	Stochastic Gradient Descent
SHAP	SHapley Additive exPlanations
SMOTE	Synthetic Minority Over-sampling Technique
SSD	Single Shot MultiBox Detector
STAR	Smart Tissue Autonomous Robot
SVM	Support Vector Machine
TPU	Tensor Processing Unit
TREWS	Targeted Real-Time Early Warning System
USMLE	United States Medical Licensing Examination
VAE	Variational Autoencoder
VDC	Virtual Dental Clinic
ViT	Vision Transformer
VOA	Virtual Operative Assistant
VR	Virtual Reality
VUS	Variants of Uncertain Significance
WHO	World Health Organization
WSI	Whole Slide Imaging
XAI	Explainable Artificial Intelligence
XGBoost	Extreme Gradient Boosting
YOLO	You Only Look Once

Chapter 1
Introduction of Artificial Intelligence in Healthcare

In this chapter, we introduced Artificial Intelligence (AI) in health care and explored its capabilities in advancing clinical outcomes and operational efficiency. The chapter investigated the general functions of AI in health care, including diagnostic processes, personalized medicine, patient monitoring through wearables, and the more efficient operation of health care organizations. We stressed the collaborative nature of the approach, where computer scientists and engineers work together with medical scientists and service providers to deploy AI solutions into established health care systems to advance these capabilities.

We introduced Machine Learning (ML), Deep Learning (DL), Natural Language Processing (NLP), and Computer Vision (CV) as specific types or methodologies of AI with extensive applications in healthcare. In addition, we briefly outlined other important branches such as Robotics and Knowledge Representation and Reasoning (KR&R), which play a growing role in areas like surgical assistance, rehabilitation, and structured decision support in both medicine and dentistry. We also discussed performance metrics and evaluation strategies for AI models and their role in assessing reliability and usefulness. The chronological evolution of AI from early rule-based expert systems to today's data-driven approaches was also highlighted to show how technical progress and clinical needs have shaped one another over time. Finally, the chapter presented a perspective on how AI can possibly change health care by creating more effective, accurate, and accessible approaches, while opening new avenues for the integration of AI in dentistry alongside broader medical applications.

L. Tayebi et al., *Artificial Intelligence in Medicine and Dentistry*,
https://doi.org/10.1007/978-3-032-15977-9_1

1.1 Definition and Scope of AI

AI is a rapidly developing, multidisciplinary field focused on building intelligent machines to perform actions typically assumed to be done by humans. The eventual goal of AI is to replicate or mimic human cognitive processes such as perception, reasoning, learning, prediction, decision-making, and other complex mental tasks [1, 2]. The greatest strength of AI lies in its ability to extract useful and unbiased information from large and complex datasets—far beyond what an individual human mind could feasibly analyze. With unprecedented computing capacity, the development of powerful algorithms, and their implementation through open-source architectures such as frameworks, Application Programming Interfaces (APIs), and training databases, AI has proven helpful in many areas, including agriculture, autonomous vehicles and robotics, health, education, business, marketing, social media, finance, and more [3–15].

Different types of classifications were proposed to categorize AI. One common categorization is based on the AI's level of capability, including Weak AI and Strong AI [16–21]. Weak AI, also known as Narrow AI, refers to systems designed for specific tasks and have expertise in a limited domain, such as voice assistant systems like Siri and Alexa or recommendation and image recognition systems. Strong AI, also known as General AI or Artificial General Intelligence (AGI), refers to systems with human-like cognitive abilities across a spectrum of tasks. These systems would be able to understand, learn, and apply knowledge across various domains. Since Strong AI is almost exclusively theoretical at this time and has few applicable examples, this book will focus on Weak AI and its subcategories. In this context, many AI methods and techniques can aid in the advancement of healthcare applications. The next section will discuss these AI methodologies to demonstrate the function and output of each method and their potential use in medical and dental sciences.

1.2 AI Methods and Techniques

Subsets of AI are shown in Fig. 1.1. Among these subsets, ML, DL, NLP, and CV have a variety of applications in healthcare. AI also includes Robotics and KR&R. These AI techniques and algorithms are designed to enable computers to process complex data faster and with greater accuracy. Given the relevance of these areas to healthcare, the following sections will briefly review their concepts and applications.

1.2.1 Machine Learning

As a core field of AI, ML focuses on the design and implementation of complex algorithms that enable computers to learn from large datasets and subsequently make

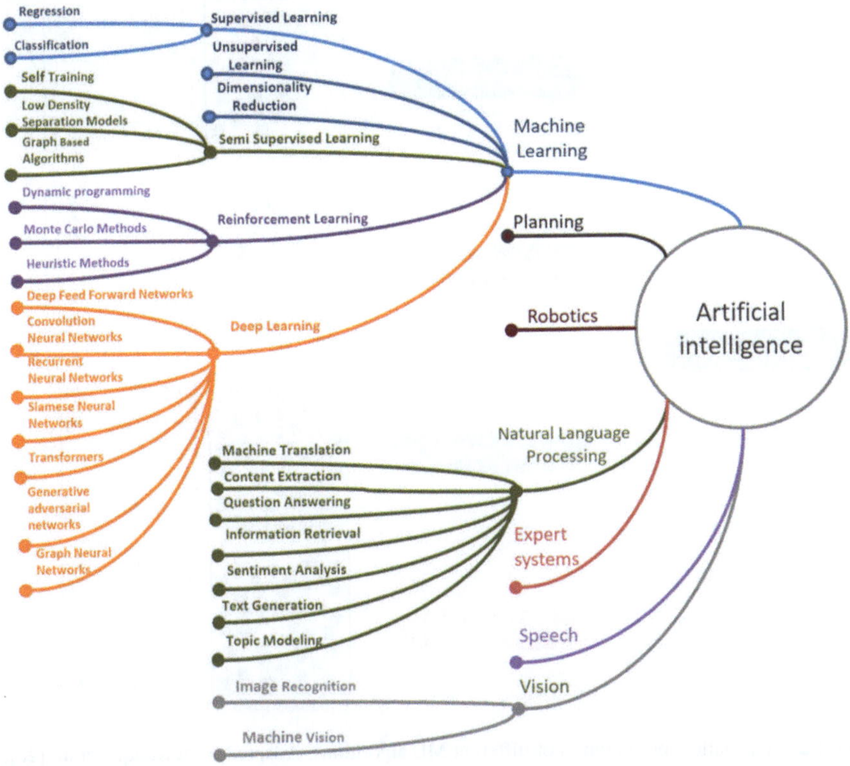

Fig. 1.1 Subsets of AI. Reproduced from Mukhamediev et al. [22], published in Mathematics 10 (2022) 2552, under the Creative Commons Attribution 4.0 International License (CC BY), (https://creativecommons.org/licenses/by/4.0/)

intelligent forecasts or decisions without being expressly programmed [23, 24]. This approach has shown considerable capability to uncover complex patterns and relationships in diverse datasets accurately. In addition, machines continuously improve themselves through continuous learning mechanisms, working interactively with experimental observations over time while dramatically improving overall performance far past what scientists imagined many years ago on early versions of these systems.

The objective of ML is to take the known data in its feature space and make predictions about unseen or unlabeled data. There are two main phases to the development of an ML model: training and testing. During the training phase, the ML model obtains knowledge from its labeled or unlabeled inputs and forms an idea of the relationships in the data. The training inputs are saved in feature space for predictions in the future. During testing, the ML model utilizes the knowledge gained in training phase to produce the appropriate output to the new input data. The degree to which an ML model is useful is based on how well it has been trained. It is also

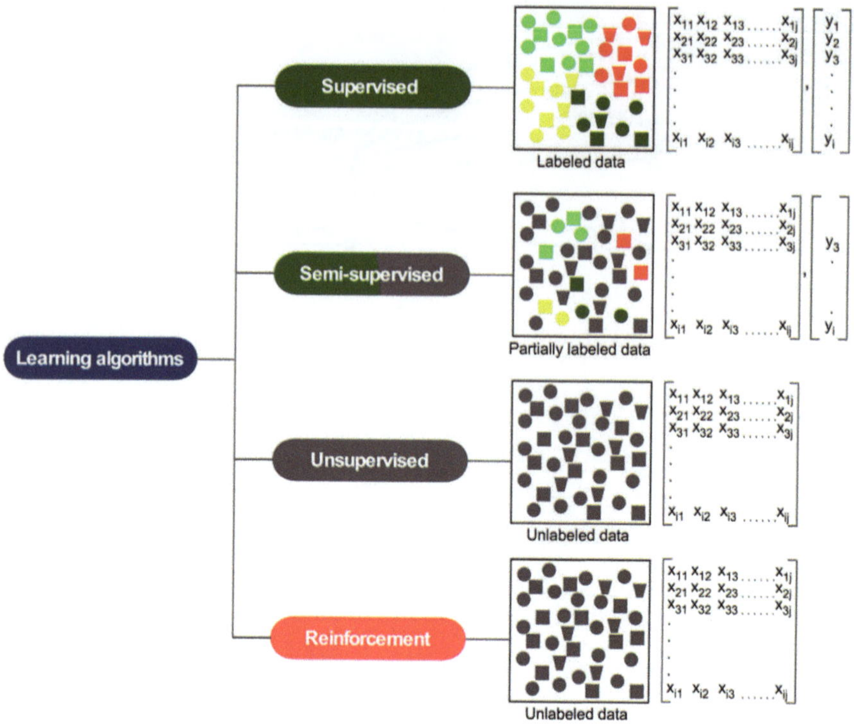

Fig. 1.2 Schematic representation of different ML algorithms. Adapted from Rafique et al. [26], published in Computational and Structural Biotechnology Journal 19 (2021) 4003–4017, under the Creative Commons Attribution 4.0 International License (CC BY), (https://creativecommons.org/licenses/by/4.0/)

important to note that the ML model can improve its accuracy and effectiveness through continued training and improvement.

According to Fig. 1.2, ML algorithms include four main categories: Supervised, Unsupervised, Semi-supervised, and Reinforcement Learning (RL) [25]. Each includes multiple common algorithms that are widely used in ML applications. A summary of these learning types is presented in Table 1.1 to provide a concise description of each, their model-building approach, and the key advantages and limitations associated with each type.

1.2.1.1 Supervised Learning

Supervised learning is a key type of ML where a model learns from labeled pairs of inputs coupled with corresponding outputs. Labeling is the means by which the model understands the relationship between the features and the target outputs. The essence of supervised learning is to learn a predictive function that generalizes to

Table 1.1 Types of ML algorithms. Adapted from Pugliese et al. [25], published in Data Science and Management 4 (2021) 19–29, under the Creative Commons Attribution 4.0 International License (CC BY), (https://creativecommons.org/licenses/by/4.0/)

Learning type	Description	Model building	Pros and cons
Supervised learning	Data are labeled with classes and outcomes (task-driven approach)	Models learn from labeled data. This type of learning comprises classification, regression, Naïve Bayes classification, random forests, and neural networks	Pros: exact idea about the classes in the training data; find out exactly how many classes are there before giving the data for training; helpful in classification problems; predict a numerical target value from given data and labels Cons: limited in a variety of sense so that it cannot handle some of the complex tasks in machine learning; it cannot cluster or classify data by discovering its features on its own; training and classification need a lot of computation time, especially if the data set is very large, which will test the machine's efficiency
Unsupervised learning	Data are not labeled. The algorithm optimally separates the samples into different classes on the basis of the features of the training data alone, without corresponding labels (data-driven approach)	Models learn from unlabeled data. This type of learning comprises *k*-means clustering, hierarchical clustering, and Principal Component Analysis (PCA)	Pros: It can detect what human eyes cannot understand; the potential of hidden patterns can be powerful for the business as it can detect fraud detection; output can determine the unexplored territories and new ventures for businesses; the outcome of an unsupervised task can yield an entirely new business vertical or venture Cons: It is expensive as it might require human intervention to understand the patterns and correlate them with the domain knowledge; it is not always certain that the obtained results will be useful since there is no label or output measure to confirm its usefulness; it is heavily dependent on the model and in turn, on the machine, and the results often have lesser accuracy

(continued)

Table 1.1 (continued)

Learning type	Description	Model building	Pros and cons
Semi-supervised learning	The algorithm works with labeled and unlabeled data	Models are built using combined labeled and unlabeled data. This type of learning includes both classification and clustering	Pros: It is easy to understand; it reduces the amount of annotated data used Cons: Iteration results are not stable; it is not applicable to network-level data; it has low accuracy
Reinforcement learning	The algorithm operates sequentially to automatically evaluate the optimal behavior in a particular context or environment to improve its efficiency (environment-driven approach)	Models are based on reward or penalty. This type of learning uses classification	Pros: It can be used to solve complex problems that cannot be solved by other techniques; it is preferred to achieve long-term results, which are very difficult to achieve; its model is very similar with the learning of human beings; the model can correct the errors that occurred during the training process Cons: Too much reinforcement learning can lead to an overload of states, which can diminish the results; it needs a lot of data and a lot of computation

unseen data so that it can make accurate classifications or predictions based on learned patterns. Supervised learning is very common in different real-world applications, such as healthcare and finance, as it is an expressive, tractable method for handling structured data.

Supervised learning typically consists of a dataset of input variables (features) and output variables (labels). The supervised learning algorithm learns by iteratively understanding the relationship between features and labels by minimizing a loss function, which is defined as the degree to which predicted values differ from actual values. Supervised learning approaches are commonly divided into two broad families, including classification and regression [27].

i. **Classification**: The model learns how to sort the input data into specific categories. For example:

    medical diagnostics: AI models are trained on labeled patient data to classify diseases, such as diabetes or cancer [28, 29],
    spam detection: the model learns to classify emails as spam or not spam using labeled email datasets [30],
    image recognition: classifying medical images as normal or abnormal, such as identifying pneumonia in chest X-rays [31].

ii. **Regression**: The model predicts continuous numerical values as outputs rather than discrete classes. For example:

predicting patient recovery time based on clinical parameters [32],
predicting blood glucose levels from continuous glucose monitoring data [33],
forecasting stock prices using historical market data [34].

Different algorithms are used in supervised learning, each with unique characteristics and use cases. In what follows, we briefly present some common supervised learning algorithms that are widely used in healthcare applications. Readers may refer to [35, 36] for further details on different supervised learning algorithms and their applications.

- **Linear Regression (LinReg)**: LinReg is one of the most basic and yet effective algorithms for regression tasks. It describes the relationship between independent variables ($x_1, x_2, \ldots, x_k$) and a dependent variable (y) as [37]:

$$y = \beta_0 + \beta_1 x_1 + \beta_2 x_2 + \cdots + \beta_k x_k + \epsilon \tag{1.1}$$

where k is the number of regressors or predictor variables, $\beta_0, \beta_1, \beta_2, \ldots, \beta_k$ are the regression coefficients learned from the data, and ϵ is the error term. LinReg has several applications, such as estimation of healthcare costs [38] and blood pressure deterioration trends [39].

- **K-Nearest Neighbor (K-NN)**: The K-NN algorithm is a basic, non-parametric, instance-based ML algorithm used for both classification and regression [27, 40]. K-NN is different from many parametric models because it does not make specific assumptions about data distribution but rather uses the training dataset itself to guide predictions. The general idea is to judge how similar a new, unlabeled data entry is to existing samples in feature space by calculating distances. K-NN then predicts a label for this new data entry based on the labels of the k closest neighbors.

In classification situations, the K-NN model classifies the observations by voting among the k nearest labeled neighbors and choosing the class that has the highest proportion. In the case of regression, it usually takes the mean (or a weighted mean) of that neighborhood's target values. The variable k is an important hyperparameter that can affect the performance of the model. If you have too few neighbors (e.g., $k = 1$), it can easily lead to overfitted results with high variance, while a large k (as k approaches the total number of training samples) will lead to overly averaged results that may wash out meaningful distinctions or oversimplify class boundaries. Selecting an appropriate k-value is critical to providing the highest probability of having neither overfitted nor underfitted results.

Another important consideration in K-NN is how neighbors are weighted. A neighbor can be given an arbitrary weight based on distance to their target value. Intuitively, we expect points that are closer to share more similarity than points that are farther away. In cases where the features are heterogeneous, it is also important to normalize or scale your features. An attribute with larger values can dominate the calculation of distance to a given point. For example, if one feature goes from 1 to 100 and all of the others go from 0 to 1, the larger-valued feature will dominate unless all features are scaled.

K-NN can be computationally expensive for large datasets since it does not create a separate training model; instead, distances are computed during inference time. For each new query, we need to compare the query point against all points in the existing dataset; this can take a long time in the case of large or high-dimensional datasets. But K-NN is easy to understand, implement, and update with new data because it is simple and does not have parameters, and predictions are explained transparently because inference is based on observed "neighbors" rather than learned, abstract parameters.

K-NN has been successfully applied across a vast number of healthcare disciplines because of its ease and ability to accommodate structured and unstructured medical data simultaneously. It is often helpful for disease diagnosis, for example, to assess the probability of heart disease [41] and/or diabetes [42, 43] by analyzing patient data. K-NN is widely useful for medical image classification, as it can detect abnormalities—for example, diagnosis and/or tumor detection by evaluating radiology scan data in MRI and CT images [44–46]. K-NN can also be effective for genomic studies, where it can predict gene expressions and identify genetic markers associated with diseases [47, 48]. In drug response prediction, K-NN models analyze patient data to suggest tailored treatment plans based on patient data and their historical response patterns [49]. In the case of Electronic Health Record (EHR) analysis, K-NN can assist with patient risk stratification and help identify high-risk patients for timely preventive interventions, resulting in optimized hospital resource allocation [50]. Overall, K-NN is a powerful tool in healthcare applications because of its flexibility, ability to handle complex datasets with few parameters, and generally lower requirements for ML applications. For these reasons, K-NN continues to be very useful in healthcare applications across all categories, particularly where interpretability and real-time decision-making are needed.

- **Decision Tree (DT)**: DTs split data into subsets based on one or more features and depict that split in a visual, tree-like representation where each interior node represents a decision made based on a feature, each branch corresponds to the possible values or outcomes of that decision, and each leaf node is a final prediction or classification. For numerical features, DTs typically split data at specific threshold values. In contrast, categorical features are divided into groups along different branches. Once trained, the model traverses the tree from root to leaf and makes predictions based on that traversal. DTs are highly interpretable and are often used in applications such as medical diagnosis [51–53], assessing financial risk [54], and approving loans [55].
- **Random Forest (RF)**: RFs work in much the same way as DTs, with the added advantage of robustness. RFs improve upon DTs by making a group of trees and then using a combination of each tree's predictions to yield one average final prediction (in the case of regression) or majority vote (in the case of classification).

Each tree in a RF is based on a random subset of the data and uses different random groups of features. RFs have been used in genetic analysis [56], detection of tumors [57], and in drug discovery [58].

- **Support Vector Machine (SVM)**: SVM is a powerful supervised ML algorithm used mainly in supervised classification and regression tasks. Its advantage lies in its strength in high-dimensional spaces. SVM is also a very suitable approach for cases where the number of labeled samples is less than the number of features [59]. An SVM does this by constructing an optimal hyperplane that separates the classes in the dataset in a way that maximizes the margin between the closest data points, known as support vectors. The learning approach using margins allows for robust generalization performance. SVM has found applications in many areas in health care due to its robustness in complex and high-dimensional biomedical data. In particular, SVM has had successes in the field of biomedical imaging in finding anomalies in MRI and CT scans, including tumor classification and lesion segmentation [60]. Likewise, SVM is very common for breast cancer detection in screening mammograms [61], brain tumor classification [62], and lung disease detection from radiological images [63].
- **Neural Network (NN)**: One of the most important building blocks of modern AI and ML are NNs, which are based on how our brains work. NNs consist of layers of interconnected processing units, called neurons, forming an adaptive system capable of learning from data. Each neuron takes in information, processes and weights it, applies an activation function, and outputs a value. NNs operate through different layers of neurons that make up the network. Each network learns patterns based on the weightings assigned during its training. The training itself uses some form of learning algorithm, such as backpropagation, which adjusts the weights in the NN to minimize error and improve accuracy.

The most common types of NNs include Feedforward Neural Networks (FNNs), Recurrent Neural Networks (RNNs), and Radial Basis Function (RBF) networks. FNNs, the most basic type of NNs, are commonly used for problems such as pattern recognition, signal processing, and classification. In an FNN, starting with input data, the data travels through multiple hidden layers before reaching the output layer, following a one-directional path. RNNs are designed for sequential data processing, as they include loops that allow access to previous data time frames. RNNs are particularly well-suited to healthcare applications involving time-series data, including analysis of electrocardiogram (ECG) and electroencephalogram (EEG) signals [64, 65], detection of cardiac arrhythmias [66], analysis of brain activity [67], and monitoring patient vitals over extended periods [68]. One of the more widely used RNNs is the Long Short-Term Memory (LSTM) network, which addresses the issue of vanishing gradients and enables long-term dependencies in medical records and clinical predictions [69].

In addition, RBF networks are commonly used, though they differ from typical NNs. RBF networks contain radial basis functions that serve as activation functions. These networks offer useful and accurate solutions to a range of problems, such as function approximation and classification tasks. In healthcare, RBF networks have been used for disease progression modeling and early-stage identification of diseases like Alzheimer's [70] and Parkinson's [71].

In healthcare, NNs have been pivotal for automating complex decisions and enhancing the accuracy of medical diagnoses. For example, NNs have been used in the interpretation of medical signals, helping doctors analyze physiological data from wearable sensors and monitoring devices [72]. Additionally, they are applied in bioinformatics for analyzing gene expression to classify diseases and personalize treatment strategies [73]. They have also been implemented in medical decision support systems that coordinate clinical workflows and optimize resource allocation in hospitals [74].

Even though NNs have become commonplace in society, they still pose challenges regarding interpretability and computational requirements. Unlike traditional statistical models, NNs are often considered black-box models due to their lack of explainability. This presents a significant concern in high-stakes applications like medicine, where transparency is crucial. While foundational NNs offer impressive predictive capabilities, researchers are working to make them more interpretable through methods such as attention-based mechanisms and rule-extraction techniques, aiming to foster transparency and trust in AI-assisted healthcare applications [75].

Additionally, NNs require substantial computational resources and large datasets to generate effective, accurate, and meaningful results, which may exclude smaller medical institutions that cannot afford such infrastructure. Hardware accelerators, such as Graphics Processing Units (GPUs) and Tensor Processing Units (TPUs), have helped improve training and inference efficiency. Readers may refer to [76, 77] for further details on NN algorithms and their applications.

1.2.1.2 Unsupervised Learning

Unsupervised learning is an important form of ML that allows models to examine unlabeled data in order to find patterns, relationships, and structures without predefined categories. In contrast to supervised learning with labeled data, unsupervised learning studies the data to reveal its intrinsic properties, which is useful in various areas like healthcare, genomics, and medical imaging. The categories of unsupervised learning are clustering and association [27].

i. **Clustering**: Clustering is perhaps the most fundamental unsupervised learning technique, as it categorizes data points by similarity. Clustering can be applied in healthcare applications such as identifying disease subtypes, assigning risk levels to patients, and recommending personalized treatments. For example, Khalid et al. [78] used clustering algorithms to examine patient pain patterns during the weeks following knee replacement surgery by grouping patients into subgroups based on their post-surgery pain outcomes. Similarly, Bose & Radhakrishnan [79] employed hierarchical clustering and *k*-means clustering to categorize heart failure patients into risk categories based on telehealth data. Important clustering algorithms include:

- **K-Means Clustering**: This algorithm categorizes data into k clusters by assigning points based on their proximity to cluster centroids. K-means clustering is often used for patient segmentation and disease classification. For example, Sarker et al. [80] used k-means clustering to segment and classify lung tumors from 3D CT images.
- **Mean Shift Clustering**: This algorithm does not require the number of clusters to be determined a priori. It works by continuously moving centroids toward areas with the highest data density, which correspond to the peaks (modes) in a kernel-estimated density function. This algorithm has been applied to medical imaging [81].
- **Density-Based Spatial Clustering of Applications with Noise (DBSCAN)**: DBSCAN clusters dense regions of points and identifies outliers, which is useful for anomaly detection in EHRs [82] and fraudulent billing in healthcare [83]. This approach has also been applied to anomaly detection in heart disease [84].

ii. **Association**: Association learning determines relationships between variables in large datasets and is frequently used in medical research and clinical decision support systems. It identifies associations in healthcare data, such as co-occurring diseases, medication interactions, and risk factors. For instance, Manolitsis et al. [85] used association learning to reveal patterns of antimicrobial resistance in patients with stone disease, which aided clinicians in determining which antibiotics work against specific bacterial infections. Examples of association algorithms include:

- **Apriori Algorithm**: This algorithm finds frequent itemsets and develops association-based on user-defined thresholds (support and confidence). The apriori algorithm has been used in drug interaction analysis to help clinicians predict adverse drug reactions by reviewing historical prescription data [86].
- **Eclat Algorithm**: This algorithm is very similar to apriori, but it uses a depth-first search approach to improve the efficiency of rule mining. It has been used to predict comorbid conditions in patients with chronic diseases, assisting physicians in crafting early intervention methods [87].
- **FP-Growth Algorithm**: This algorithm employs a more scalable approach compared to apriori because it does not require candidate generation. It has been used in studies on drug interactions in hospital settings to suggest combinations of prescription medications that avoid drug interactions and reduce the risks of adverse drug reactions [88].

Unsupervised learning methods, such as clustering and association, have transformed the landscape of healthcare analytics. These techniques are increasingly leveraged to improve precision medicine, patient risk stratification, and models of disease progression. With the expanding availability of EHRs, genomic data, and wearable health monitoring systems, the use of unsupervised learning in healthcare is expected to grow rapidly, providing increasingly data-driven and personalized healthcare solutions.

1.2.1.3 Semi-Supervised Learning

Semi-supervised learning is a ML paradigm that incorporates aspects of both supervised and unsupervised approaches. Semi-supervised learning uses a small number of labeled inputs alongside a large number of unlabeled inputs to help train the model. This is particularly important when using labeled inputs is infeasible due to cost, time, or other constraints. Unlike supervised learning, where the model relies solely on labeled datasets, semi-supervised learning allows the system to recognize and learn from the properties of the unlabeled data. In this way, the system can make predictions even when annotated data represents only a small fraction of the overall training data. Semi-supervised learning is useful in fields where labeled datasets are scarce, such as medical imaging, genomic sequencing, and cybersecurity.

Semi-supervised learning can generally be divided into two groups: semi-supervised classification and semi-supervised clustering [27]. Semi-supervised classification focuses on improving prediction accuracy when only part of the training set is labeled, while semi-supervised clustering uses limited labels to guide the grouping of unlabeled data into meaningful clusters. These categories describe how semi-supervised learning algorithms utilize both labeled and unlabeled data to enhance learning performance.

i. **Semi-Supervised Classification**: Semi-supervised classification methods aim to improve supervised classification problems using unlabeled data. These methods rely on the assumption that decision boundaries align with the inherent structure of the data, allowing similar data points to belong to the same class. Multiple semi-supervised classification methods have been developed:

    - **Self-Training (Pseudo-Labeling)**: A classifier is first trained on a small set of labeled data, then applied to unlabeled samples. The most confidently predicted samples are assigned pseudo-labels and iteratively added back into the training set. While simple and effective, this method can suffer from error propagation. This method is commonly used in radiology, where AI-assisted diagnostic systems learn from expert-annotated scans while making predictions on unlabeled new images [89].
    - **Co-Training**: Co-training trains two classifiers on distinct feature subsets ("views") of the same dataset. Each classifier labels unlabeled samples for the other, expanding the training pool. This approach assumes that the two views are conditionally independent and sufficient for classification. Co-training has been applied in speech recognition and text classification using different data types (e.g., audio and text) [90].
    - **Graph-Based Semi-Supervised Learning**: This method models data as a graph, where nodes are data points and edges represent relationships and similarities. Labels are propagated across the graph under the smoothness assumption that connected nodes should share similar labels. It has been successfully used in cancer diagnostics, where labeled biopsy samples are used to infer malignancy in unlabeled histopathological images [91].

- **Generative Models**: Generative approaches learn the joint distribution of labeled and unlabeled data, enabling the model to generate synthetic labeled samples or exploit distributional structure. Variational Autoencoders (VAEs) and semi-supervised Generative Adversarial Network (GANs) have shown strong performance in image recognition, medical imaging, and text analysis [92–94].

ii. **Semi-Supervised Clustering**: Semi-supervised clustering methods group similar data points into clusters and transfer labels from a small sample of labeled points to the entire cluster. These methods rely on the assumption that data points in the same cluster share similar properties and belong to the same class. Semi-supervised clustering can incorporate supervision in different ways. For example, there may be must-link constraints, which specify that two samples belong to the same cluster, or cannot-link constraints, which indicate that two samples should be placed in different clusters [95]. In some cases, partial cluster assignments may also be known in advance. One way of using such information is through cluster seeding. Basu et al. [96] suggested initializing clusters based on data points with known assignments. In their method, the centroid of each cluster in the k-means algorithm is set to the mean feature values of the labeled points assigned to that cluster. They also introduced an alternative version where the cluster assignments of labeled points remain fixed during the k-means procedure. Semi-supervised clustering represents a smaller area of research compared to semi-supervised classification.

Semi-supervised learning has enabled entirely new healthcare applications. In MRI, CT, and X-ray image analysis, labeled images are often scarce. Methods such as self-training and graph-based approaches can classify and segment medical images accurately, enabling earlier diagnosis and detection of disease [89]. In cancer pathology, where labeled histopathological images are limited, semi-supervised models have helped detect tumors using both labeled and unlabeled data [97]. In gene expression datasets, which often contain a mix of labeled and unlabeled samples, semi-supervised algorithms can assist in gene classification and function prediction using clustering and classification [98].

Semi-supervised learning bridges the gap between supervised and unsupervised learning. It offers a powerful means to utilize large volumes of unlabeled medical data. As computational power and data availability continue to grow, semi-supervised learning will play an increasingly significant role in transforming healthcare analytics and personalized medicine.

1.2.1.4 Reinforcement Learning

RL is a core paradigm of AI that advances sequential decision-making in complex and evolving environments [99–101]. Unlike supervised learning methods, RL does not require labeled input–output pairs. Instead, an agent interacts with an environment through trial-and-error and gradually improves its performance. In this approach, the

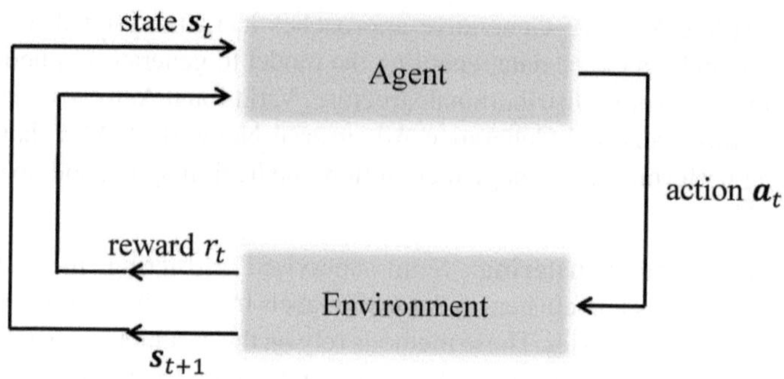

Fig. 1.3 Schematic representation of the RL framework. At each time step t, the agent observes the current state (s_t), selects an action (a_t), and receives a reward (r_t) from the environment along with the next state (s_{t+1}). This interaction cycle enables the agent to refine its behavior over time in order to maximize long-term cumulative reward. Reproduced from Kim et al. [109], published in Fluids 9 (2024) 216, under the Creative Commons Attribution 4.0 International License (CC BY), (https://creativecommons.org/licenses/by/4.0/)

agent observes the current state (s_t) of the environment (for example, a patient's vital signs in healthcare) at each time step t, selects an action (a_t) (such as adjusting a drug dosage), and then receives a reward or penalty (r_t) that reflects the quality of that decision (for instance, whether the patient's condition improves or worsens). The environment also transitions into a new state (s_{t+1}). This feedback cycle of states, actions, and rewards, illustrated in Fig. 1.3, guides the agent to refine its behavior over time, with the objective of maximizing long-term cumulative reward. RL approaches are commonly divided into two broad families, including model-based RL and model-free RL [102].

i. **Model-Based RL**: In these methods, the agent either has access to or learns a model of the environment. This model predicts how actions lead to new states and rewards. With this model, the agent can plan by simulating possible future outcomes before making real decisions. Two main subgroups are usually distinguished:

   - **Model-Given (Planning)**: In this scenario, the full model of the environment is already known. A clear example is board games such as chess or Go, where the rules specify exactly how each move affects the game. These methods are highly efficient in structured environments but impractical in domains like healthcare, where the rules governing patient responses are complex and uncertain.
   - **Model-Learning (Learned Models)**: In many real-world settings, the environment model is not known in advance. Here, the agent must learn the model by observing data. For example, in healthcare, a model might be trained to predict how a patient's condition changes in response to different treatments.

ii. **Model-Free RL**: In contrast, model-free methods do not try to learn or use a model of the environment. Instead, the agent learns directly from experience by focusing on which actions lead to higher rewards. The main subgroups include:

- **Value-Based Methods**: These methods estimate numerical values that tell the agent how good different situations and choices are expected to be over time. The state-value function, denoted as $V(s)$, measures the expected long-term reward of being in a particular state s. For example, if s represents a patient's current condition, $V(s)$ reflects how favorable that condition is in terms of expected recovery if the same treatment strategy continues. The action-value function, denoted as $Q(s,a)$, goes one step further by estimating the expected reward of taking a specific action a in a given state s, followed by continuing with the strategy. In the healthcare example, $Q(s,a)$ could represent the outcome of adjusting a medication dose for a patient in a particular condition. The agent then makes decisions by choosing the action with the highest estimated value. One of the most widely known algorithms in this group is Q-learning, which directly learns the action-value function without needing a model of the environment [103]. Q-learning has been successfully applied in healthcare to optimize sepsis treatment strategies and design adaptive drug dosing policies [104, 105].
- **Policy-Based Methods**: These methods directly learn a policy—a mapping from states to actions—without relying on explicit value estimates. These policies are often parameterized with NNs and optimized using gradient-based methods. Policy-based methods are especially useful in continuous action spaces (e.g., adjusting the exact angle of a surgical robot's arm), where evaluating discrete action values becomes infeasible. In medicine, policy-based RL has been used in prosthetic limb control, learning optimal movement strategies for amputee patients [104].
- **Actor–Critic Methods**: These methods combine the two previous approaches. Here, the actor updates the policy by proposing actions, while the critic evaluates those actions using value functions. This interaction reduces instability and improves learning efficiency. Well-known algorithms in this family include Advantage Actor–Critic (A2C), Proximal Policy Optimization (PPO), and Deep Deterministic Policy Gradient (DDPG). In healthcare, actor–critic methods have been used in robotic prosthetics [106], ventilator control [107], and adaptive rehabilitation [108], where real-time adaptation and stability are crucial.

With modern algorithms and available computing power, RL has seen remarkable success across various domains, including game playing [110], autonomous control systems [111], advertising and recommendation systems [112], energy management systems [113], healthcare [114, 115], and optimization problems [116]. Intelligent machines using RL are effective and rapid decision-makers, enabling solutions that are often not achievable through traditional approaches. State-of-the-art research is also exploring its role in emerging areas like quantum ML, where RL could facilitate advanced scientific simulations and more efficient data processing [117].

Overall, RL demonstrates its potential to address some of today's most significant challenges—from promoting sustainable energy use to developing smarter cities—while respecting individual autonomy and upholding ethical standards for AI applications. Interested readers may refer to [100, 118] for further insights into RL algorithms.

1.2.2 Deep Learning

One of the most technical and important sub-disciplines of ML is DL, which focuses on developing innovative and powerful methods for training Artificial Neural Networks (ANNs). Functionally, DL systems train NNs to process large amounts of complex data and uncover intricate patterns within it. These networks, called deep because of their multiple stacked layers, are capable of learning hierarchical representations of raw input data.

The benefit of the hierarchical representation in DL architectures is their ability to progressively translate low-level features (e.g., pixel values) into high-level abstract features (e.g., shapes, objects, or semantic meaning). This makes DL architecture far more powerful than traditional shallow models in terms of representational capacity. DL also differentiates itself from traditional ML methods, which often relied on user experience or intermediary knowledge, by leveraging raw data to derive inference. Accordingly, this methodological shift means DL requires less reliance on user expertise and prior knowledge [119].

Several methods of DL exist to address different tasks. However, FNNs are especially important because they form the foundational algorithm for DL [120]. In Fig. 1.4, we see that an FNN has an input layer, one or more hidden layers, and an output layer. Each layer consists of nodes, or neurons, which are interconnected to perform mathematical computations and send the result to the next layer of neurons. This structure represents the flow of data through the network, enabling FNNs to solve complex tasks. While FNNs are foundational, many other algorithms have driven major advances in specific domains—for example, Convolutional Neural Networks (CNNs), RNNs, LSTM Networks, and GANs [121].

DL has transformed AI by achieving breakthrough performance compared to other methods, particularly in its ability to develop complex models for image recognition and speech processing. With broad applications, DL remains at the cutting edge, enabling innovations in diverse AI applications and improving decision-making in impactful ways already present in daily life. For more information on DL algorithms, readers are directed to [121, 122].

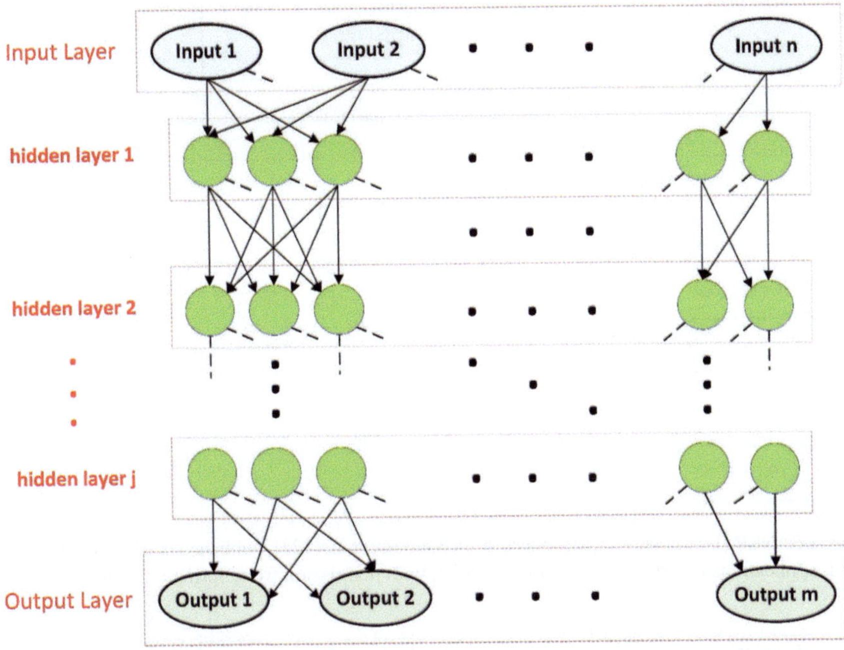

Fig. 1.4 Schematic illustration of FNNs

1.2.3 Natural Language Processing

Recently, NLP has become an active and exciting area of study due to growing interest in interactive and user-friendly computer systems. Understanding what humans mean or intend to communicate involves numerous complex patterns of human communication. The ultimate goal of NLP research is to develop algorithms that allow for seamless communication between computers and humans. The aim is to produce robust models for machines that can comprehensively identify, understand, and express language.

As shown in Fig. 1.5, NLP is typically divided into two components: Natural Language Understanding (NLU) and Natural Language Generation (NLG). NLU analyzes and interprets text or speech input, while NLG produces text that is both readable and meaningful. Linguistics, the scientific study of language, plays an important role in NLP. It includes several sub-disciplines: Phonology (the study of sounds in speech), Morphology (the study of word formation), Syntax (the study of sentence structure), Semantics (the study of meaning), and Pragmatics (the study of language in context). NLG transforms the internal representation into meaningful phrases, sentences, and paragraphs. Its objective is to generate human-like, coherent output.

The literature utilizes a variety of NLP methods including SVM, Naïve Bayes, Conditional Random Fields (CRFs), RFs, Maximum Entropy (MaxEnt), DTs, deep

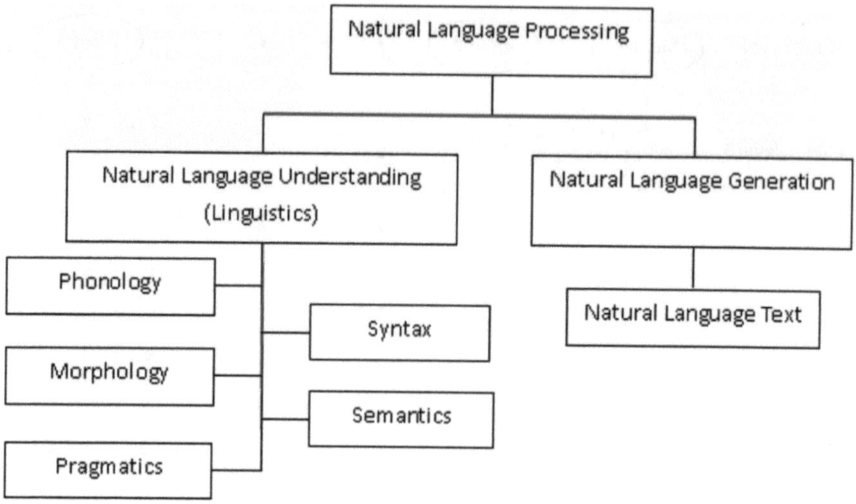

Fig. 1.5 NLP classification. Reproduced from Khurana et al. [123], published in Multimedia Tools and Applications 82 (2023) 3713–3744, © 2022, with permission from Springer Nature

NNs, Logistic Regression (LogReg), and rule-based approaches [124]. Additionally, NLP's applications cross industry boundaries, from language translation services enabling globalization efforts to chatbots providing 24/7 customer service on e-commerce sites. Techniques for sentiment analysis developed through NLP research can provide insights into consumer behavior, while voice assistants are common in homes across the globe, allowing for efficient management of daily tasks.

With rapid advancements in technology, researchers are working to improve existing NLP solutions or develop new ones based on datasets obtained from various sources, such as social media posts or transcripts from recorded conversations. Readers interested in more details about NLP methods should find useful information in [125, 126].

1.2.4 Computer Vision

In the field of AI, CV is an evolving area that allows machines to perceive and analyze visual data, such as images and videos. CV systems replicate how the human visual system performs, transforming raw visual data into identifiable patterns so that data-driven decisions can be made. CV often combines image processing techniques, ML, and deep NNs—particularly CNNs—to achieve high performance in perception. The application of CV has only become widespread with the advent of big data and high-performance computing, making it one of the most significant areas of AI within modern industries.

CV can be viewed as a sequence of several steps: image acquisition, preprocessing, feature extraction, and interpretation. Image acquisition involves capturing visual information from cameras, sensors, or medical imaging equipment (e.g., X-rays, MRI, CT imaging). Preprocessing refers to image filtering, denoising, and normalization to improve image quality and eliminate noise that could reduce AI performance. Feature extraction is the step at which important visual characteristics, such as edges, shapes, and textures, are identified. Interpretation is performed by an AI model to classify images, detect objects, or determine medical conditions based on recognized patterns [127–129].

To enhance CV applicability, numerous computational techniques, algorithms, and AI methods have been developed. While traditional image processing techniques—such as edge detection (Sobel and Canny filters), histogram equalization, and feature descriptors (SIFT, SURF, ORB)—focused on well-understood problems, the arrival of AI and modern DL models has begun to overtake conventional methods. Some existing approaches and algorithms that constitute CV include:

- **CNNs**: CNNs are specialized NNs designed for image recognition and classification tasks. They consist of convolutional layers that extract features from images hierarchically by detecting edges, textures, and patterns that become more complex as the network deepens. CNN architectures such as ResNet, VGG, and EfficientNet are among the most successful in achieving high classification accuracy in image datasets [130].
- **Vision Transformers (ViTs)**: ViTs are a recent technology that employs self-attention mechanisms to model how different regions of an image relate to one another. Unlike CNNs, which rely on spatial hierarchies, ViTs process entire images in parallel, making them effective in applications including medical image segmentation and multimodal analysis [131].
- **Object Detection Algorithms**: Algorithms such as YOLO (You Only Look Once) and Faster R-CNN (Region-based Convolutional Neural Network) are popular methods for detecting objects in images and videos [130]. These frameworks have been used in security surveillance, autonomous vehicles, and real-time traffic monitoring applications.
- **Image Segmentation Models**: U-Net, Mask R-CNN, and DeepLab are popular DL architectures used for the segmentation of medical images, allowing for accurate outlines of organs, tumors, and lesions in medical imaging [130, 132].

CV has been widely adopted across multiple sectors, transforming the way machines interact with visual data. Figure 1.6 presents some of the most important use cases for CV. It is used in applications such as self-driving cars [133] and medical imaging [130], among others. CV will continue to shape the future of technology.

CV technology has the potential to transform healthcare. Innovations in medical imaging, diagnostics, and surgical assistance are happening everywhere. Advanced DL architectures like CNNs and ViTs are being used for the early detection and classification of tumors utilizing MRI and CT scans [134]. These models have demonstrated improved accuracy, reduced interpretation time, and enabled radiologists to

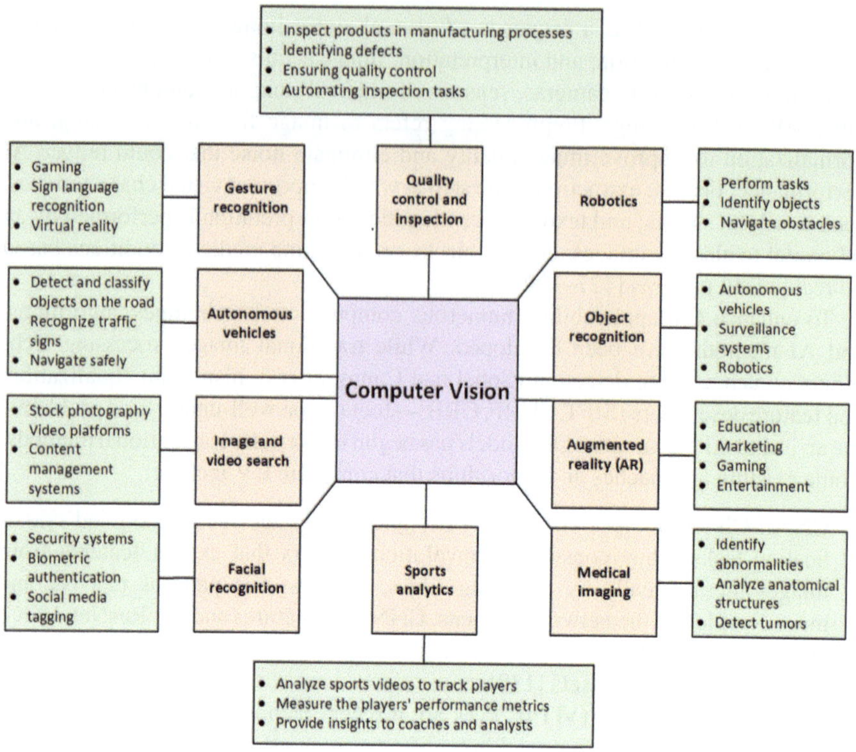

Fig. 1.6 Some applications of CV

make accurate decisions, compared to traditional manual examination in each individual study. Recent studies have used DL-based CV models to identify and classify lung disease in COVID-19 patients by examining chest X-rays and CT scans [135]. Innovative approaches to AI-based image segmentation have also enabled the automated assessment of cardiac MRIs to identify heart diseases in cardiology [136]. These applications help to minimize human error and improve the diagnosis of potential diseases.

Histopathological image analysis is yet another area where CV has achieved exciting possibilities. The computer-aided analysis of histopathological slides, with AI-based image processing methods, allows pathologists to identify malignancies, grade tumors, and categorize tissue abnormalities with high precision. The use of Whole Slide Imaging (WSI) and CNNs has eliminated many manual actions in pathology labs while enhancing reproducibility, which improves classification and reporting of information [137]. In dermatology, CNN-based models are used to assess skin lesions and identify melanoma with diagnostic performance comparable to dermatologist evaluation [138]. These AI-based methods provide real-time analysis, helping clinicians make timely treatment recommendations; improved treatment onset, in turn, improves patient survival rates.

AI-mediated screeners and CV have made disease detection cheaper and more accessible. For example, AI diabetic retinopathy screening automatically identifies retinal abnormalities in images, leading to timely and early diagnosis and treatment [139, 140]. Likewise, automated analysis of mammography for early breast cancer detection improves the prognosis for patients diagnosed with early breast cancer [141].

CV is also approaching surgical planning and intra-operative guidance in new ways. AI-enabled systems apply CV technologies to process preoperative medical images to help surgeons plan for minimally invasive procedures more precisely than ever before. Using 3D reconstructions generated from CT and MRI, virtual surgical simulations can be performed, allowing the surgeon to observe and anticipate complications before an actual operation is conducted [142]. Augmented Reality (AR), enhanced by CV, also supports higher surgical accuracy by providing real-time imaging overlaid on the patient's body during the operation. Robotic-assisted surgery, such as the da Vinci Surgical System, also uses CV to enable greater surgical precision, smaller incisions, and faster recovery [143].

Despite the advancements made in CV and its utilization in healthcare, there are still challenges and limitations to be addressed. There are data quality and standardization issues across different healthcare settings, which can limit AI model performance and effectiveness. Variability in imaging modality, scanner resolution, and inconsistency in annotations can all negatively affect the generalizability of models. Ongoing work is being done to further develop domain adaptation techniques and self-supervised learning models to mitigate these issues [144].

Another challenge is the interpretability of AI models. Many DL-powered image analysis systems are black boxes, making them inscrutable for clinicians who have no way to understand how decisions are made. Strategies from explainable AI (XAI), such as attention-based techniques and gradient-based visualizations, are being developed to improve transparency and clinical trustworthiness [75].

With ongoing improvements to CV, the future of medical image analysis appears promising. Continued advancements in AI-powered CV tools will improve diagnostic accuracy, inform real-time clinical decision-making, provide personalized treatment strategies, and enhance patient outcomes while decreasing healthcare costs.

1.2.5 Robotics

Robotics is an interdisciplinary area of study that combines elements from AI, mechanical engineering, and electronics to create intelligent machines called robots. The integration of AI techniques into robots provides them with the capabilities to perceive their environment and adapt to new situations through experience, as well as seek new knowledge and make decisions autonomously and intelligently based on their understanding. Robotic AI allows robots to perceive their environment using sensors such as cameras, lidar, radar, or tactile sensors. AI processes sensory data to recognize objects, comprehend visual scenes, identify obstacles, and understand the environment. Beyond sensing, robots learn from their interactions and experiences. They use ML techniques—supervised, unsupervised, or RL—to improve and develop over time. With data to exploit, robots learn to adapt to new contexts, reason about their actions, and improve their ability to choose.

With AI, robots can also reason. They use techniques such as logical reasoning, probabilistic reasoning, or symbolic reasoning to infer, conclude, or derive insights from the available data. This reasoning capability allows a robot to identify relationships, predict outcomes, and choose actions. Where there is data, AI enables robots to make data-driven decisions independently, based on perception, learning, and reasoning. Not only can a robot evaluate the possible choices available, but it can also consider constraints and objectives to determine the best course of action for a specific task. As part of AI, robots can make decisions before and during task execution, enabling them to operate in dynamic, unstructured environments that do not always allow for constant human involvement or intervention.

The use of AI methods in robotics enables more intelligent and adaptive robots that can perform an increasing number of tasks with improved efficiency, accuracy, and autonomy. This technology has opened up new frontiers for drones, autonomous mobile robots, and industrial robots—often focusing on complex applications such as surveillance, the assembly of goods within manufacturing industries, and the provision of care services in healthcare organizations, all autonomously. Robotics has the potential to be applied across a range of sectors, creating new use cases. These include agriculture, where robotic devices assist with tasks such as crop monitoring and harvesting [145], and space exploration, where unmanned probes travel hundreds of thousands of kilometers on missions without human intervention [146], among many others. Several examples of AI applications in robotics across various fields and industries are illustrated in Fig. 1.7. Some recently published papers covering the application of AI in robotics are listed in the recommendations [147, 148].

1.2.6 Knowledge Representation and Reasoning

The depiction and manipulation of knowledge to perform reasoning and resolve problems is a highly technical subfield of AI. These systems often feature advanced formal techniques that create schemas for storing and structuring data, allowing AI tools to perform logical deduction, inference, or analysis of complex patterns. The capability of an intelligent system to reason based on the information processed in a specific domain has steadily increased through approaches like expert systems and more recent methods such as knowledge graphs and ML models. Machines are handling increasingly complex tasks, such as decision-making and resolving intricate issues, due to the approach of representing knowledge using machine-readable schemas to process large amounts of structured data through properly designed algorithms.

For KR&R, various approaches are used—for example, logical representation [149], semantic networks [150], frames and ontologies [151–153], probabilistic models [154], and others. The progress made with KR&R has enabled intelligent

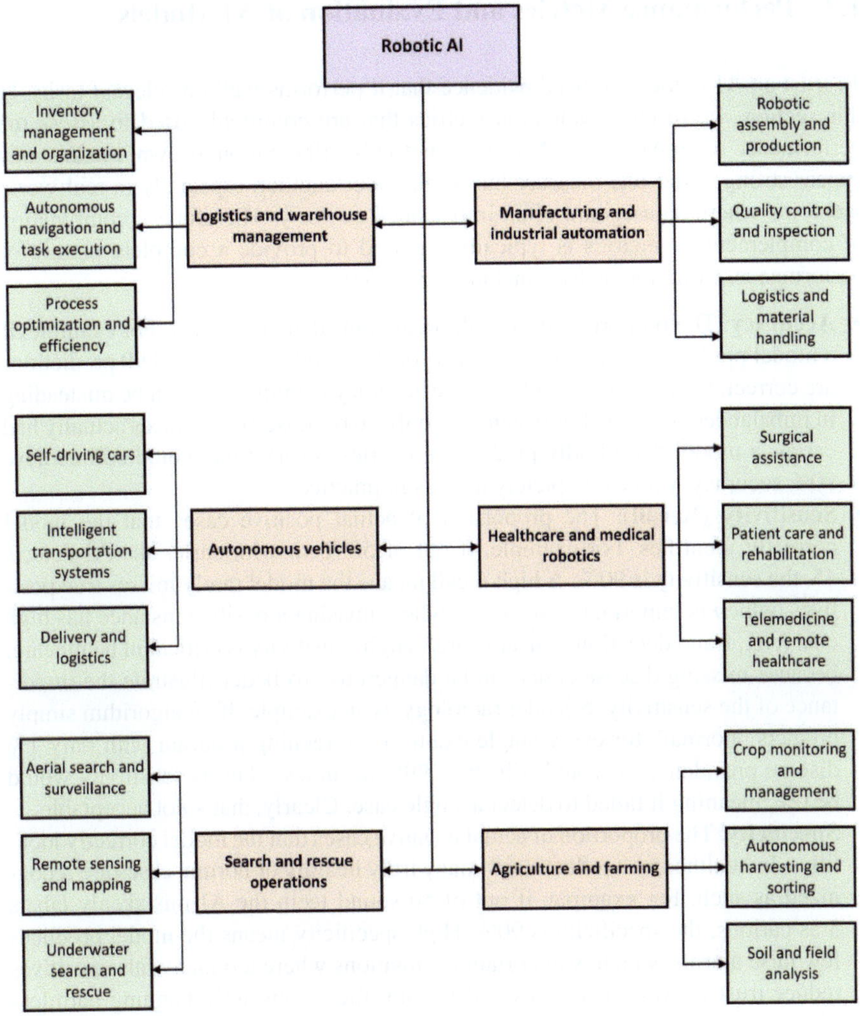

Fig. 1.7 Some different applications of robotic AI

systems to make decisions and solve problems. By applying reasoning to structured data, intelligent systems have the potential to solve complex problems and provide solutions and recommendations. However, KR&R itself has not progressed at the same pace as other areas of AI such as DL. As AI continues to advance, so too will the development of better and more flexible KR&R approaches. The combination of various methods, the inclusion of domain-specific knowledge, and the power of new learning techniques may eventually lead to greater reasoning capacity in intelligent systems and the ability to address increasingly complex challenges across different fields. Readers interested in KR&R algorithms can find further reading dedicated to this topic [155].

1.3 Performance Metrics and Evaluation of AI Models

To trust an AI model, we need evidence that it performs well on relevant tasks. In this section, we discuss evaluation metrics that are commonly used to assess the performance of an AI system. No single metric is sufficient on its own; models may appear strong under one measure but weak under another, especially in real-world scenarios where datasets are often imbalanced or noisy. Therefore, a combination of complementary metrics is typically reported to provide a complete picture of performance. Common metrics include [156, 157]:

- **Accuracy**: The proportion of overall predictions that are correct. For example, if a model predicts "caries" or "no caries" on 100 tooth surfaces and 90 predictions are correct, the accuracy is 90%. While accuracy is intuitive, it can be misleading in imbalanced datasets. For instance, if only 10 of those 100 surfaces actually had caries, a model that blindly predicts "no caries" every time would still achieve 90% accuracy, yet be completely useless in practice.
- **Sensitivity (Recall)**: The proportion of actual positive cases that the model correctly identifies. For example, if out of 50 teeth with caries the AI detects 45, the sensitivity is 90%. A high recall means the model rarely misses true positives, which is important in scenarios where missing a positive instance has high cost (e.g., fraud detection or healthcare). High sensitivity is critical in healthcare, because missing disease cases can be dangerous. To better illustrate the importance of the sensitivity, consider radiology as an example. If an algorithm simply predicts "normal" for every single exam in a screening program with only 1% disease prevalence, it would still show 99% accuracy—but its sensitivity would be 0%, meaning it failed to detect a single case. Clearly, that's not acceptable.
- **Specificity**: The proportion of actual negative cases that the model correctly identifies. In healthcare, it reflects how many truly healthy or normal cases are recognized as such. For example, if out of 50 sound teeth the AI mistakenly labels 5 as carious, the specificity is 90%. High specificity means the model produces few false alarms, which is important in situations where too many false positives reduce trust or waste resources—like spam filters constantly flagging harmless emails. In medicine, specificity helps prevent overtreatment; for example, an AI that flags every stain as a cavity may look cautious but is ultimately unhelpful. Often, there's a trade-off: increasing sensitivity can lower specificity, and vice versa, so finding the right balance is key.
- **Precision (Positive Predictive Value, PPV)**: The proportion of predicted positive cases that are actually correct. For example, if the AI marked 20 teeth as having caries and 15 truly did, the PPV is 75%. Precision reflects the reliability of a model's positive predictions. High precision is especially important when false positives come at a cost—for instance, wrongly flagging a legitimate transaction as fraudulent. In healthcare, it underpins clinical confidence: if an AI frequently raises false alarms, clinicians will soon stop relying on it, no matter how sophisticated it is.

- **Negative Predictive Value (NPV)**: The proportion of predicted negative cases that are truly negative. PPV and NPV together provide a balanced view of how trustworthy predictions are in both directions.
- **F1-Score**: The harmonic mean of precision and recall (sensitivity). This metric is valuable when there is a need to balance false negatives and false positives, especially in imbalanced datasets where accuracy alone may be misleading.
- **Area Under the Receiver Operating Characteristic Curve (AUC-ROC)**: This metric captures a model's performance across all possible sensitivity/specificity trade-offs. The ROC curve plots true positive rate (sensitivity) vs. false positive rate (1-specificity) as the decision threshold varies. The area under a curve (AUC) provides a single numerical summary of this relationship, representing the model's overall ability to distinguish between the two classes. A higher AUC indicates better performance. An AUC of 1.0 is perfect, 0.5 is random guessing. A high AUC means the model can achieve both high sensitivity and specificity with appropriate thresholding.
- **Confusion Matrix**: A structured table showing the counts of true positives, false positives, true negatives, and false negatives. It provides a detailed breakdown of errors and helps identify systematic weaknesses (e.g., a model consistently confusing one class with another). In multi-class settings, the confusion matrix is particularly useful for diagnosing where the model struggles.

When AI models are evaluated in studies, they are often tested against an expert "gold standard." For example, a set of radiographs may be labeled by the consensus of three experienced dentists, and the AI's detections are then compared to that consensus to compute sensitivity, specificity, and other metrics. In some cases, studies directly compare AI with human performance, such as reporting that "AI had an accuracy of 86%, while the average of five dentists was 82% on the same task." It's also important to test AI on diverse, external datasets (not just the data it was trained on) to ensure it generalizes.

Thus far, many AI models show very high "lab performance"—e.g., caries detection sensitivities >90% and specificities around 80–90%. But one challenge is that these performance stats sometimes drop in real-world use due to differences in X-ray machines, patient populations, etc. Therefore, continuous monitoring and validation of AI in the field is an important practice challenge.

1.4 Chronological Evolution of AI in Medicine and Dentistry

The historical evolution of AI in medicine and dentistry has moved from theory to present-day practice, now impacting healthcare directly. AI began in the mid-twentieth century when a cadre of computer scientists initiated the theoretical pursuit of intelligent machines capable of imitation and human reasoning. AI in healthcare first emerged as expert systems—rule-based programs designed to replicate and simulate physicians' decision-making capabilities. Several notable systems were developed, including MYCIN in the 1970s, which was used to diagnose bacterial infections and suggest antibiotic therapy. While MYCIN exposed AI's potential to the healthcare field, its clinical value remained limited due to hardware constraints, lack of physician acceptance, and the state of digital health capabilities at the time [158].

Advancements in computational power and data storage during the 1980s and 1990s led to a resurgence of AI research in medicine. Improvements in ML algorithms allowed AI to evolve from rule-based systems to statistical models capable of detecting patterns in previously unseen datasets. Highlights from this period include the development of ANNs and their DL applications. Classification models were created for predicting cardiovascular morbidity and detecting cancers at early stages [159]. AI research in dentistry was reported in the late 1990s, primarily focusing on computer-aided radiography and the detection of oral pathologies [160].

The twenty-first century has clearly marked the era of AI in healthcare, driven by exponential advances in computation and the digitization of patient charts and medical records. The introduction of DL models has fundamentally transformed medical image analysis by enabling AI systems to interpret complex visual data with unprecedented accuracy. In this regard, CNNs have been applied to radiologic diagnosis, with AI models developed to detect abnormalities in X-ray, CT, and MRI scans [134]. Similarly, AI diagnostic tools in dentistry have emerged alongside architectural advances in AI models for diagnosing abscesses, automated caries detection, and disease prediction based on quantified periodontal disease models. Related developments include AI-assisted prosthodontics and orthodontics, where algorithms help design and validate custom dental implants and make predictions about malocclusion treatment (e.g., class I, II, III) [160, 161].

As AI technologies advanced, their integration into clinical practice became more common. The widespread adoption of EHRs created an abundance of data for AI predictive analytics to assist in the early identification of high-risk patients and the development of individualized treatment plans. AI-driven chatbots and virtual assistants were developed to engage patients for symptom assessment and triage services [162]. In general practice, AI technology has begun assisting with treatment planning by using pre-treatment images to model orthodontic movements and complete prosthetic fittings, reducing the need for clinicians to make manual adjustments [163, 164].

Continuous advances will drive AI technologies to profound levels of sophistication in medicine and dentistry. Open platforms based on cloud computing, combined with the Internet of Things (IoT), have enabled physicians to provide real-time monitoring of patients with chronic illnesses [165]. Wearable health devices enhanced by AI algorithms for monitoring vital signs, anomaly detection, and alerting healthcare providers to potential medical emergencies are increasingly entering clinical practice. Notably, some devices, such as glucose monitoring apps, have received the U.S. Food and Drug Administration (FDA) approval, reflecting their transition into regulated medical use [166]. In dentistry, enhanced imaging procedures using AI algorithms—such as 3D Cone-Beam Computed Tomography (CBCT)—have improved the specificity and accuracy of surgical planning for dental implants and maxillofacial procedures [167].

The adoption of AI in medical and dental practice has progressed to the point where it enhances clinician decision-making and improves patient outcomes. AI has been widely adopted in surgery, with robotic systems such as the da Vinci Surgical System facilitating minimally invasive procedures beyond human capabilities [143]. AI predictive models are also in place to monitor disease outbreaks and allocate resources for interventions, improving community preparedness for public health emergencies [168].

While AI has transformed various domains of clinical practice, the implementation of AI tools into everyday use has been slow due to regulatory hurdles, data privacy concerns, and the need for substantial validation studies. Ethical issues around algorithmic bias and explainability are also significant challenges to ensuring AI systems are fair and trustworthy. AI models must be continually evaluated to support valid and unbiased recommendations. If there is bias in the training dataset, it can lead to inequities in healthcare delivery. Therefore, collaboration between developers and clinicians is essential to improve AI-based diagnostic and treatment systems. Concerns about patient data privacy and security must also be addressed, as AI relies on large volumes of medical data to function effectively.

AI is already having a deep impact on medicine and is poised to do even more. Ongoing research aims to improve AI models' accuracy, interpretability, and adaptability to broader patient populations. Moreover, with AI's integration into emerging technologies such as blockchain for secure medical record-keeping and quantum computing for enhanced computation, AI tools are expected to become increasingly widespread. The more capable these tools become, the greater their future use in delivering more accurate diagnoses, less invasive treatment options, and improved overall health outcomes. AI is being steadily adopted into clinical practice nationwide, indicating a cultural shift toward data-driven, evidence-based healthcare that ultimately benefits both providers and patients.

1.5 Current Trends and Future Outlook

The integration of AI into healthcare is continually evolving at a staggering rate, with developing technologies shaping the future of patient care, evaluation, and treatment options. The use of AI-related processes such as predictive analytics, ML, and virtual healthcare assistants is changing the healthcare landscape. AI's ability to deliver improved diagnostic and treatment plans, monitor patients, and accelerate health research has fundamentally changed the medical field by solidifying its place as a crucial technology for personalized medicine and healthcare operations. As AI continues to develop across healthcare platforms, it is also beginning to impact healthcare accessibility, cost-effectiveness, and patient experience and outcomes.

Recent developments in AI technologies have allowed healthcare providers to make more accurate and timely diagnoses. AI-based imaging systems leveraging

DL algorithms are now helping radiologists identify anomalies in medical images, including early-stage cancers, cardiovascular diseases, and neurological disorders [134, 169–171]. Another major trend is the use of predictive analytics, whereby AI models access large-scale datasets—including EHRs and genomic information—to identify high-risk patients and predict disease progression [172]. These predictive capabilities can improve early intervention and offer better disease management.

One of the most prominent trends in AI-enabled healthcare is the move toward personalized medicine. AI models, using patient-centered data such as genetic information, individual lifestyles, and medical histories, develop individualized treatment protocols [173]. This approach improves therapeutic efficacy and minimizes side effects by selecting treatments specifically suited to an individual's unique biological profile. In oncology, for example, AI models help physicians select from a number of chemotherapy regimens based on the molecular characteristics of a patient's tumor to maximize survival while minimizing treatment complications [174].

Another transformative trend is AI's disruptive potential in drug discovery. Traditional drug development is often lengthy and costly. AI speeds up this process by rapidly predicting molecular interactions and narrowing compound selection. Pharmaceutical companies are increasingly relying on AI algorithms to identify drug candidates, analyze clinical trial data, and explore new uses for existing drugs [175]. AI-enabled drug discovery has already shown promise in developing and repurposing treatments for neurodegenerative diseases and rare genetic conditions, thereby shortening the path to research and regulatory approval [176, 177].

One of the most exciting and promising applications of AI is in virtual healthcare assistants and telemedicine. With various options available, AI-enabled chatbots and virtual assistants can provide medical advice in seconds, schedule appointments, and monitor patient symptoms in real time [162]. These applications are especially useful in rural and underserved areas where access to healthcare professionals is limited. Virtual assistants enhance patient engagement and adherence to treatment plans using NLP, empowering patients to take responsibility for their own health and reducing hospital readmissions and overall healthcare costs.

The future of AI in healthcare is bright, with several new developments on the horizon. AI-guided robotic surgery is expected to enhance value by increasing precision and lowering the rate of human error in complex procedures. The increased precision of AI-enhanced robots will improve surgical outcomes. Robots guided by AI algorithms will help improve accuracy in minimally invasive surgeries, leading to faster healing and fewer post-surgical complications. Furthermore, wearable devices supported by AI technology will enhance remote monitoring and facilitate early diagnosis and interventions.

In the coming years, AI is expected to address many issues related to healthcare access while also helping reduce inequities in global healthcare delivery. AI-powered mobile applications and new digital diagnostics will enable individuals to engage in their own health management without needing to rely solely on traditional healthcare systems. AI-enabled translation services will also enhance communication among providers, patients, and even family members or caregivers who speak different languages, enabling inclusive communication during medical consultations.

The economic considerations surrounding the integration of AI in healthcare remain an important topic. AI has the potential to decrease healthcare costs while improving patient outcomes by reducing administrative burdens, minimizing diagnostic errors, and enhancing treatment planning. Predictive analytics and AI-enabled workflow automation may improve hospital operations, making them more efficient and allowing for better resource allocation. However, organizations must carefully weigh the cost of implementing AI against ongoing patient care and backend operational expenses.

While technological advances are beginning to address some of the barriers to AI adoption in healthcare, several persistent challenges remain. One of the most significant concerns is data privacy. AI is highly dependent on large amounts of patient data. For AI to function effectively, access to many data points is crucial, which raises ethical and legal concerns about data security and privacy. Regulations such as the Health Insurance Portability and Accountability Act (HIPAA) and the General Data Protection Regulation (GDPR) attempt to clarify requirements for data protection, but AI systems—like any technology—are still subject to breaches and misuse. Gaining and maintaining patient trust will require the most rigorous encryption protocols and secure data-sharing practices.

Another challenge is the inconsistent deployment of AI across healthcare institutions. Differences in data collection methods, AI model training processes, and regulatory approvals can hinder the implementation of AI systems. Without standardized approaches, AI-generated insights may vary across institutions, potentially affecting clinical decisions and patient outcomes. Integrating AI into clinical workflows requires collaboration among healthcare providers, AI developers, and policymakers to establish agreed-upon norms and practices. A critical concern is algorithmic bias: AI models trained on biased datasets may produce skewed or inaccurate results, exacerbating healthcare disparities [178]. Addressing this issue will require ensuring diversity in training datasets and embedding ethical AI principles throughout the development process. These strategies are essential to promote health equity in AI-driven solutions.

In conclusion, AI is dramatically transforming healthcare delivery. It is enabling predictive analytics, personalized medicine, virtual healthcare assistants, and AI-powered drug discovery, among many other innovations. Uncertainty remains about how future data privacy regulations may affect AI adoption or how emerging standards and research will shape its ethical use. However, its potential to influence patient care, improve access, and reduce costs is substantial. Collaborative, interdisciplinary efforts—alongside progressive regulation and ongoing research—will be essential to fully realize AI's promise and create a more efficient, equitable, and patient-centered healthcare system.

References

1. Y. Xu, X. Liu, X. Cao, C. Huang, E. Liu, S. Qian, X. Liu, Y. Wu, F. Dong, C.W. Qiu, J. Qiu, K. Hua, W. Su, J. Wu, H. Xu, Y. Han, C. Fu, Z. Yin, M. Liu, R. Roepman, S. Dietmann, M. Virta, F. Kengara, Z. Zhang, L. Zhang, T. Zhao, J. Dai, J. Yang, L. Lan, M. Luo, Z. Liu, T. An, B. Zhang, X. He, S. Cong, X. Liu, W. Zhang, J.P. Lewis, J.M. Tiedje, Q. Wang, Z. An, F. Wang, L. Zhang, T. Huang, C. Lu, Z. Cai, F. Wang, J. Zhang, Artificial intelligence: a powerful paradigm for scientific research. The Innovation **2**, 100179 (2021). https://doi.org/10.1016/J.XINN.2021.100179
2. D.A. Hashimoto, G. Rosman, D. Rus, O.R. Meireles, Artificial intelligence in surgery: promises and perils. Ann. Surg. **268**, 70–76 (2018). https://doi.org/10.1097/SLA.0000000000002693
3. E.P.V. Le, Y. Wang, Y. Huang, S. Hickman, F.J. Gilbert, Artificial intelligence in breast imaging. Clin. Radiol. **74**, 357–366 (2019). https://doi.org/10.1016/J.CRAD.2019.02.006
4. A. Zhavoronkov, Artificial intelligence for drug discovery, biomarker development, and generation of novel chemistry. Mol. Pharm. **15**, 4311–4313 (2018). https://doi.org/10.1021/ACS.MOLPHARMACEUT.8B00930/ASSET/IMAGES/LARGE/MP-2018-00930N_0001.JPEG
5. A. Pannu, Artificial intelligence and its application in different areas. Artif. Intell. **4**, 79–84 (2015)
6. L. Benos, A.C. Tagarakis, G. Dolias, R. Berruto, D. Kateris, D. Bochtis, Machine learning in agriculture: a comprehensive updated review. Sensors **21** (2021). https://doi.org/10.3390/S21113758
7. G. Bathla, K. Bhadane, R.K. Singh, R. Kumar, R. Aluvalu, R. Krishnamurthi, A. Kumar, R.N. Thakur, S. Basheer, Autonomous vehicles and intelligent automation: applications, challenges, and opportunities. Mob. Inf. Syst. **2022** (2022)
8. M. Hengstler, E. Enkel, S. Duelli, Applied artificial intelligence and trust—the case of autonomous vehicles and medical assistance devices. Technol. Forecast. Soc. Change **105**, 105–120 (2016)
9. O. Zawacki-Richter, V.I. Marín, M. Bond, F. Gouverneur, Systematic review of research on artificial intelligence applications in higher education–where are the educators? Int. J. Educ. Technol. High. Educ. **16**, 1–27 (2019)
10. F. Königstorfer, S. Thalmann, Applications of artificial intelligence in commercial banks–a research agenda for behavioral finance. J. Behav. Exp. Finance **27**, 100352 (2020)
11. H. Pallathadka, E.H. Ramirez-Asis, T.P. Loli-Poma, K. Kaliyaperumal, R.J.M. Ventayen, M. Naved, Applications of artificial intelligence in business management, e-commerce and finance. Mater. Today Proc. **80**, 2610–2613 (2023)
12. R.E. Bawack, S.F. Wamba, K.D.A. Carillo, S. Akter, Artificial intelligence in E-commerce: a bibliometric study and literature review. Electron. Mark. **32**, 297–338 (2022)
13. A. Haleem, M. Javaid, M.A. Qadri, R.P. Singh, R. Suman, Artificial intelligence (AI) applications for marketing: a literature-based study. Int. J. Intell. Netw. (2022)
14. A.M.A. Musleh Al-Sartawi, K. Hussainey, A. Razzaque, The role of artificial intelligence in sustainable finance. J. Sustain. Financ. Invest. 1–6 (2022)
15. A. Capatina, M. Kachour, J. Lichy, A. Micu, A.-E. Micu, F. Codignola, Matching the future capabilities of an artificial intelligence-based software for social media marketing with potential users' expectations. Technol. Forecast. Soc. Change **151**, 119794 (2020)
16. W. Wang, K. Siau, Artificial intelligence, machine learning, automation, robotics, future of work and future of humanity: a review and research agenda. J. Database Manag. (JDM) **30**, 61–79 (2019)
17. W.J. Park, J.-B. Park, History and application of artificial neural networks in dentistry. Eur. J. Dent. **12**, 594–601 (2018)
18. R. Fjelland, Why general artificial intelligence will not be realized. Humanit. Soc. Sci. Commun. **7**, 1–9 (2020)
19. H.R. Tizhoosh, L. Pantanowitz, Artificial intelligence and digital pathology: challenges and opportunities. J Pathol Inform **9**, 38 (2018)

20. A.I. Strong, Applications of artificial intelligence and associated technologies. Science [ETEBMS-2016] **5** (2016)
21. G.W. Ng, W.C. Leung, Strong artificial intelligence and consciousness. J. Artif. Intell. Conscious. **7**, 63–72 (2020)
22. R.I. Mukhamediev, Y. Popova, Y. Kuchin, E. Zaitseva, A. Kalimoldayev, A. Symagulov, V. Levashenko, F. Abdoldina, V. Gopejenko, K. Yakunin, Review of artificial intelligence and machine learning technologies: classification, restrictions, opportunities and challenges. Mathematics **10**, 2552 (2022)
23. I.H. Sarker, Machine learning: algorithms real-world applications and research directions. SN Comput. Sci. **2**, 160 (2021). https://doi.org/10.1007/s42979-021-00592-x
24. A.S. Ahuja, The impact of artificial intelligence in medicine on the future role of the physician. PeerJ **7**, e7702 (2019)
25. R. Pugliese, S. Regondi, R. Marini, Machine learning-based approach: global trends, research directions, and regulatory standpoints. Data Sci. Manag. **4**, 19–29 (2021). https://doi.org/10.1016/J.DSM.2021.12.002
26. R. Rafique, S.M.R. Islam, J.U. Kazi, Machine learning in the prediction of cancer therapy. Comput. Struct. Biotechnol. J. **19**, 4003–4017 (2021)
27. A. Aldahiri, B. Alrashed, W. Hussain, Trends in using IoT with machine learning in health prediction system. Forecasting **3**, 181–206 (2021)
28. N.A. Azit, S. Sahran, V.M. Leow, M. Subramaniam, S. Mokhtar, A.M. Nawi, Prediction of hepatocellular carcinoma risk in patients with type-2 diabetes using supervised machine learning classification model. Heliyon **8** (2022)
29. N. Al-Azzam, I. Shatnawi, Comparing supervised and semi-supervised machine learning models on diagnosing breast cancer. Ann. Med. Surg. **62**, 53–64 (2021)
30. D.K. Renuka, T. Hamsapriya, M.R. Chakkaravarthi, P.L. Surya, Spam classification based on supervised learning using machine learning techniques, in *2011 International Conference on Process Automation, Control and Computing* (IEEE, 2011), pp. 1–7
31. B. Antin, J. Kravitz, E. Martayan, Detecting pneumonia in chest X-Rays with supervised learning. Semanticscholar. Org **2017** (2017).
32. T. Da Silva, P. Macaskill, K. Mills, C. Maher, C. Williams, C. Lin, M.J. Hancock, Predicting recovery in patients with acute low back pain: a clinical prediction model. Eur. J. Pain **21**, 716–726 (2017)
33. M. Zanon, M. Riz, G. Sparacino, A. Facchinetti, R.E. Suri, M.S. Talary, C. Cobelli, Assessment of linear regression techniques for modeling multisensor data for non-invasive continuous glucose monitoring, in *2011 Annual International Conference of the IEEE Engineering in Medicine and Biology Society* (IEEE, 2011), pp. 2538–2541
34. U. Khan, F. Aadil, M.A. Ghazanfar, S. Khan, N. Metawa, K. Muhammad, I. Mehmood, Y. Nam, A robust regression-based stock exchange forecasting and determination of correlation between stock markets. Sustainability **10**, 3702 (2018)
35. F.Y. Osisanwo, J.E.T. Akinsola, O. Awodele, J.O. Hinmikaiye, O. Olakanmi, J. Akinjobi, Supervised machine learning algorithms: classification and comparison. Int. J. Comput. Trends Technol. (IJCTT) **48**, 128–138 (2017)
36. V. Nasteski, An overview of the supervised machine learning methods. Horizons. b **4**, 56 (2017)
37. D.C. Montgomery, E.A. Peck, G.G. Vining, *Introduction to Linear Regression Analysis* (John Wiley & Sons, 2021)
38. A.I. Taloba, R.M. Abd El-Aziz, H.M. Alshanbari, A.-A.H. El-Bagoury, Estimation and prediction of hospitalization and medical care costs using regression in machine learning. J. Healthc Eng. **2022**, 7969220 (2022)
39. Y.-Y. Hsieh, C.-D. Wu, S.-S. Lu, Y. Tsao, A linear regression model with dynamic pulse transit time features for noninvasive blood pressure prediction, in *2016 IEEE Biomedical Circuits and Systems Conference (BioCAS)* (IEEE, 2016), pp. 604–607
40. Z. Zhang, Introduction to machine learning: k-nearest neighbors. Ann Transl Med **4**, 218 (2016)

41. M. Shouman, T. Turner, R. Stocker, Applying k-nearest neighbour in diagnosing heart disease patients. Int. J. Inf. Educ. Technol. **2**, 220–223 (2012)
42. M. Panwar, A. Acharyya, R.A. Shafik, D. Biswas, K-nearest neighbor based methodology for accurate diagnosis of diabetes mellitus, in *2016 Sixth International Symposium on Embedded Computing and System Design (ISED)* (IEEE, 2016), pp. 132–136
43. A. Oza, A. Bokhare, Diabetes prediction using logistic regression and K-nearest neighbor, in *Congress on Intelligent Systems: Proceedings of CIS 2021*, vol 2 (Springer, 2022), pp. 407–418
44. R.J. Ramteke, K.Y. Monali, Automatic medical image classification and abnormality detection using k-nearest neighbour. Int. J. Adv. Comput. Res. **2**, 190 (2012)
45. R.H. Ramdlon, E.M. Kusumaningtyas, T. Karlita, Brain tumor classification using MRI images with K-nearest neighbor method, in *2019 International Electronics Symposium (IES)* (IEEE, 2019), pp. 660–667
46. P. Thamilselvan, J.G.R. Sathiaseelan, An enhanced k nearest neighbor method to detecting and classifying MRI lung cancer images for large amount data. Int. J. Appl. Eng. Res. **11**, 4223–4229 (2016)
47. R.M. Parry, W. Jones, T.H. Stokes, J.H. Phan, R.A. Moffitt, H. Fang, L. Shi, A. Oberthuer, M. Fischer, W. Tong, K-Nearest neighbor models for microarray gene expression analysis and clinical outcome prediction. Pharmacogenomics J. **10**, 292–309 (2010)
48. S.M. Ayyad, A.I. Saleh, L.M. Labib, Gene expression cancer classification using modified K-Nearest Neighbors technique. Biosystems **176**, 41–51 (2019)
49. A.A. Kashif, B. Bakhtawar, A. Akhtar, S. Akhtar, N. Aziz, M.S. Javeid, Treatment response prediction in hepatitis C patients using machine learning techniques. Int. J. Technol. Innov. Manag. (IJTIM) **1**, 79–89 (2021)
50. D.J. Peterson, N.P. Ostberg, D.W. Blayney, J.D. Brooks, T. Hernandez-Boussard, Machine learning applied to electronic health records: identification of chemotherapy patients at high risk for preventable emergency department visits and hospital admissions. JCO Clin. Cancer Inform. **5**, 1106–1126 (2021)
51. J. Gupta, The accuracy of supervised machine learning algorithms in predicting cardiovascular disease, in *2021 International Conference on Artificial Intelligence and Computer Science Technology (ICAICST)* (IEEE, 2021), pp. 234–239
52. W.-J. Kuo, R.-F. Chang, D.-R. Chen, C.C. Lee, Data mining with decision trees for diagnosis of breast tumor in medical ultrasonic images. Breast Cancer Res. Treat. **66**, 51–57 (2001)
53. A.T. Azar, S.M. El-Metwally, Decision tree classifiers for automated medical diagnosis. Neural Comput. Appl. **23**, 2387–2403 (2013)
54. L. Tong, G. Tong, A novel financial risk early warning strategy based on decision tree algorithm. Sci. Program. **2022**, 4648427 (2022)
55. M. Alaradi, S. Hilal, Tree-based methods for loan approval, in *2020 International Conference on Data Analytics for Business and Industry: Way Towards a Sustainable Economy (ICDABI)* (IEEE, 2020), pp. 1–6
56. X. Chen, H. Ishwaran, Random forests for genomic data analysis. Genomics **99**, 323–329 (2012)
57. R. Anitha, D. Siva Sundhara Raja, Development of computer-aided approach for brain tumor detection using random forest classifier. Int. J. Imaging Syst. Technol. **28**, 48–53 (2018)
58. G. Cano, J. Garcia-Rodriguez, A. Garcia-Garcia, H. Perez-Sanchez, J.A. Benediktsson, A. Thapa, A. Barr, Automatic selection of molecular descriptors using random forest: application to drug discovery. Expert Syst. Appl. **72**, 151–159 (2017)
59. R. Guido, S. Ferrisi, D. Lofaro, D. Conforti, An overview on the advancements of support vector machine models in healthcare applications: a review. Information **15**, 235 (2024)
60. S. Ruan, S. Lebonvallet, A. Merabet, J.-M. Constans, Tumor segmentation from a multispectral MRI images by using support vector machine classification, in *2007 4th IEEE International Symposium on Biomedical Imaging: From Nano to Macro* (IEEE, 2007), pp. 1236–1239
61. Y. Rejani, S.T. Selvi, *Early Detection of Breast Cancer Using SVM Classifier Technique.* ArXiv:0912.2314 (2009)

62. A.K. Mandle, S.P. Sahu, G. Gupta, Brain tumor segmentation and classification in MRI using clustering and kernel-based SVM. Biomed. Pharmacol. J. **15**, 699–716 (2022)
63. L.N. Mahdy, K.A. Ezzat, H.H. Elmousalami, H.A. Ella, A.E. Hassanien, Automatic x-ray covid-19 lung image classification system based on multi-level thresholding and support vector machine. MedRxiv 2020–2023 (2020)
64. E.D. Übeyli, Recurrent neural networks employing Lyapunov exponents for analysis of ECG signals. Expert Syst. Appl. **37**, 1192–1199 (2010)
65. N.F. Güler, E.D. Übeyli, I. Güler, Recurrent neural networks employing Lyapunov exponents for EEG signals classification. Expert Syst. Appl. **29**, 506–514 (2005)
66. Z. Xiong, M.P. Nash, E. Cheng, V.V. Fedorov, M.K. Stiles, J. Zhao, ECG signal classification for the detection of cardiac arrhythmias using a convolutional recurrent neural network. Physiol. Meas. **39**, 094006 (2018)
67. S. Mao, E. Sejdić, A review of recurrent neural network-based methods in computational physiology. IEEE Trans. Neural. Netw. Learn. Syst. **34**, 6983–7003 (2022)
68. E. Choi, A. Schuetz, W.F. Stewart, J. Sun, Using recurrent neural network models for early detection of heart failure onset. J. Am. Med. Inform. Assoc. **24**, 361–370 (2017)
69. S.M. Al-Selwi, M.F. Hassan, S.J. Abdulkadir, A. Muneer, E.H. Sumiea, A. Alqushaibi, M.G. Ragab, RNN-LSTM: from applications to modeling techniques and beyond—systematic review. J. King Saud Univ.-Comput. Inf. Sci. 102068 (2024)
70. C.R. Parra, A.P. Torres, J.M. Sotos, A.L. Borja, Classification of moderate and advanced Alzheimer's patients using radial basis function based neural networks initialized with fuzzy logic. Irbm **44**, 100795 (2023)
71. S. Anita, P.A. Priya, Three dimensional analysis of SPECT images for diagnosing early Parkinson's disease using Radial Basis Function kernel−extreme learning machine. Curr Med Imaging Rev **15**, 461–470 (2019)
72. B. Rim, N.-J. Sung, S. Min, M. Hong, Deep learning in physiological signal data: a survey. Sensors **20**, 969 (2020)
73. S. Vadapalli, H. Abdelhalim, S. Zeeshan, Z. Ahmed, Artificial intelligence and machine learning approaches using gene expression and variant data for personalized medicine. Brief. Bioinform. **23**, bbac191 (2022)
74. N. Shahid, T. Rappon, W. Berta, Applications of artificial neural networks in health care organizational decision-making: a scoping review. PLoS ONE **14**, e0212356 (2019)
75. N. Rane, S. Choudhary, J. Rane, *Explainable Artificial Intelligence (XAI) in Healthcare: Interpretable Models for Clinical Decision Support*, Available at SSRN 4637897 (2023)
76. J.A. Freeman, D.M. Skapura, *Neural Networks: Algorithms, Applications, and Programming Techniques* (Addison Wesley Longman Publishing Co., Inc, 1991)
77. M.A. Rao, J. Srinivas, *Neural Networks: Algorithms and Applications* (Alpha Science Int'l Ltd., 2003)
78. S. Khalid, A. Judge, R. Pinedo-Villanueva, An unsupervised learning model for pattern recognition in routinely collected healthcare data, in: *11th International Conference on Health Informatics (HEALTHINF 2018)* (Scitepress, 2018)
79. E. Bose, K. Radhakrishnan, Using unsupervised machine learning to identify subgroups among home health patients with heart failure using telehealth, CIN: computers, Informatics. Nursing **36**, 242–248 (2018)
80. P. Sarker, M.M.H. Shuvo, Z. Hossain, S. Hasan, Segmentation and classification of lung tumor from 3D CT image using K-means clustering algorithm, in *2017 4th International Conference on Advances in Electrical Engineering (ICAEE)* (IEEE, 2017), pp. 731–736
81. D.M. Mahalakshmi, S. Sumathi, Brain tumour segmentation strategies utilizing mean shift clustering and content based active contour segmentation. ICTACT J. Image Video Process. **9**, 2002–2008 (2019)
82. M. Ayaz, M.F. Pasha, T.Y. Le, T.J. Alahmadi, N.N.B. Abdullah, Z.A. Alhababi, A framework for automatic clustering of EHR messages using a spatial clustering approach, in *Healthcare* (MDPI, 2023), p. 390

83. W. Zhang, X. He, An anomaly detection method for medicare fraud detection, in *2017 IEEE International Conference on Big Knowledge (ICBK)* (IEEE, 2017), pp. 309–314
84. Y.A. Nanehkaran, Z. Licai, J. Chen, A.A.M. Jamel, Z. Shengnan, Y.D. Navaei, M.A. Aghbolagh, Anomaly detection in heart disease using a density-based unsupervised approach. Wirel. Commun. Mob. Comput. **2022**, 6913043 (2022)
85. I. Manolitsis, G. Feretzakis, L. Tzelves, D. Kalles, E. Loupelis, S. Katsimperis, T. Kosmidis, A. Anastasiou, D. Koutsouris, S. Kofopoulou, Using association rules in antimicrobial resistance in stone disease patients, in *Advances in Informatics, Management and Technology in Healthcare* (IOS Press, 2022), pp. 462–465
86. Y. Noguchi, A. Ueno, M. Otsubo, H. Katsuno, I. Sugita, Y. Kanematsu, A. Yoshida, H. Esaki, T. Tachi, H. Teramachi, A new search method using association rule mining for drug-drug interaction based on spontaneous report system. Front. Pharmacol. **9**, 197 (2018)
87. Z. Ding, J. Zhu, Y. Ding, C. Zhu, Comorbidities in congenital heart disease: different patterns in childhood and adulthood. BMC Cardiovasc. Disord. **23**, 613 (2023)
88. R. Anggrainingsih, N.R. Khoirudin, H. Setiadi, Discovering drugs combination pattern using FP-growth algorithm, in *2017 4th International Conference on Electrical Engineering, Computer Science and Informatics (EECSI)* (IEEE, 2017), pp. 1–4
89. K. Chaitanya, E. Erdil, N. Karani, E. Konukoglu, Local contrastive loss with pseudo-label based self-training for semi-supervised medical image segmentation. Med. Image Anal. **87**, 102792 (2023)
90. S. Xie, H. Lin, Y. Liu, Semi-supervised extractive speech summarization via co-training algorithm, in *Interspeech* (2010), pp. 2522–2525
91. Z. Song, X. Yang, Z. Xu, I. King, Graph-based semi-supervised learning: a comprehensive review. IEEE Trans. Neural. Netw. Learn. Syst. **34**, 8174–8194 (2022)
92. A. Madani, M. Moradi, A. Karargyris, T. Syeda-Mahmood, Semi-supervised learning with generative adversarial networks for chest X-ray classification with ability of data domain adaptation, in *2018 IEEE 15th International Symposium on Biomedical Imaging (ISBI 2018)* (IEEE, 2018), pp. 1038–1042
93. D.P. Kingma, D.J. Rezende, S. Mohamed, M. Welling, Semi-supervised learning with deep generative models. Adv. Neural. Inf. Process. Syst. **27** (2014)
94. A. Odena, *Semi-Supervised Learning with Generative Adversarial Networks*, ArXiv:1606.01583 (2016)
95. J.E. Van Engelen, H.H. Hoos, A survey on semi-supervised learning. Mach. Learn. **109**, 373–440 (2020)
96. S. Basu, A. Banerjee, R.J. Mooney, Semi-supervised clustering by seeding, in *Proceedings of the Nineteenth International Conference on Machine Learning* (2002), pp. 27–34
97. J.-N. Eckardt, M. Bornhäuser, K. Wendt, J.M. Middeke, Semi-supervised learning in cancer diagnostics. Front. Oncol. **12**, 960984 (2022)
98. J. Oyelade, I. Isewon, F. Oladipupo, O. Aromolaran, E. Uwoghiren, F. Ameh, M. Achas, E. Adebiyi, Clustering algorithms: their application to gene expression data. Bioinform. Biol. Insights. 10, BBI-S38316 (2016)
99. L.P. Kaelbling, M.L. Littman, A.W. Moore, Reinforcement learning: a survey. J. Artif. Intell. Res. **4**, 237–285 (1996)
100. R.S. Sutton, A.G. Barto, *Reinforcement Learning: An Introduction* (MIT Press, 2018)
101. R.S. Sutton, Dyna, an integrated architecture for learning, planning, and reacting. ACM Sigart. Bulletin **2**, 160–163 (1991)
102. A.S. Polydoros, L. Nalpantidis, Survey of model-based reinforcement learning: applications on robotics. J. Intell. Robot. Syst. **86**, 153–173 (2017)
103. C.J.C.H. Watkins, P. Dayan, Q-learning. Mach. Learn. **8**, 279–292 (1992)
104. H. Ali, Reinforcement learning in healthcare: optimizing treatment strategies, dynamic resource allocation, and adaptive clinical decision-making. Int. J. Comput. Appl. Technol. Res. **11**, 88–104 (2022)
105. E.M. Tosca, A. De Carlo, D. Ronchi, P. Magni, Model-informed reinforcement learning for enabling precision dosing via adaptive dosing. Clin. Pharmacol. Ther. **116**, 619–636 (2024)

106. R. Wu, Z. Yao, J. Si, H.H. Huang, Robotic knee tracking control to mimic the intact human knee profile based on actor-critic reinforcement learning. IEEE/CAA J. Autom. Sin. **9**, 19–30 (2021)
107. C. Yu, G. Ren, Y. Dong, Supervised-actor-critic reinforcement learning for intelligent mechanical ventilation and sedative dosing in intensive care units. BMC Med. Inform. Decis. Mak. **20**, 124 (2020)
108. X. Huang, F. Naghdy, H. Du, G. Naghdy, C. Todd, Reinforcement learning neural network (RLNN) based adaptive control of fine hand motion rehabilitation robot, in *2015 IEEE Conference on Control Applications (CCA)* (IEEE, 2015), pp. 941–946
109. I. Kim, Y. Jeon, J. Chae, D. You, Deep reinforcement learning for fluid mechanics: control, optimization, and automation. Fluids **9**, 216 (2024)
110. O. Vinyals, I. Babuschkin, W.M. Czarnecki, M. Mathieu, A. Dudzik, J. Chung, D.H. Choi, R. Powell, T. Ewalds, P. Georgiev, Grandmaster level in StarCraft II using multi-agent reinforcement learning. Nature **575**, 350–354 (2019)
111. A. Folkers, M. Rick, C. Büskens, Controlling an autonomous vehicle with deep reinforcement learning, in *2019 IEEE Intelligent Vehicles Symposium (IV)* (IEEE, 2019), pp. 2025–2031
112. X. Zhao, L. Xia, J. Tang, D. Yin, Deep reinforcement learning for search, recommendation, and online advertising: a survey, ed. by X. Zhao, L. Xia, J. Tang, D. Yin, M. Vesely as coordinator (ACM Sigweb Newsletter, 2019), pp. 1–15
113. P. Bijapur, P. Chakradhar, M. Rishab, S. Srinivas, B.S. Nagabhushana, Reinforcement learning for energy storage optimization in the smart grid, in *2020 IEEE International Conference on Power Electronics, Smart Grid and Renewable Energy (PESGRE2020)* (IEEE, 2020), pp. 1–6
114. A. Coronato, M. Naeem, G. De Pietro, G. Paragliola, Reinforcement learning for intelligent healthcare applications: a survey. Artif. Intell. Med. **109**, 101964 (2020)
115. R.K. Jha, S. Bag, D. Koley, G.R. Bojja, S. Barman, An appropriate and cost-effective hospital recommender system for a patient of rural area using deep reinforcement learning. Intell. Syst. Appl. **18**, 200218 (2023)
116. K. Li, T. Zhang, R. Wang, Deep reinforcement learning for multiobjective optimization. IEEE Trans. Cybern. **51**, 3103–3114 (2020)
117. P. Wittek, *Quantum Machine Learning: What Quantum Computing Means to Data Mining* (Academic Press, 2014)
118. C. Szepesvári, *Algorithms for Reinforcement Learning* (Springer Nature, 2022)
119. X. Du, Y. Cai, S. Wang, L. Zhang, Overview of deep learning, in *2016 31st Youth Academic Annual Conference of Chinese Association of Automation (YAC)* (IEEE, 2016), pp. 159–164
120. M.H. Sazlı, A brief review of feed-forward neural networks. Commun. Fac. Sci. Univ. Ank. Ser. A2-A3 Phys. Sci. Eng. **50** (2006)
121. S. Pouyanfar, S. Sadiq, Y. Yan, H. Tian, Y. Tao, M.P. Reyes, M.-L. Shyu, S.-C. Chen, S.S. Iyengar, A survey on deep learning: algorithms, techniques, and applications. ACM Comput. Surv. (CSUR) **51**, 1–36 (2018)
122. A. Shrestha, A. Mahmood, Review of deep learning algorithms and architectures. IEEE Access **7**, 53040–53065 (2019)
123. D. Khurana, A. Koli, K. Khatter, S. Singh, Natural language processing: state of the art, current trends and challenges. Multimed. Tools. Appl. **82**, 3713–3744 (2023)
124. S. Sheikhalishahi, R. Miotto, J.T. Dudley, A. Lavelli, F. Rinaldi, V. Osmani, Natural language processing of clinical notes on chronic diseases: systematic review. JMIR Med. Inform. **7**, e12239 (2019)
125. J. Eisenstein, *Introduction to Natural Language Processing* (MIT press, 2019)
126. P.M. Nadkarni, L. Ohno-Machado, W.W. Chapman, Natural language processing: an introduction. J. Am. Med. Inform. Assoc. **18**, 544–551 (2011)
127. M. Nixon, A. Aguado, *Feature Extraction and Image Processing for Computer Vision* (Academic press, 2019)
128. J. Chaki, N. Dey, *A Beginner's Guide to Image Preprocessing Techniques* (CRC Press, 2018)
129. B. Chitradevi, P. Srimathi, An overview on image processing techniques. Int. J. Innov. Res. Comput. Commun. Eng. **2**, 6466–6472 (2014)

130. E. Elyan, P. Vuttipittayamongkol, P. Johnston, K. Martin, K. McPherson, C.F. Moreno-García, C. Jayne, M.M.K. Sarker, Computer vision and machine learning for medical image analysis: recent advances, challenges, and way forward. Artif. Intell. Surg. **2**, 24–45 (2022)
131. S. Khan, M. Naseer, M. Hayat, S.W. Zamir, F.S. Khan, M. Shah, Transformers in vision: a survey. ACM Comput. Surv. (CSUR) **54**, 1–41 (2022)
132. L.-C. Chen, G. Papandreou, I. Kokkinos, K. Murphy, A.L. Yuille, Deeplab: semantic image segmentation with deep convolutional nets, atrous convolution, and fully connected crfs. IEEE Trans. Pattern Anal. Mach. Intell. **40**, 834–848 (2017)
133. J. Janai, F. Güney, A. Behl, A. Geiger, Computer vision for autonomous vehicles: problems, datasets and state of the art. Found. Trends® Comput. Graph. Vis. **12**, 1–308 (2020)
134. X. Jiang, Z. Hu, S. Wang, Y. Zhang, Deep learning for medical image-based cancer diagnosis. Cancers (Basel) **15**, 3608 (2023)
135. S. Goyal, R. Singh, Detection and classification of lung diseases for pneumonia and Covid-19 using machine and deep learning techniques. J. Ambient. Intell. Humaniz. Comput. **14**, 3239–3259 (2023)
136. D.B. Olawade, N. Aderinto, G. Olatunji, E. Kokori, A.C. David-Olawade, M. Hadi, Advancements and applications of Artificial Intelligence in cardiology: Current trends and future prospects. J. Med., Surg., Public Health 100109 (2024)
137. J. Höhn, E. Krieghoff-Henning, T.B. Jutzi, C. von Kalle, J.S. Utikal, F. Meier, F.F. Gellrich, S. Hobelsberger, A. Hauschild, J.G. Schlager, Combining CNN-based histologic whole slide image analysis and patient data to improve skin cancer classification. Eur. J. Cancer **149**, 94–101 (2021)
138. T.J. Brinker, A. Hekler, A.H. Enk, C. Berking, S. Haferkamp, A. Hauschild, M. Weichenthal, J. Klode, D. Schadendorf, T. Holland-Letz, Deep neural networks are superior to dermatologists in melanoma image classification. Eur. J. Cancer **119**, 11–17 (2019)
139. A. Grzybowski, P. Brona, G. Lim, P. Ruamviboonsuk, G.S.W. Tan, M. Abramoff, D.S.W. Ting, Artificial intelligence for diabetic retinopathy screening: a review. Eye **34**, 451–460 (2020)
140. A. Grzybowski, P. Singhanetr, O. Nanegrungsunk, P. Ruamviboonsuk, Artificial intelligence for diabetic retinopathy screening using color retinal photographs: from development to deployment. Ophthalmol. Ther. **12**, 1419–1437 (2023)
141. J. Tang, R.M. Rangayyan, J. Xu, I. El Naqa, Y. Yang, Computer-aided detection and diagnosis of breast cancer with mammography: recent advances. IEEE Trans. Inf. Technol. Biomed. **13**, 236–251 (2009)
142. L. Soler, H. Delingette, G. Malandain, N. Ayache, C. Koehl, J.-M. Clément, O. Dourthe, J. Marescaux, An automatic virtual patient reconstruction from CT-scans for hepatic surgical planning. Stud. Health Technol. Inform. **70**, 316–322 (2000)
143. T. Haidegger, S. Speidel, D. Stoyanov, R.M. Satava, Robot-assisted minimally invasive surgery—surgical robotics in the data age. Proc. IEEE **110**, 835–846 (2022)
144. J. Xu, L. Xiao, A.M. López, Self-supervised domain adaptation for computer vision tasks. IEEE Access **7**, 156694–156706 (2019)
145. A. Krishnan, S. Swarna, Robotics, IoT, and AI in the automation of agricultural industry: a review, in *2020 IEEE Bangalore Humanitarian Technology Conference (B-HTC)* (IEEE, 2020), pp. 1–6
146. R. Doyle, T. Kubota, M. Picard, B. Sommer, H. Ueno, G. Visentin, R. Volpe, Recent research and development activities on space robotics and AI. Adv. Robot. **35**, 1244–1264 (2021)
147. R.R. Murphy, *Introduction to AI Robotics* (MIT press, 2019)
148. M. Soori, B. Arezoo, R. Dastres, Artificial intelligence, machine learning and deep learning in advanced robotics, a review. Cogn. Robot. **3**, 54–70 (2023)
149. S. Chen, J. Liu, Y. Xu, A logical reasoning based decision making method for handling qualitative knowledge. Int. J. Approx. Reason. **129**, 49–63 (2021)
150. R. Bernardo, J.M.C. Sousa, P.J.S. Gonçalves, A novel framework to improve motion planning of robotic systems through semantic knowledge-based reasoning. Comput. Ind. Eng. **182**, 109345 (2023)

151. Y.-J. Chen, Development of a method for ontology-based empirical knowledge representation and reasoning. Decis. Support. Syst. **50**, 1–20 (2010)
152. J. Gómez-Romero, M.A. Patricio, J. García, J.M. Molina, Ontology-based context representation and reasoning for object tracking and scene interpretation in video. Expert. Syst. Appl. **38**, 7494–7510 (2011)
153. P. Zangeneh, B. McCabe, Ontology-based knowledge representation for industrial megaprojects analytics using linked data and the semantic web. Adv. Eng. Inform. **46**, 101164 (2020)
154. L. De Raedt, A. Kimmig, Probabilistic (logic) programming concepts. Mach. Learn. **100**, 5–47 (2015)
155. R. Brachman, H. Levesque, *Knowledge Representation and Reasoning* (Elsevier, 2004)
156. H.-J. Kim, K.D. Kim, D.-H. Kim, Deep convolutional neural network-based skeletal classification of cephalometric image compared with automated-tracing software. Sci. Rep. **12**, 11659 (2022)
157. S. Faghani, B. Khosravi, K. Zhang, M. Moassefi, J.M. Jagtap, F. Nugen, S. Vahdati, S.P. Kuanar, S.M. Rassoulinejad-Mousavi, Y. Singh, Mitigating bias in radiology machine learning: 3 Performance metrics. Radiol Artif. Intell. **4**, e220061 (2022)
158. E. Shortliffe, *Computer-Based Medical Consultations* (MYCIN, Elsevier, 2012)
159. W.G. Baxt, Use of an artificial neural network for data analysis in clinical decision-making: the diagnosis of acute coronary occlusion. Neural Comput. **2**, 480–489 (1990)
160. H. Ding, J. Wu, W. Zhao, J.P. Matinlinna, M.F. Burrow, J.K.H. Tsoi, Artificial intelligence in dentistry—a review. Front. Dent. Med. **4**, 1085251 (2023)
161. A. Ossowska, A. Kusiak, D. Świetlik, Artificial intelligence in dentistry—narrative review. Int. J. Environ. Res. Public Health **19**, 3449 (2022)
162. C. de Cock, M. Milne-Ives, M.H. van Velthoven, A. Alturkistani, C. Lam, E. Meinert, Effectiveness of conversational agents (virtual assistants) in health care: protocol for a systematic review. JMIR Res Protoc **9**, e16934 (2020)
163. G. Dipalma, A.D. Inchingolo, A.M. Inchingolo, F. Piras, V. Carpentiere, G. Garofoli, D. Azzollini, M. Campanelli, G. Paduanelli, A. Palermo, Artificial intelligence and its clinical applications in orthodontics: a systematic review. Diagnostics **13**, 3677 (2023)
164. A.A.F. Alshadidi, A.A. Alshahrani, L.I.N. Aldosari, S. Chaturvedi, R.S. Saini, S.A. Bin Hassan, M. Cicciù, G. Minervini, Investigation on the application of artificial intelligence in prosthodontics. Appl. Sci. **13**, 5004 (2023)
165. S. Basheer, A.S. Alluhaidan, M.A. Bivi, Real-time monitoring system for early prediction of heart disease using Internet of Things. Soft. Comput. **25**, 12145–12158 (2021)
166. D. Dias, J. Paulo Silva Cunha, Wearable health devices—vital sign monitoring, systems and technologies. Sensors **18**, 2414 (2018)
167. S. Kurt Bayrakdar, K. Orhan, I.S. Bayrakdar, E. Bilgir, M. Ezhov, M. Gusarev, E. Shumilov, A deep learning approach for dental implant planning in cone-beam computed tomography images. BMC Med Imaging **21**, 86 (2021)
168. T. Zhang, F. Rabhi, X. Chen, H. Paik, C.R. MacIntyre, A machine learning-based universal outbreak risk prediction tool. Comput. Biol. Med. **169**, 107876 (2024)
169. N. Nazir, A. Sarwar, B.S. Saini, Recent developments in Denoising medical images using deep learning: an overview of models, techniques, and challenges. Micron, 103615 (2024)
170. M. Hamdi, S. Bourouis, K. Rastislav, F. Mohmed, Evaluation of neuro images for the diagnosis of Alzheimer's disease using deep learning neural network. Front. Public Health **10**, 834032 (2022)
171. A.A.-A. Valliani, D. Ranti, E.K. Oermann, Deep learning and neurology: a systematic review. Neurol. Ther. **8**, 351–365 (2019)
172. C.K. Fisher, A.M. Smith, J.R. Walsh, Machine learning for comprehensive forecasting of Alzheimer's Disease progression. Sci. Rep. **9**, 13622 (2019)
173. M. Ghanem, A.K. Ghaith, M. Bydon, Artificial intelligence and personalized medicine: transforming patient care, in *The New Era of Precision Medicine* (Elsevier, 2024), pp. 131–142

174. Z. Dlamini, F.Z. Francies, R. Hull, R. Marima, Artificial intelligence (AI) and big data in cancer and precision oncology. Comput. Struct. Biotechnol. J. **18**, 2300–2311 (2020)
175. A. Blanco-Gonzalez, A. Cabezon, A. Seco-Gonzalez, D. Conde-Torres, P. Antelo-Riveiro, A. Pineiro, R. Garcia-Fandino, The role of AI in drug discovery: challenges, opportunities, and strategies. Pharmaceuticals **16**, 891 (2023)
176. M.A. Alghamdi, From molecules to medicines: the role of AI-driven drug discovery against Alzheimer's disease and other neurological disorders. Pharmaceuticals **18**, 1041 (2025)
177. L. Cortial, V. Montero, S. Tourlet, J. Del Bano, O. Blin, Artificial intelligence in drug repurposing for rare diseases: a mini-review. Front. Med. (Lausanne) **11**, 1404338 (2024)
178. N. Jothi, W. Husain, Data mining in healthcare–a review. Procedia. Comput. Sci. **72**, 306–313 (2015)

Chapter 2
AI in Medical Diagnostics

The second chapter discusses the expanding roles of Artificial Intelligence (AI) in revolutionizing diagnostic medicine. The first part discusses the use of AI in radiology and imaging. It describes how sophisticated pattern recognition algorithms assist in the detection, segmentation, and identification of various anatomical features, as well as pathological processes such as tumors and fractures. The chapter continues to reference the importance of AI in cancer, cardiovascular disease, and other chronic disorders in predictive analytics, genetic risk prediction, early disease detection, and large-scale screening programs. Outstanding case studies reveal the life-altering potential enabled by preventive measures made viable through AI systems in diagnostic processes.

The last subsection addresses the utilization of AI for pathology, most notably with digitized slides and how computational models transform diagnosis at the cellular scale. This includes automated malignancy detection, grading of histologic tumors, and prediction of molecular profiling from tissue samples. Along the chapter, the emphasized problems involve accuracy in diagnosis, workflow and productivity improvement, augmented clinical decision-making support, and numerous more crucial matters regarding the utilization of AI in everyday medicine.

2.1 Introduction

Precise medical diagnoses are crucial to effective healthcare, as they form the basis for clinical decision-making, treatment planning, and patient management. Once a diagnosis has been correctly made, appropriate and timely interventions can prevent disease from progressing and also limit morbidity and mortality rates. Incorrect diagnostic judgments lead to inappropriate treatments, unnecessary procedures, increased costs to healthcare systems, and, most consequentially, poor outcomes for patients. Studies have started to show that diagnostic process inaccuracies account for almost

L. Tayebi et al., *Artificial Intelligence in Medicine and Dentistry*,
https://doi.org/10.1007/978-3-032-15977-9_2

10–15% of all medical errors [1]. Thus, they are a major part of any discussion of diagnostic process errors occurring in modern healthcare systems.

The importance of accurate diagnoses goes beyond the clinical care of an individual patient or a single disease/diagnosis category. In healthcare, earlier is better—especially for the treatment of diseases such as infection, cancer, and cardiovascular conditions. For example, if cancer is diagnosed early, survival rates improve, as localized tumors can often be treated without the complex considerations required for tumors that have metastasized. Effective accumulated diagnostic measures, for infectious diseases such as tuberculosis and, more recently, COVID-19, allow for early and rapid triage to isolation, increasing treatment options and ultimately reducing both disease transmission and virus-induced mortality. In the case of chronic, progressive diseases, developing accurate, high-quality diagnostic tools can help clinicians create tailored treatment plans, maximizing therapeutic benefit while reducing complications.

Although medical diagnostic systems have advanced remarkably, the methods of human assessment still have substantial constraints. Medical practitioners must use complex medical data, sometimes in scenarios of time pressure or cognitive limitation, and therefore, mistakes can be made that may lead to misinterpretation, misdiagnosis, or delayed diagnosis altogether. In addition to human interpretation variability from practitioner to practitioner, there is also variability from specialty to specialty. The greatest potential predictive variability is found in specialties like radiology, pathology, and dermatology because practitioners in these fields often have to rely on subjective interpretation. The same could be said for specialists in fields that rely more on medical history and/or laboratory testing as opposed to imaging. For example, studies have examined interobserver variability among radiologists interpreting standard mammograms [2, 3]. Ultimately, if there is variability due to the human aspect of diagnostics, there is a need to develop standard, automated assessments that augment human abilities—or better, augment the reliability of human clinical decision-making. Conversely, as we continue to discover and learn more about advances in epidemiology and health sciences, we are also learning about increasingly complex diseases and a greater amount of patient data, in order to facilitate diagnostic assessments either precisely or rapidly.

In recent years, AI has become a disruptive technology in medical diagnosis, complementing human expertise and overcoming barriers posed by traditional diagnosis. AI-based diagnostic systems provide better accuracy, greater speed, and better decision support than existing methods, ultimately improving healthcare effectiveness and accessibility as a whole. AI-based systems use Machine Learning (ML) algorithms, Deep Learning (DL) networks, and Natural Language Processing (NLP) capabilities that process large amounts of medical information with improved accuracy and efficiency. They can process imaging scans, lab results, and clinical documents to identify patterns that may not be observed by humans. For instance, AI diagnostic algorithms in radiology have been developed to identify abnormalities from X-rays, CT scans, and MRIs with accuracy levels similar to experienced human radiologists. This advantage becomes particularly beneficial when access to specialists is limited, as AI could potentially fill that gap and thereby improve health equity.

AI is also revolutionizing the field of pathology, which relies on histopathological interpretation of tissue specimens to facilitate diagnoses of several cancers and infectious diseases. Digital pathology, combined with AI-enabled image analysis, increasingly improves the accuracy and efficiency of diagnosing conditions including breast cancer, prostate cancer, and melanoma. In this aspect of its utility for patient care, AI can assist the pathologist in identifying cellular changes that indicate abnormality, classifying tumor grade, and predicting patient prognosis. Research has shown that AI approaches to pathology achieved the same or better performance than pathologists for specific tasks in certain conditions [4]. Most importantly, diagnostic work in pathology can be performed as real-time analysis of pathology slides, expediting diagnostic workflow and allowing for quicker clinical decisions.

In addition to imaging and pathology, the role of AI in laboratory medicine and clinical decision support is essential. ML algorithms are being applied to blood tests, genetic information, and biomarker profiles to provide disease detection earlier than before. As an example, ML predictive models have been trained to recognize early physiologic changes in critically ill patients to predict the onset of sepsis and offer timely interventions that helped save lives [5, 6]. Continuing the focus on predictions, ML algorithms have also been applied to genomic analysis and can aid our understanding of underlying genetic susceptibilities to dementia, neurodegenerative pathology, and hereditary cancers [7, 8]. With AI-enabled genomic diagnostic testing, clinicians can now generate precision therapies targeting an individual's genomic susceptibilities, which collectively improves the efficacy of precision medicine.

Clinical Decision Support Systems (CDSS), enabled by AI capabilities, are yet another important development in many aspects of diagnostic medicine. CDSS leverage information from a patient's history, labs, and imaging studies to help providers with evidence-based diagnostics and treatment decisions. They have also shown that they can improve accuracy in the diagnostic process by confirming a patient's information against medical databases to identify diagnostic errors (when providers overlook or misdiagnose an illness or disease). AI-enabled systems may also suggest other relevant sources of data for providers to rule out disease or confirm a diagnosis. In the case of emergency medicine, AI-powered triage systems have the potential to be used to analyze symptoms in real time, much like a triage nurse would assess a patient's condition, prioritizing the severity of illness or disease to improve resource allocation in hospitals for life-threatening conditions and injuries. As CDSS are applied in this manner, it leads to better outcomes for patients and improved efficiency in healthcare.

As AI keeps improving and adapting, it is becoming clearer that it has the potential to disrupt medical diagnostics. When combined with emerging technological capabilities such as the Internet of Things (IoT) or health wearables, it is anticipated to improve real-time disease monitoring and predictive diagnostics. AI-enabled wearables can collect biometric data continuously over time, detecting early physiological changes and alerting health providers to possible risks before acute conditions develop. We see a chance for healthcare to shift from reactive to proactive; it facilitates prevention and earlier intervention against many common health concerns.

Given the importance of accurate diagnostics in healthcare overall, as well as AI's power to revolutionize the diagnostic process, this chapter will outline the intersection of AI and diagnostics in medicine. AI's application in diagnostic medicine is not simply an improvement to an existing process, but rather a necessity—it addresses many of the constraints of traditional diagnostics, advances decision-making, and optimizes patient care. AI has changed the availability of medical data for analysis; it enables more relevant pattern recognition and evidence-based recommendations. AI is becoming an indispensable part of healthcare today. Additionally, advances in ML, DL, and overall computational capabilities have created a new way to perform diagnostic processing that is often cheaper, faster, and more accessible than traditional methods.

The following sections of this chapter will further describe AI's use in various diagnostic applications. Section 2.2 will show how AI has been widely deployed in radiology and medical imaging, detailing how AI algorithms detect patterns and anomalies associated with individual presentations across X-rays, CT scans, and MRIs. It will also discuss the advantages, particularly in how AI improves diagnostic accuracy and efficiency, alongside challenges such as false-positive rates, false-negative rates, and data dependency. Following that, Sect. 2.3 will cover early disease detection through AI, explaining predictive analytics, genomics analysis, and AI-supported screening programs, where early diagnosis and treatment of life-threatening diseases like cancer and cardiovascular conditions are possible. The chapter will also describe AI workflows that enhance pathology (Sect. 2.4), where AI improves digital pathology and enables automated disease diagnosis. Finally, the chapter will conclude with an in-depth exploration of the implications for the future of AI in diagnostics, emphasizing how AI-oriented innovations will have a lasting impact on medical judgment and enhance healthcare value.

2.2 AI Algorithms and Applications in Radiology and Imaging

Today, radiologists utilize a number of AI algorithms, mainly to analyze images for disease detection purposes (such as diagnosis or cancer detection), general segmentation of images for anatomical parts of the body, and anomaly detection. In this section, we provide the reader with an overall overview of the fundamental AI techniques used in radiology, including Convolutional Neural Networks (CNNs), Recurrent Neural Networks (RNNs), Transformer models, and Generative Adversarial Networks (GANs), and how these models can be deployed in practice. It will include a summary of data preprocessing strategies, examples from applied literature (including brief case studies), strategies for evaluation metrics, explainability, algorithm rankings based on task and degree of success, and challenges (bias, interpretability, and computational limits). The objective of this structured overview is to give the audience—healthcare personnel and AI researchers—a straightforward overview of how these AI algorithms work and how they can be applied to medical imaging.

2.2.1 *Key AI Techniques in Radiology and Medical Imaging*

2.2.1.1 CNNs in Medical Imaging

CNNs form the basis of DL architectures used for image analysis. A CNN consists of layers of convolutional filters (kernels) that convolve across images to detect local patterns (edges, textures, or recognizable shapes). A convolution is mathematically described as an operation where filters (or filter matrices) are multiplied element-wise with a region of the image and summed up to form a feature response. Each filter is trained to recognize a specific feature (for example, a filter may activate for regions that look like tumors or lung nodules). Multiple layers of convolutions allow the network to learn a hierarchy of complex features, going from low-level edges in the first convolutional layers to high-level anatomical structures in the deeper layers. This sense from each local area is useful for understanding the complexity of medical images. CNN architecture also includes pooling layers (to reduce spatial resolution and provide invariance to small translations) and fully connected layers or classifiers at the end of the predicted output.

In the field of radiology, CNNs have had remarkable success in accomplishing tasks such as image classification, object detection/localization, and segmentation [9, 10]. For example, CNN-based models are able to correctly and automatically identify pneumonia on chest X-rays or classify breast lesions on mammograms by learning differences in texture that are imperceptible to human readers. The U-Net architecture (an encoder-decoder structure of a CNN) led to significant advancements in the segmentation of medical images and remains the best conventional (or fallback) solution for delineation of organs and/or pathologies with high accuracy [10]. Figure 2.1 provides an example of a standard U-Net CNN architecture for segmenting the femur, tibia, and fibula in MRI scans. The encoder-decoder structure, coupled with the presence of skip connections, facilitates effective feature extraction and anatomical segmentation with the required accuracy. Thus, CNNs can utilize complex structures and patterns in imaging data to successfully detect anomalies (like tumors or fractures), segment organs or lesions, and improve the speed and consistency of image interpretation. In summary, CNNs have improved the precision, efficiency, and automation of diagnostic tasks in radiology, ultimately enhancing patient care [9].

A traditional CNN is trained using a backpropagation routine to optimize a loss function (e.g., the cross-entropy loss for classification). This CNN has many weights associated with convolutional filters, and backpropagation adjusts these weights using gradient descent to minimize the difference between predicted probability (output from the Neural Network (NN) layers) and true labels (e.g., ground truth). For

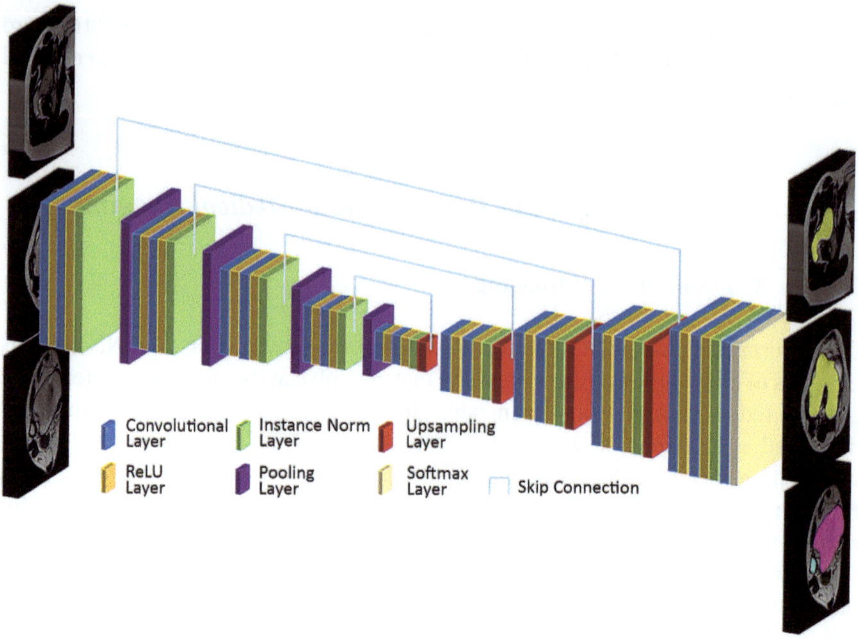

Fig. 2.1 U-Net architecture for bone structure segmentation in MRI scans. Reproduced from Schock et al. [11], published in Scientific Reports 11 (2021) 23,244, under the Creative Commons Attribution 4.0 International License (CC BY), (https://creativecommons.org/licenses/by/4.0/). Font style and text size were adjusted for improved readability; the figure content is unchanged

example, suppose a CNN predicts "no tumor" when the ground truth label provided by the user's diagnostic says "tumor present," effectively increasing the loss; the optimizer will update the filter weights in the direction where the CNN will be more likely to detect the presence of a tumor next time. Convolutional layers enhance learning by taking advantage of the spatial structure of images using relatively small receptive fields and weight sharing, so CNNs have a built-in inductive bias in reconstructing locality and translation invariance, which in effect gives them some advantages with respect to data efficiency and training time in higher-dimensional datasets compared to other recent architectures [10]. Modern CNNs (e.g., ResNet, VGG, DenseNet) have several million parameters, so they typically employ regularization methods such as dropout, weight decay, or data augmentation to avoid overfitting. CNNs tend to reach convergence levels faster than other architectures for image tasks, and they are also relatively robust when trained on small data sizes—partially due to the inductive biases included in the model architecture and the decades of Computer Vision (CV) research informing these architectures [10].

Almost all successful radiology AI products that exist today utilize CNNs at their core for the purpose of image analysis. For example, one system utilizing a CNN for analysis of chest radiographs achieved an Area Under a Curve (AUC) of 0.99

for detecting pulmonary tuberculosis [12]—an accuracy comparable to expert radiologists. CNNs are used to detect lung nodules in CT scans, differentiate malignant from benign lesions in mammograms, and segment tumors or organs on MRI for treatment planning. CNNs excel at tasks where spatial patterns in the pixel data are associated with pathology. In fact, CNN models have been FDA-cleared for a variety of applications in radiology, from flagging strokes on head CT to detecting pneumothorax on chest X-ray, with real-world examples such as the lung nodules study mentioned earlier [13].

2.2.1.2 RNNs and Long Short-Term Memories (LSTMs) for Sequential Data

While CNNs are effective at handling spatial information in a single image, RNNs apply to sequences of data that have temporal structure. RNNs commonly process inputs in order and recursively update their hidden state at each time step to encode relevant information from previous time steps. Thus, an RNN can be utilized for medical data that follows an inherent order or time frame. In radiology, RNNs are primarily used in scenarios involving temporal and sequential images (e.g., ultrasound video frames, cardiac MRI sequences, or treating individual slices from stacked CT scans as a sequence). RNNs can be used to encode either the temporal dependencies between frames or incorporate context and information from all of the previous frames [9]. In cardiac imaging, an RNN could recognize changes in heart chamber sizes as they relate to the cardiac cycle, or in oncologic imaging, an RNN may consider tumor changes across successive follow-up scans.

A fundamental issue for RNNs is the ability to remember long-term dependencies (RNNs can face both vanishing and exploding gradients as sequences become longer), which is why they are not more widely used. LSTM networks and Gated Recurrent Units (GRUs) are used in practice. While LSTMs have gates that control the flow of information—so the network can learn what to keep, write, or delete from the cell state—the LSTM architecture allows it to represent complex, longer-term temporal dynamics more effectively than simpler RNN structures [9].

In the field of radiology, RNNs and their variants have been used for tasks such as:

- **Video Analysis**: For example, classifying ultrasound video clips or endoscopic videos by disease-type patterns, where the LSTM processes the video frames as CNN features in order to identify events or abnormalities over time.
- **Longitudinal Studies**: For example, predicting disease progression when analyzing a series of imaging studies. An LSTM can learn trends, such as lung nodule growth across several CT scans, to predict malignancy risk or estimate time until an adverse event occurs.
- **Multi-Modal Time-Series**: For example, combining imaging with other sequential data (e.g., vitals or lab trends). CNNs are used to extract features from images, while RNNs can combine those imaging features with time-dependent clinical data to strengthen prognostic models.

RNNs have also been combined with CNNs in hybrid models where a CNN encodes each image in a series, and the RNN (or LSTM) then takes the encodings as sequential input. This combines both spatial and temporal representations, accounting for and preserving the fine details of the image in each frame and the changes over time. In a recent study, CNN and LSTM were used together to classify sequential histopathology images of breast cancer. The CNN extracted features, and the LSTM acted on these features as a sequence, which increased classification robustness [14]. RNNs (and especially LSTMs) are generally important when using sequential or time-series medical imaging data. They provide the ability to recognize patterns in a sequence of time points. RNNs can be particularly effective for predicting a patient's condition timeline (e.g., predicting how a patient's disease at time T will change at time $T + 1$ based on previous imaging scans). RNNs are also used in areas outside of imaging (e.g., predicting radiology text report strings or modeling sequences of Electronic Health Record (EHR) events in imaging studies). RNNs represent a temporal dimension to radiologic AI, providing researchers with the ability to model a time-dependent process that cannot be expressed in a static (single time point) image model.

2.2.1.3 Transformers in Medical Imaging Domain

Transformers are a newer family of DL architecture that is gaining traction due to their application and success in NLP and, more recently, in CV. Instead of convolutions or recurrence, Transformers are built on a fundamental unit of self-attention. Self-attention provides the model with the ability to weigh the various components of the input relative to each other. For images, Vision Transformers (ViTs) divide an image into patches (e.g., 16×16 pixels) and linearly project them into an embedding space. The Transformer then processes the patches using self-attention layers that allow it to model global relationships: each patch can attend to every other patch, regardless of their spatial distance from each other. This global approach is quite different from that of CNNs, which can only see a local neighborhood in the earlier layers of the model and must stack many layers to achieve long-range context.

The main strength of Transformers in imaging is their large effective receptive field—they can integrate data from the entire image (or even multiple images) in one layer [10]. In radiology, this implies that the Transformer could learn that a faint finding in the lung apex may be equally reflected in another finding in the lower lung, or that, when considering the presence of an abnormality, it must be done in relation to much of the surrounding anatomy. The most obvious benefit of this type of learning is in more complex images, where context matters. For example, a classifier responsible for differentiating tumor tissue from normal tissue will need to evaluate the border as well as the surrounding tissue types. Similarly, disease diagnostic reasoning may require scanning the entire image to detect subtle cues from other areas. Again, the global context naturally encapsulated in the Transformer model makes it ideal for such scenarios. Early research has demonstrated that Transformers are able to match or even exceed CNN performance on medical image classification and segmentation

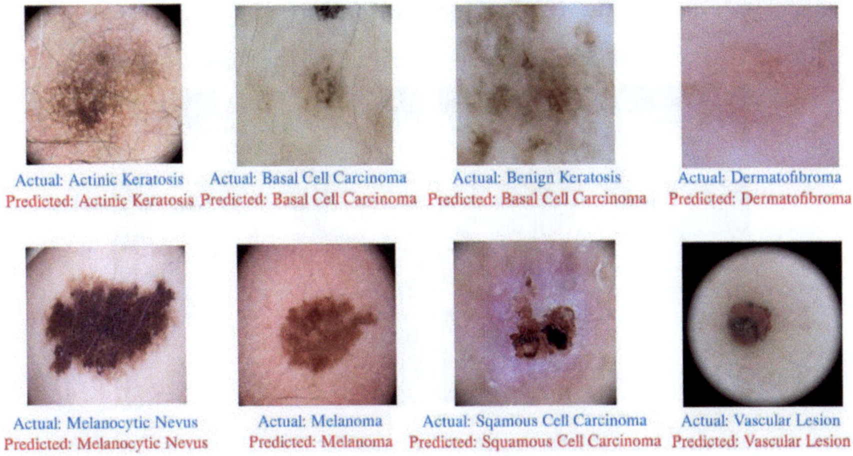

Fig. 2.2 Examples of skin disease detection using ViTs. Reproduced from Saha et al. [17], published in Informatics in Medicine Unlocked 47 (2024) 101,495, © 2024, with permission from Elsevier

tasks when enough training data is available [15]. They have been employed to classify images of skin lesions [16, 17] (seen in Fig. 2.2), detect diseases on chest X-rays [18–20] (seen in Fig. 2.3), and segment organs from MRI/CT [21] (seen in Fig. 2.4), often matching or exceeding CNN performance—particularly when the global context of the image is important.

However, Transformers face significant hurdles in medical imaging. They have many more parameters than CNNs and don't have the built-in biases (such as locality and translational invariance) that CNNs do [10]. This means you need much bigger datasets and more computing power to train Transformers well. In medical imaging, data can be scarce (it's tougher to get thousands of labeled MRI scans than millions of regular photos), and privacy issues make it hard to share data. Because of this, a Transformer might not work well if you just apply it to a small set of radiology images where a CNN would do fine. Scientists tackle this problem by using pre-training (often on large general image databases or medical data from multiple institutions) and by creating hybrid models that mix CNN and Transformer parts. For instance, a common method for medical image segmentation is TransUNet, which uses a CNN encoder to capture basic features and a Transformer module to model global interactions followed by a decoder for segmentation [22]. These hybrids use CNNs to make the most of limited data and Transformers to understand the big picture.

In conclusion, Transformers in radiology are an exciting technology with very high potential. They have been used successfully in image classification, segmentation, detection, and image reconstruction and enhancement tasks. Transformers afford flexibility and global reasoning in medical imaging; however, they are also more data- and compute-hungry. Though Transformers may offer advantages, they are more compute-intensive and typically require Graphics Processing Unit (GPU)

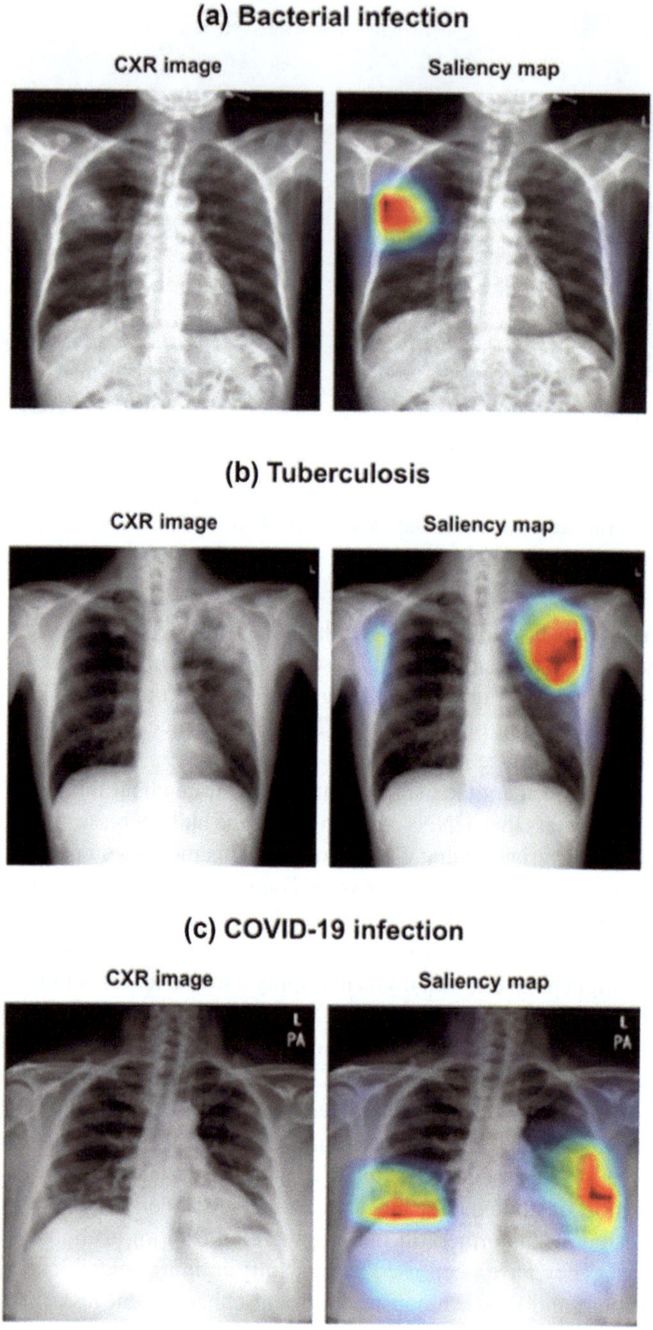

Fig. 2.3 Examples of disease detection in chest X-rays using ViTs. Reproduced from Park et al. [20], published in Medical Image Analysis 75 (2022) 102,299, © 2022, with permission from Elsevier

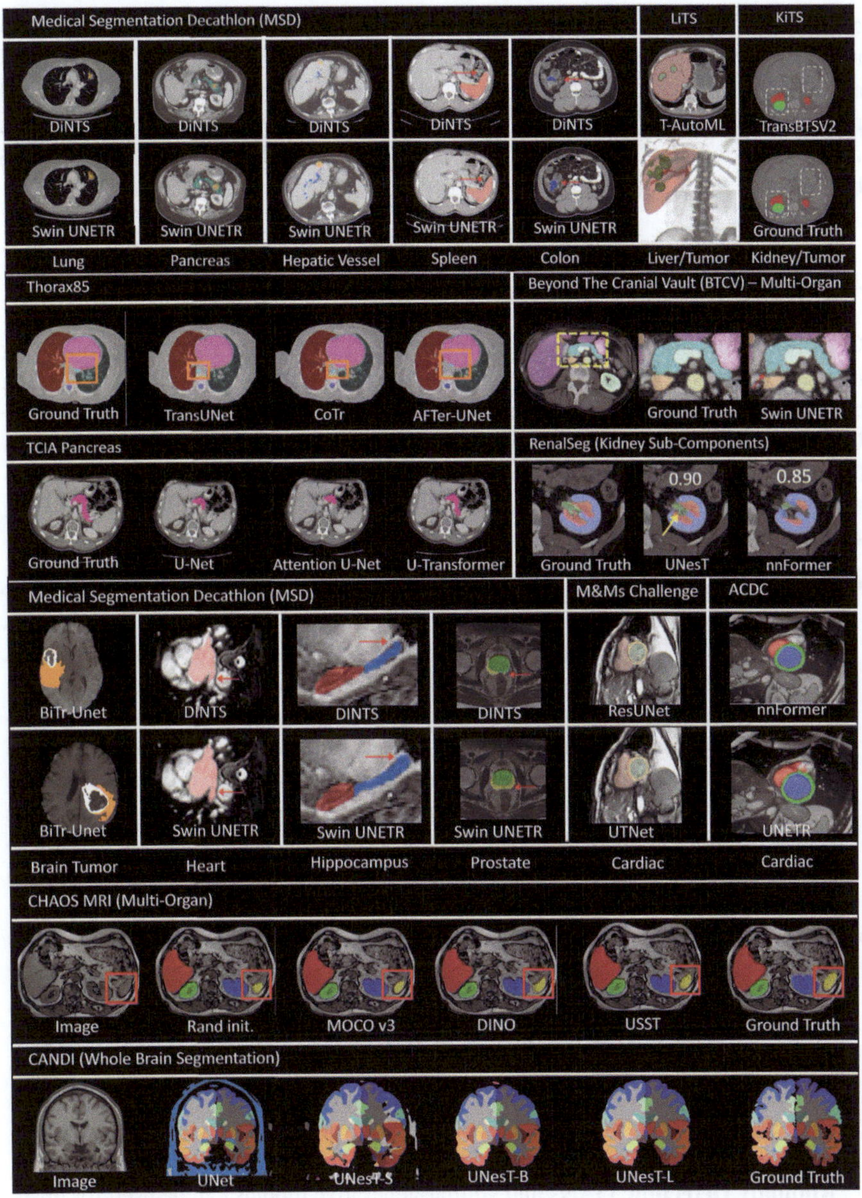

Fig. 2.4 Segmentation of organs in MRI/CT using Transformer-based models. Reproduced from Li et al. [10], published in Medical Image Analysis 85 (2023) 102,762, © 2023, with permission from Elsevier

acceleration and longer training times than CNNs. Whether or not they will actually "transform" radiology remains to be seen. Nevertheless, in the current literature, Transformers can reach (or exceed) state-of-the-art results in a variety of medical imaging tasks, as long as the appropriate amount of data is provided. As more methodologically annotated datasets and Federated Learning (FL) consortia become available in radiology, the role of Transformers will continue to increase.

2.2.1.4 GANs in Radiology

GANs are a specific type of AI algorithm that is well-suited for creating or enhancing images. A GAN consists of two NNs—a Generator and a Discriminator—which compete in a game-like scenario: the Generator aims to produce realistic fake images, while the Discriminator learns to identify fakes versus real images. With this adversarial training approach, the Generator becomes better and better at generating data that resembles real distribution. In radiology, GANs can be applied in several important ways:

- **Data Augmentation and Synthesis**: GANs are capable of generating realistic synthetic medical images to augment limited datasets [9]. For example, if a training set has few examples of a rare tumor, a GAN could generate additional plausible tumor images for the CNN to learn from. This helps address class imbalance and counteracts data scarcity. GAN-generated images (when done successfully) closely resemble real images, which is confirmed by both visual inspection and statistical evaluation. By adding synthetic images to an existing dataset, GANs have been shown to improve the accuracy of diagnostic models performing tasks such as lesion classification or abnormality detection. One study used GAN to generate diverse synthetic medical IoT data (including imaging data) and found that models trained on this augmented dataset performed better [23].
- **Image-to-Image Translation**: GANs (especially conditional GANs or CycleGANs) can translate images between domains. In radiology, this is useful for converting low-dose CT images to higher quality ones or for cross-modality tasks [24]. For example, a model called DU-GAN was proposed to denoise low-dose CT images; it incorporates a GAN with dual U-Net discriminators, producing CT images with considerably less noise and improved image quality [25]. GANs have also been used to synthesize MRI scans from CT (or vice versa), providing additional information or compensating for missing modalities [26–28].
- **Anomaly Detection**: GANs and similar generative models can be used for unsupervised anomaly detection. The idea is to train a GAN only on normal images, so the Generator learns the distribution of normal anatomy. When making predictions, if a new image contains areas the model cannot reconstruct well (i.e., high reconstruction error), those regions are likely anomalies. This allows for flagging unusual findings without explicit labels. For instance, an adversarial autoencoder (a kind of GAN) trained on healthy images was able to detect diseases like breast

cancer or lung lesions by identifying areas with the highest reconstruction error—regions that did not match normal anatomy [29]. GAN-based anomaly detectors may prove useful in screening contexts, where they highlight "something atypical" for the radiologist—even if the model has never seen that type of pathology before.

- **Synthetic Data to Train Other Models**: GANs have also been used to generate synthetic training data for models predicting clinical outcomes. Kadri et al. [30], for instance, used a GAN to synthesize training samples (to simulate patients) for predicting length of stay in an emergency department. These simulated patients helped address limited training data and improved the model's performance. In another study, GAN-generated images were used to fine-tune a CNN in a semi-supervised learning setting; classification accuracy improved when GAN-labeled images were used alongside a small number of real labeled images from an unlabeled set [31].

Training a GAN is typically framed as a minimax optimization problem: the Generator attempts to minimize loss (e.g., binary cross-entropy), reflecting how well it fooled the Discriminator, while the Discriminator attempts to maximize that loss (or equivalently, Generator minimizes the negative of the loss) to correctly distinguish real from fake. In practice, Discriminator and Generator take turns updating via gradient descent. If balanced properly, their performance improves iteratively—Discriminator gets better at detecting fakes, and Generator gets better at producing realistic outputs. A well-trained GAN should capture the underlying data distribution. The "realism" of a GAN-synthesized medical image is judged both by visual inspection and by objective metrics such as Frechet Inception Distance (FID), or by measuring how well a trained classifier performs using GAN-generated images. In radiology, it is especially important that synthetic images retain medically meaningful features (e.g., a GAN-generated chest X-ray showing tuberculosis must clearly display characteristic infiltrates). Some studies have reported that GANs can produce such medically plausible variations [23].

In conclusion, GANs can be seen as auxiliary tools in radiology AI. They supplement and enhance training data, indirectly improving the performance of discriminative models [9]. They also address specific needs in image processing (e.g., denoising and modality transformation) and facilitate semi-supervised and unsupervised learning. While GANs do present training challenges (such as instability and sensitivity to hyperparameter tuning), their ability to "daydream" new medical images give them unique power in the field of medical imaging.

2.2.2 *Training, Optimization, and Hyperparameters*

For an AI model in radiology to function adequately, the training of the model is important. The training process involves giving labeled imaging data to the model and iteratively adjusting the model's parameters to reduce prediction errors. This section will cover some of the other mathematical and practical implementations involved in training DL models, which include optimization methods, loss functions, and hyperparameter tuning.

2.2.2.1 Optimization and Loss Functions

Most DL models are trained through a gradient-based optimization procedure. There is a loss function $L(\theta)$ defined for the model that quantifies how far off the predictions are from the ground truth labels as a function of the model parameters θ. Some common loss functions used in radiology include: binary cross-entropy or categorical cross-entropy for classification (measuring the disparity between model-predicted probabilities and true label classes), Mean Square Error (MSE) for regression problems (predicting a continuous value), and other specific losses for segmentation problems like Dice coefficient loss and Intersection-over-Union (IoU) loss (these losses directly optimize the overlap between predicted and true masks). The model is trained in the following way: the model computes predictions in a forward pass, which are then used to evaluate the loss function. Next, a backpropagation step computes the gradient of the loss with respect to each parameter, followed by an optimizer that adjusts the parameters in the direction that lowers the loss [32]. This is usually done using variants of Stochastic Gradient Descent (SGD).

- **SGD**: The classic optimizer, which updates weights by small amounts based on the negative gradient. In practice, mini-batch SGD is used, where the gradient is estimated from a batch of, e.g., 16 or 32 images at a time (i.e., trading off noise versus compute efficiency).
- **Adaptive optimizers**: In the literature, Adam (Adaptive Moment Estimation) is very popular in radiology AI [11]. Adam adjusts the learning rate for each parameter dynamically, based on estimates of the first and second moments of the gradients, and can lead to faster convergence than basic SGD. Other optimizers include RMSProp, Adagrad, etc. The choice of optimizer and learning rate remains somewhat of an art—if the learning rate is too high, the model may diverge; if too low, it may converge slowly or get stuck in a local minimum.
- **Regularization**: To avoid overfitting (in which the model memorizes training images rather than generalizing), techniques such as dropout (randomly zeroing out neurons during training) and L2 weight decay (penalizing large weights in the loss function) are applied. Early stopping is also helpful, where training is paused once validation loss stops improving. Regularization helps the model better reflect the data's complexity by adding either constraints or noise during training.

2.2.2.2 Hyperparameter Tuning

Hyperparameters are the external parameters of the learning process—meaning they are parameters of the model that are not directly learned from the data. Hyperparameters include the learning rate, number of layers in the network, number of filters, kernel size, batch size, number of training epochs, and more. Hyperparameter tuning is necessary to achieve the best model performance [33]. In the context of radiology, an optimized hyperparameter tuning can be the difference between average model performance and state-of-the-art performance.

Researchers employ a number of hyperparameter optimization approaches. The simplest method is manual tuning, based on experience and trial-and-error. More systematic methods include grid search (searching all combinations of a predefined set of values for each hyperparameter) and random search (randomly sampling the hyperparameter space), both of which are widely used [34]. For example, we may use grid search learning rates of $\{0.1, 0.01, 0.001\}$ and batch sizes of $\{16, 32\}$, etc., to find the best combination that yields the best performance. Random search can sometimes find suitable configurations more efficiently than grid search, especially when some hyperparameters are not very sensitive.

More sophisticated methods in the academic literature—such as Bayesian optimization and evolutionary algorithms—are also used for hyperparameter tuning, though they tend to be computationally expensive. Similarly, there is increasing interest in Automated ML (AutoML) and neural architecture search, but these approaches have seen limited adoption in radiology due to their high computational cost and the need for oversight to ensure clinical validity.

It is worth mentioning that hyperparameters should be tuned only on training and validation data—not on the test data—to avoid biased evaluation. Hyperparameter tuning can introduce data leakage (i.e., accidentally using test data during the tuning process), which may lead to overly optimistic results that do not reflect performance on truly unseen. Hyperparameter searches should be conducted without any access to the test set, and also default configurations used in other publications may not be suitable for new datasets [34].

2.2.2.3 Monitoring Training (Overfitting vs. Underfitting)

During training, the loss on the training set will typically decrease over time, but we need to monitor the loss and accuracy on a held-out validation set during training as well. If the validation loss is also decreasing—meaning both training and validation loss are going down—your model is improving generalization. However, if the validation loss starts to increase while the training loss is still decreasing, then your model is likely overfitting; it is learning spurious details from the training data that do not generalize. If that happens, then in practice, one would stop training (early stopping) or increase regularization. If both training and validation loss are high and neither is improving, then it is likely your model is underfitting (too simple or not trained enough) [35]. If your model is underfitting, some things you could do are: train longer, pick a more complex model (e.g., add more layers or parameters), or tune hyperparameters such as the learning rate. Radiology datasets can be very complex, so achieving the right model capacity and training time is challenging.

In conclusion, training DL models for radiology is all about finding a balance between learning enough and not overfitting. This is a careful process that requires a combination of good initialization (often using pre-trained models from either ImageNet or large medical datasets), a loss function that aligns with the goals of the task, a robust optimization algorithm, and thoughtful tuning of hyperparameters. Reporting the exact training specifics, such as optimizer type, learning rates, and the criteria for decreasing or stopping the learning rate is crucial, as these details are essential for reproducing the reported performance in any research study.

2.2.3 *Frameworks and Implementation*

Implementing AI algorithms for radiology tasks is facilitated by powerful open-source frameworks. As shown in Fig. 2.5, Python is the leading programming language, primarily because of its array of DL libraries with easy-to-use functionality. Important frameworks include:

- **TensorFlow**: TensorFlow is an end-to-end open-source platform that was developed by Google for ML. TensorFlow is extremely popular in both research and production. It has a natural layered structure, which allows it to offer high-level Application Programming Interface (APIs) that run on top of lower-level APIs, such as Keras—an easy-to-use frontend for rapid prototyping—as well as lower-level APIs when deeper control is required. TensorFlow offers strong production capabilities for deploying models with TensorFlow Serving, TFLite for mobile, and more generally, excellent distributed training features.

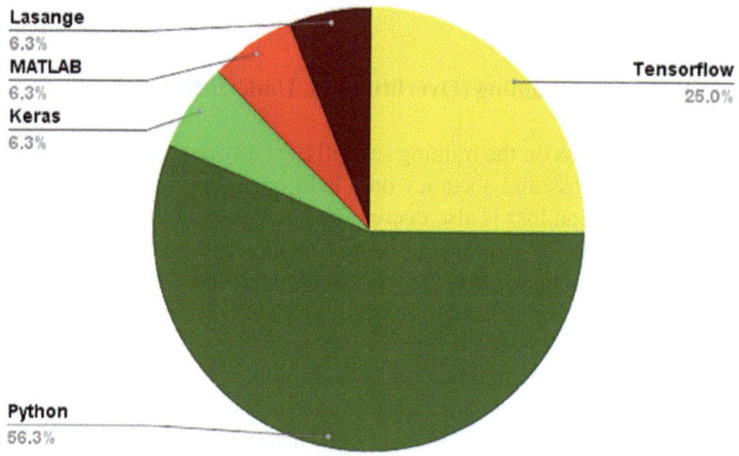

Fig. 2.5 Programming languages used in learning algorithms used for medical image analysis. Reproduced from Li et al. [9], published in Frontiers in Public Health 11 (2023) 1,273,253, under the Creative Commons Attribution 4.0 International License (CC BY), (https://creativecommons.org/licenses/by/4.0/)

- **PyTorch**: PyTorch is an open-source DL library initially developed by Facebook AI Research (FAIR), now part of Meta. It has become exceptionally popular in research due to its dynamic computation graph (eager execution), which removes a level of abstraction and makes debugging and development feel more intuitive. PyTorch is also highly extensible, and many radiology AI researchers gravitate toward it because of its flexibility and the abundance of model zoos (pre-trained models). It is also gaining adoption in production with tools like TorchServe and features such as quantization and ONNX export.
- **Other frameworks**: While other libraries like Keras (now part of TensorFlow), MXNet, and JAX are also available, TensorFlow and PyTorch remain the dominant frameworks. A recent literature review showed that, in the implementation of medical image analysis models, none of the other options were as widely used as Python (with these two libraries). The authors cited simplicity and the availability of ML-specific libraries as key reasons for Python's predominance [9].

The framework support provided by these libraries includes optimized routines for GPU acceleration, which is critical given the size of 3D medical images and the complexity of some deep networks. Model training on a standard Central Processing Unit (CPU) can be costly and time-consuming—sometimes taking weeks—but leveraging GPU-accelerated hardware (such as NVIDIA GPUs) or Tensor Processing Units (TPUs) available on modern cloud platforms can reduce training time to a few hours or days. In modern radiology AI, models are often trained on thousands of images, which can include large volumetric scans. Simply put, it is no longer practical to train on CPUs. These frameworks automatically utilize GPUs, and multi-GPU distributed training is available for handling larger workloads.

These AI frameworks have many features, making them well-suited to radiology. An important feature is pre-trained models and transfer learning. Both PyTorch and TensorFlow have model catalogs (e.g., torchvision.models, TensorFlow Hub) containing networks that have been pre-trained on ImageNet or other large datasets. For radiology projects, a common practice is to load the pre-trained weights and then fine-tune the model on medical images—this is generally referred to as transfer learning. This practice can lead to much better performance in many cases, especially when the medical dataset is small. For example, by using a ResNet50 model that has already been trained on ImageNet database as the starting point to classify chest X-rays, one can expect the learning to converge faster and achieve better accuracy than training the model with randomly initialized weights, as the model already knows how to detect generic visual information.

Furthermore, high-level APIs such as Keras (in TensorFlow) and PyTorch Lightning offer interfaces that simplify coding for training loops, logging, checkpointing, etc. This allows researchers (some of whom may be clinicians) to implement complex models without developing all of the underlying code. As a result, we see rapid prototyping in radiology AI—models can be built by stacking layers together, like Lego toys.

The robust community support and widespread availability of tutorials continue to propel AI's advancement in radiology. For example, a radiologist who wishes to apply a 3D CNN to MRI-based tumor segmentation can often find open-source code or repositories from others to build from, expediting experimentation and validation.

In summary, Python-based DL frameworks (TensorFlow, PyTorch) are the foundation of radiology AI development [9]. They provide the tools needed to implement sophisticated algorithms, leverage high-performance hardware for training, and ultimately deploy solutions. Their user-friendly design has significantly increased their utilization in research in this field. Additionally, the ecosystem offers strong support for data manipulation (through libraries such as NumPy, OpenCV, SimpleITK for medical images, etc.) and visualization (e.g., Matplotlib), creating the most robust and suitable environment for AI in imaging. Moreover, these frameworks continue to improve, ensuring that building robust and practical radiology AI remains accessible.

2.2.4 Data Preprocessing and Augmentation

High quality data is the foundation of any successful AI project. In the case of radiology, there are raw images that come from multiple modalities (e.g., X-ray, CT, MRI, ultrasound), which often require preprocessing before they can be fed into a NN. The types of training data utilized also greatly affect the model's performance, depending on the variety and how balanced the data are. This section will highlight how radiology data is processed.

2.2.4.1 Image Normalization

Medical images may have different intensity scales and resolutions depending on the devices that produce them. For example, MRI intensities are not standardized, and there may be different intensity ranges either across scanner vendors or among different scanner sequences. CT numbers, expressed in Hounsfield Units (which have physical meaning), may still require windowing (i.e., contrast adjustment). Digital radiography images also have varying ranges of pixel values. Normalization is a necessary step to ensure that the input data follow a consistent distribution. Some common practices include:

- Rescaling pixel intensities to a standard range (e.g., 0 to 1, or −1 to 1). For example, CT images can first be clipped to a specific Hounsfield range to highlight areas such as soft tissue or lung and then normalized using min–max scaling.
- Z-score normalization, where the mean intensity of the image is subtracted from each voxel's intensity, and the result is divided by the image's standard deviation [36]. This is usually performed per image or per patient. This process transforms the image so that its overall intensity distribution has a mean of 0 and a standard deviation of 1, producing standardized voxel intensities. This approach is particularly useful for MRI, where relative intensity (contrast) is meaningful, but absolute values are not.

- Spatial normalization, where images are resized to a fixed resolution or size. If a CNN expects images of 224 × 224 pixels (as many pre-trained networks do), a 512 × 512 CT slice may be resampled or cropped to that size, while preserving aspect ratio and anatomical integrity. Alternatively, 3D volumes may be cropped or padded to a standard dimension (e.g., extracting a central 128 × 128 × 128 cube from an MRI).

Normalization facilitates faster and more stable model convergence by reducing variability that is irrelevant to the prediction task. It also addresses differences in image bit depth and ensures that values from the same tissue type have consistent intensities across the dataset [9] (e.g., ensuring that "bone" appears bright in all X-rays presented to the model, and not bright in some and medium in others due to prior image processing differences).

2.2.4.2 Data Augmentation

To aid in model generalizability, data augmentation is used widely in radiology AI. The standard practice of augmenting data involves creating transformed copies of training images based on transformations that realistically simulate variability. Medical imaging has especially benefited from this, as it is generally costly or impossible to collect more data (we cannot simply request more cases of a rare disease), and slight variations in imaging should not alter the diagnosis. Augmentation helps mitigate overfitting by preventing the model from relying solely on pixel-wise memorization. The most common types of augmentations include:

- **Geometric transformations**: Random rotations (e.g., ±10 degrees), flips (horizontal or vertical for some modalities), scaling and/or zooming, translations (shifting the image), and elastic deformations. For example, a chest X-ray can easily be rotated or translated due to natural variation in patient orientation. A brain MRI can be flipped left–right because either orientation is plausible—though care must be taken if laterality is clinically important for the task. Elastic deformation (small, random shape warps) is often used in segmentation tasks to account for anatomical variability in the shape of organs or lesions.
- **Intensity transformations**: Modifying brightness and contrast, adding random noise, or simulating artifacts. A typical MRI image may include random bias field distortions (simulating coil inhomogeneity), while CT images might be augmented with Poisson noise to simulate lower radiation dose. Adding noise or blurring can help models become robust to these phenomena in real-world images.
- **Cropping and patching**: Taking random crops from a large image or combining random patches. This ensures the model can learn from partial views while still recognizing structures. In pathology Whole Slide Images (WSIs), random patches are commonly used as augmentation due to the large size of the slides.

- **Synthetic augmentation**: Using GANs or style transfer to generate new examples (as discussed earlier). For instance, a GAN may produce a plausible alternative version of a tumor based on an existing case or change the visual style of an image (e.g., to emulate the output of a different scanner model).

Data augmentation increases dataset size and diversity at no additional manual collection cost. Evidence suggests that data augmentation can enhance model robustness and prevent overfitting—especially when dataset sizes are relatively small, as is often the case in medical imaging tasks.

2.2.4.3 Handling Class Imbalance

Class imbalance is a common characteristic of medical datasets as there may be far fewer positive cases (those with disease) than negative cases. If only 5% of all chest X-rays show a collapsed lung (pneumothorax) and 95% are normal, a model could achieve 95% accuracy simply by always predicting "normal." Special consideration must be taken when training on imbalanced data. Examples of strategies to address data imbalance include [37, 38]:

- **Data resampling**: Oversampling the minority class (e.g., including multiple copies or augmentations of images with pneumothorax so that they occur more frequently during training), or undersampling the majority class to balance class counts. Typically, oversampling is preferred in radiology because each abnormal case may contain unique features that should not be discarded. Some methods generate synthetic examples of the minority class, such as Synthetic Minority Over-sampling Technique (SMOTE), or—specifically for images—GANs or other augmentation strategies with similar effect.
- **Class-balanced loss functions**: Rather than using a standard loss, one can weight the contribution of the loss for each class so that errors on the minority class are penalized more heavily. For example, a weighted cross-entropy loss could assign a higher weight (e.g., 10×) to positive cases compared to negative ones, thereby encouraging the model to reduce false negatives. Focal loss is another example (commonly used for object detection) that emphasizes harder-to-classify examples and can also help address imbalance.
- **Evaluation beyond accuracy**: In imbalanced datasets, accuracy alone is not informative (as demonstrated by the 95% example). One should instead monitor metrics such as recall, precision, AUC, or F1-score, which better reflect performance under imbalance conditions.

It is recommended that any resampling strategy (oversampling/undersampling) be applied only to the training set [34]. If oversampling is applied to cross-validation folds or test sets, performance metrics can become artificially inflated due to duplicated data. The best practice is to perform oversampling during training at each epoch, so the model sees more instances of the minority class without affecting the original distribution of the validation and test sets.

2.2.4.4 Preprocessing Example

In a typical use case (say, lung nodule classification on CT), one may normalize all CTs to have a common voxel spacing and intensity window, crop patches around the lungs, and then augment each training patch by randomly flipping and rotating. Further, if malignant nodules comprise 1/10 of the data, one may oversample malignant nodules so that, for a batch size of 32, there are approximately 16 malignant and 16 benign nodules. This creates balanced feedback to the network, despite malignancies being underrepresented in the original dataset. For the validation set, although oversampling was applied during training, no oversampling is done during evaluation; metrics are calculated directly on the true class distribution.

In conclusion, data preprocessing and augmentation are essential steps that can ultimately affect how well the model performs. Good normalization ensures that the model is not confused by irrelevant differences. Augmentation provides the model with a greater breadth of examples, making it more resilient to variability and noise. Addressing class imbalance ensures that rare but clinically significant presentations are not lost among the majority. A number of reported failures of AI models in deployment can likely be traced back to data issues (e.g., a model may perform well in one hospital but fail in another if the intensity distribution is different, or it may fail on rare cases if it saw too few during training). Therefore, it is essential that every AI practitioner has a well-defined dataset and applies appropriate preprocessing steps before training begins.

2.2.5 Comparing Algorithms for Different Tasks

Every algorithm (CNN, RNN, Transformer, and GAN) has its strengths and is more applicable to certain types of tasks in radiology. Below is a summary of their effectiveness and common uses:

- **Classification**: CNNs have largely dominated this space. For interpreting a single image or 3D scan to provide a diagnostic output, CNN-based models have proven very effective [9]. However, Transformers are beginning to emerge as strong competitors. On very large datasets, they may slightly outperform CNNs in classification accuracy. On smaller datasets, CNNs still generally perform better due to their inductive biases and lower data requirements [10]. In fact, many recent papers propose hybrid CNN-Transformer models, yielding modest performance gains over standalone CNNs [39, 40].

  It's important to note that RNNs are not suitable for standalone image classification (as there is no inherent temporal sequence), but if a task involves a sequence of images, RNNs become applicable. GANs are not classifiers either, but they can improve classification through data augmentation or class balancing. Therefore, for tasks like identifying cancer on a single MRI, a CNN or Transformer architecture is typically used. If the dataset includes tens of thousands of scans, a ViT might yield the best performance [10]; if data is limited, a fine-tuned pre-trained CNN remains more dependable. Overall, CNNs continue to deliver high performance on many classification tasks—sometimes even surpassing human-level accuracy in narrow domains—while Transformers catch up as datasets grow larger.

- **Segmentation**: CNNs, especially encoder-decoder architectures like U-Net (or V-Net for 3D), are the gold standard in medical image segmentation [10]. These models effectively capture local and mid-level context to delineate structures. Recently, Transformers have been incorporated (e.g., TransUNet or attention-only architectures) and have shown promise in modeling global context (e.g., considering both lungs when segmenting one). However, the most successful models are typically hybrids, combining a CNN with Transformer or attention layers. Transformers may require more data to train effectively. RNNs are occasionally used when temporal consistency is needed—such as tracking heart motion across cardiac cine MRI frames—ensuring smooth evolution of the segmentation mask. A more common method is to segment each frame independently with a CNN, followed by post-processing to ensure consistency.

  GANs are typically used to refine segmentation outputs (e.g., via a discriminator that evaluates whether a predicted mask looks realistic) or to generate synthetic segmentation data. There are also conditional GANs that can treat segmentation as an image translation problem (from input image to output mask) [41], but so far, these have not outperformed standard CNN-based models like U-Net at scale. Thus, CNNs remain the dominant architecture for segmentation tasks, with Transformers and GANs offering complementary improvements in specific contexts.
- **Object Detection**: Though less common than classification or segmentation in radiology, object detection is used for tasks like localizing lung nodules, detecting polyps in colonoscopy, or identifying fractures. CNN-based detectors—like Faster R-CNN, You Only Look Once (YOLO), Single Shot MultiBox Detector (SSD)—have been successfully applied. For instance, a 3D CNN can output bounding boxes for potential lung nodules. Transformer-based detectors—like DEtection TRansformer (DETR)—are newer and show promise, but their role in radiology is still evolving. More often, segmentation-based approaches are used to localize objects, with bounding boxes derived from the segmentation masks. So CNNs again are the primary tools. RNNs do not have a role in object detection, and GANs don't either—though they may support training via synthetic anomaly generation.
- **Sequential data/time-series analysis**: This is where RNNs and LSTMs shine. For example, analyzing a cardiac echo video to estimate ejection fraction can involve a CNN to process each frame and an LSTM to model temporal change. Similarly, RNNs can be used to capture longitudinal patterns across multiple imaging time points [9]. Without RNNs, CNNs model only spatial information unless time is treated as another spatial dimension. Transformers can also model sequences using self-attention and are beginning to replace RNNs in some fields (e.g., Temporal Transformers). In medical imaging, where sequences are often short, LSTMs remain popular due to their ease of training and strong performance. In video and

longitudinal analysis, RNNs or Transformer encoders generally outperform static models.

- **Generative tasks and anomaly detection**: GANs and autoencoders are best suited for generative tasks. For example, generating synthetic MRIs from CT images is typically done using CNN-based GAN architectures or newer generative models like diffusion models. GANs are also widely used for style transfer (e.g., MRI T1-to-T2 conversion or histology stain normalization). For unsupervised anomaly detection, GANs or autoencoders trained solely on normal data can identify anomalies via reconstruction error [29]. CNNs, in general, cannot detect anomalies unless explicitly trained to do so. Therefore, generative models are the most appropriate choice for tasks like unsupervised learning and modality translation. While Transformer-based generative models exist, they are still relatively uncommon in radiology compared to GANs.
- **Performance Example**: For brain tumor detection on MRI, a CNN can achieve high classification accuracy and segment tumors with a Dice coefficient of ~0.85–0.90 using architectures like U-Net. An RNN is unnecessary unless temporal imaging is involved. A ViT may achieve similar classification accuracy if trained on a sufficiently large dataset, but CNNs generally converge faster with fewer images. For clinical prediction tasks combining imaging and EHR data, a hybrid of CNN (for image feature extraction) and RNN or Transformer (for temporal data) tend to outperform any single model type. CNNs are also more established for deployment due to lower memory and computing demands compared to Transformers. Therefore, when performance is comparable, CNNs are often chosen for clinical implementation—though this may change as hardware and optimization methods improve.

In summary, CNNs remain the most common models for radiology vision tasks such as classification, segmentation, and detection due to their balance of high performance and moderate resource demands. RNNs/LSTMs are essential for handling sequential or longitudinal data (e.g., across video frames or patient visits). Transformers can outperform CNNs in some cases—particularly with large datasets or tasks requiring global context—but are often used in conjunction with CNNs. GANs are best suited for data generation, augmentation, and anomaly detection. Many successful radiology AI systems combine these architectures: for example, a GAN to generate synthetic images, a CNN to process spatial features, and an RNN to handle temporal data—all contributing to solving the overall clinical problem.

2.2.6 *Real-World Applications and Case Studies*

AI algorithms have made great strides in many radiology subspecialties, showing performance that, in some instances, rivals expert radiologists. Below is a summary of various real-world applications of CNNs, RNNs, Transformers, and GANs in radiology:

- **Detection and classification of disease**: Perhaps the most prevalent use of AI in radiology is the automatic detection of disease in images. One notable example is CheXNet, which is a 121-layer CNN that takes a chest X-ray image as input, and outputs the probability of a pathology. CheXNet famously outperformed radiologists in detecting pneumonia on chest X-rays [42]. CheXNet is illustrated in Fig. 2.6, which shows the model's workflow, while Table 2.1 provides a performance comparison with radiologists using the F1 metric. Several examples of CheXNet applied to pneumonia detection are shown in Fig. 2.7.

  In another study, a deep CNN model developed by Lakhani and Sundaram [12] detected pulmonary tuberculosis on chest radiographs with an AUC of 0.99—an exceptionally high level of accuracy. Such performance in detecting TB suggests that AI has the potential to screen chest X-rays for infectious diseases with minimal missed detections.

  ML algorithms have shown similarly strong performance in detecting breast cancer in mammography [43]. In many published studies, AI models now

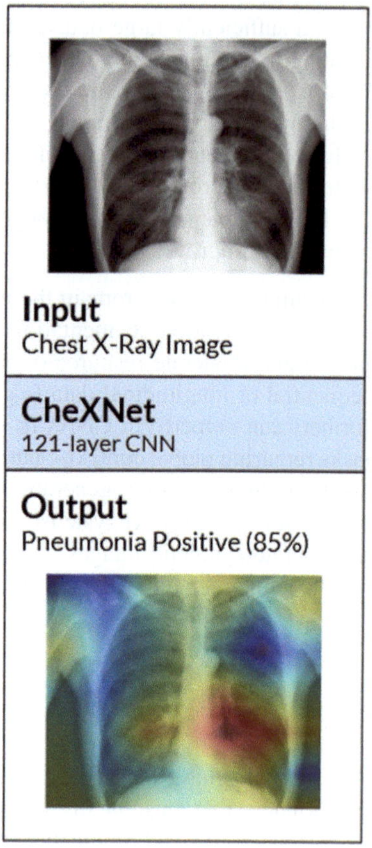

Fig. 2.6 CheXNet detects pneumonia and highlights key areas in the chest X-ray. Reproduced from Rajpurkar et al. [42], published in arXiv Preprint arXiv:1711.05225 (2017), with permission from the author

Table 2.1 The comparison between radiologists and CheXNet model on the F1 metric. Reproduced from Rajpurkar et al. [42], published in arXiv Preprint arXiv:1711.05225 (2017), with permission from the author

	F1 score (95% CI)
Radiologist 1	0.383 (0.309, 0.453)
Radiologist 2	0.356 (0.282, 0.428)
Radiologist 3	0.365 (0.291, 0.435)
Radiologist 4	0.442 (0.390, 0.492)
Radiologist Avg	0.387 (0.330, 0.442)
CheXNet	0.435 (0.387, 0.481)

routinely report sensitivity and specificity in the range of 90–95% for different imaging tasks, highlighting their growing potential for clinical application.

- **Segmentation of Anatomy and Pathology**: AI-based segmentation tools can identify and segment organs (e.g., liver, heart, brain structures) and pathologies (e.g., tumors, cysts, hemorrhages) visible on medical images. The U-Net CNN architecture and its variations have proven highly valuable in this area [10]. For example, in brain MRI, CNN-based models can segment tumors (such as gliomas) into subregions (edema, enhancing core, necrosis) with accuracy comparable to human raters, as demonstrated in the results of the MICCAI BraTS challenge [44].

  In radiation oncology, auto-segmentation is commonly used for organs at risk to accelerate treatment planning. Additionally, in a pediatric radiology case study, an AI model developed to segment lungs on neonatal chest X-rays was able to accurately quantify diseased lung area—useful for clinical management of conditions like respiratory distress syndrome [45] (see Fig. 2.8). As shown in Fig. 2.9, another AI model was developed for projective measurements, including automated MRI segmentation and torsion calculations. This model can analyze knee and hip MRI and perform bone segmentation to define anatomical reference lines [11].
- **Workflow optimization (detecting critical findings)**: AI algorithms are used as "virtual assistants" to triage studies. For example, in an emergency context, an algorithm may concurrently analyze incoming head CTs and identify those likely to demonstrate an intracranial hemorrhage. This can reduce time for treatment for critical patients. AI can catch a "needle in the haystack" finding (e.g., a tiny lung nodule amidst normal variation), acting as a second set of eyes and improving radiologist performance. In one real-world trial, AI for pneumothorax detection on chest radiographs dramatically reduced missed cases by flagging them for radiologist review [46]. Though these tools are not comprehensive, they serve as a safety net against high-risk findings.
- **Prognosis and quantitative measurements**: AI models have a role beyond detection; they can also generate quantitative biomarkers from images that assist in outcome prediction. In neuroradiology, CNN models have been developed to evaluate MRI scans of glioblastoma patients, predicting the presence of genetic markers (such as MGMT promoter methylation) and overall survival by identifying subtle imaging characteristics. One study developed a 3D CNN to predict

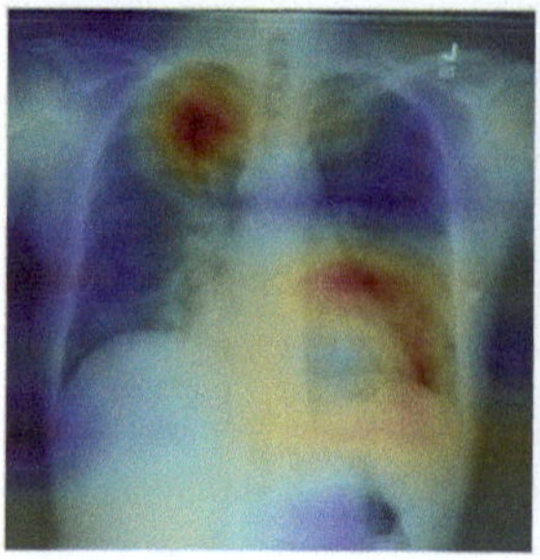

(a) Patient with multifocal community acquired pneumonia. The model correctly detects the airspace disease in the left lower and right upper lobes to arrive at the pneumonia diagnosis.

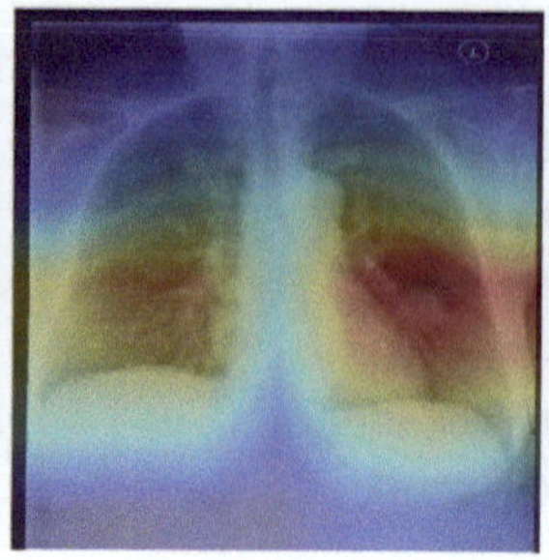

(b) Patient with a left lung nodule. The model identifies the left lower lobe lung nodule and correctly classifies the pathology.

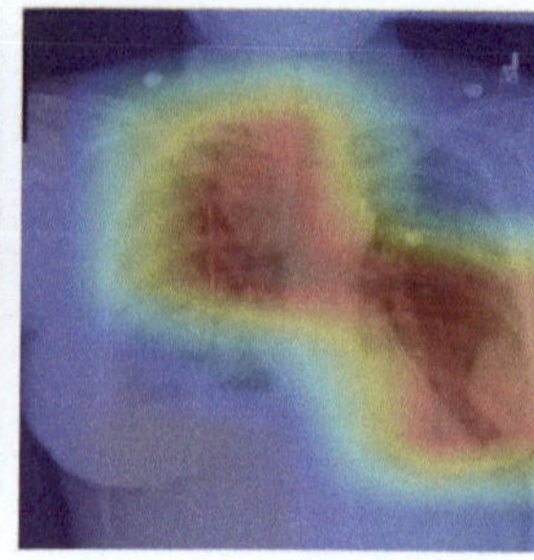

(c) Patient with primary lung malignancy and two large masses, one in the left lower lobe and one in the right upper lobe adjacent to the mediastinum. The model correctly identifies both masses in the X-ray.

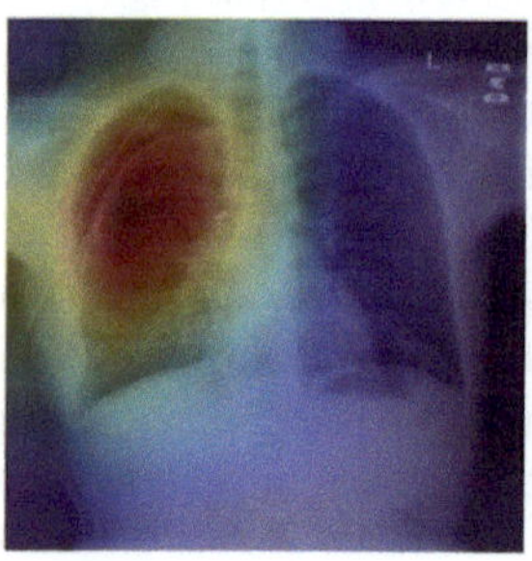

(d) Patient with a right-sided pneumothroax and chest tube. The model detects the abnormal lung to correctly predict the presence of pneumothorax (collapsed lung).

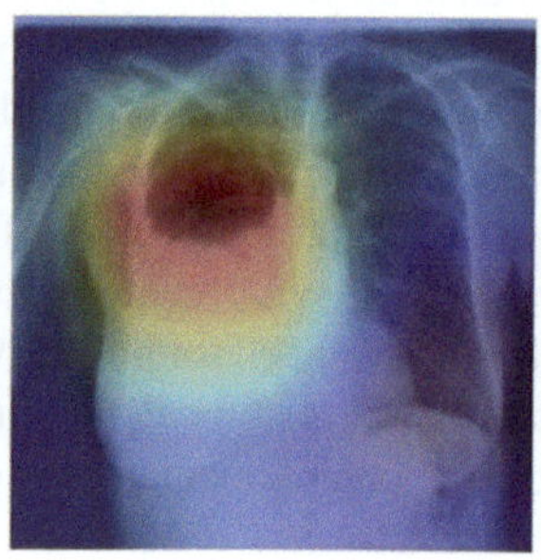

(e) Patient with a large right pleural effusion (fluid in the pleural space). The model correctly labels the effusion and focuses on the right lower chest.

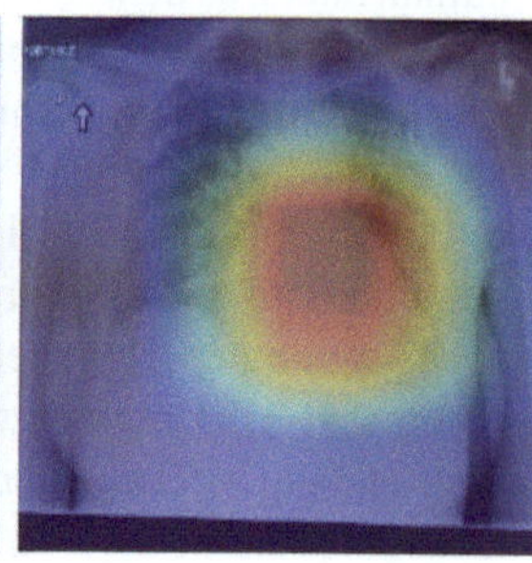

(f) Patient with congestive heart failure and cardiomegaly (enlarged heart). The model correctly identifies the enlarged cardiac silhouette.

Fig. 2.7 Visualization of CheXNet localizing disease regions with Class Activation Maps. Reproduced from Rajpurkar et al. [42], published in arXiv Preprint arXiv:1711.05225 (2017), with permission from the author

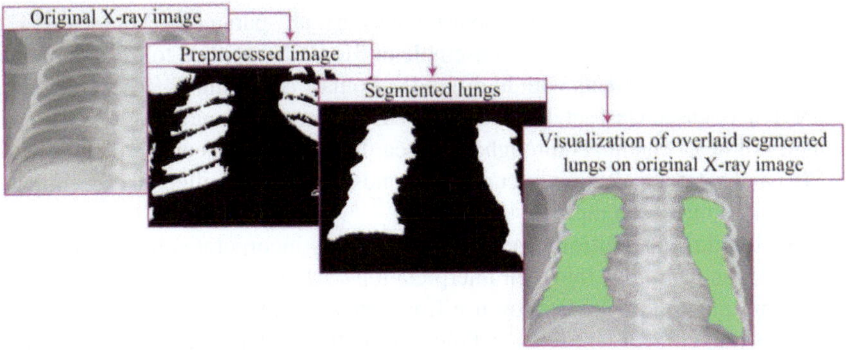

Fig. 2.8 Segmentation process and visualization of the lungs on neonatal chest X-rays. Reproduced from Prodanovic et al. [45], published in Diagnostics 14 (2024) 214, under the Creative Commons Attribution 4.0 International License (CC BY), (https://creativecommons.org/licenses/by/4.0/)

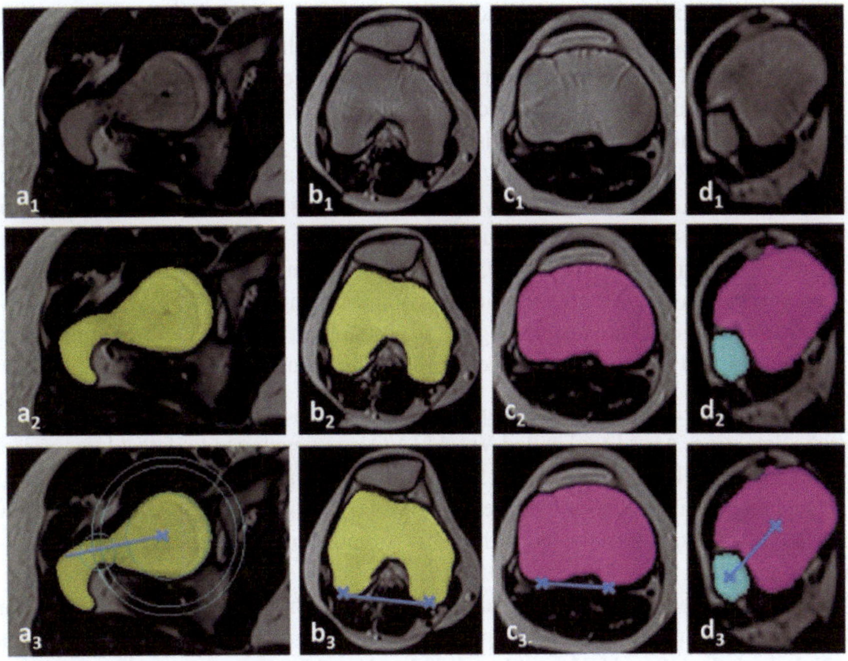

Fig. 2.9 AI-based segmentation and reference line identification in MR images of **a** proximal femur, **b** distal femur, **c** proximal tibia, and **d** distal tibia. Reproduced from Schock et al. [11], published in Scientific Reports 11 (2021) 23,244, under the Creative Commons Attribution 4.0 International License (CC BY), (https://creativecommons.org/licenses/by/4.0/)

MGMT methylation status in glioblastoma from multi-parametric MRI scans [47]. Ben Ahmed et al. [48] used an ensemble of 3D CNNs applied to MRI to predict survival time in patients with high-grade gliomas, achieving 74% accuracy on a previously unseen test set. In cardiology, DL can provide accurate volumetric estimates of heart chambers throughout the cardiac cycle from echocardiography or MRI and estimate ejection fraction in seconds—a task that often takes a clinician several minutes to complete [49].

- **Multi-modal integration**: Radiologists routinely incorporate clinical notes, lab results, and pathology into their interpretations. AI models are beginning to replicate this integration. Studies now use Transformers or hybrid models that take both images and clinical text (e.g., radiology reports or referral reasons) to generate a diagnosis or produce a report [50]. For example, a model might take a chest X-ray and lab results to output probabilities of various diagnoses, serving as a diagnostic support tool. Another application is report generation from images, where CNNs extract features and an RNN (LSTM) or Transformers generates descriptive text—similar to a radiologist dictating findings [51]. Although still in early stages, these auto-reporting systems have shown they can generate basic sentences and interpret images at a fundamental level, though they often miss the nuance that human experts would recognize.
- **Image enhancement and acquisition**: GANs have been used to enhance image quality. In MRI, accelerated imaging is an active area of research—AI models can fill in missing k-space data, allowing for faster scans. GANs and CNNs have been used to reconstruct high-quality images from under-sampled data, reducing scan time significantly [52]. Similarly, AI-based denoising has improved CT imaging, enabling ultra-low-dose scans without compromising quality [53]. These innovations support safer and faster imaging. In ultrasound, AI models can automatically select optimal frames [54], or even guide technicians during acquisition [55].

To further illustrate how these applications influence clinical practice, consider stroke detection. An AI tool called Viz.AI LVO was developed to detect large vessel occlusions on CT angiograms [56, 57]. Upon receiving a scan, the AI processes it in seconds and alerts the on-call neurologist via mobile phone, providing preview images if a blockage is detected. While it is difficult to quantify precisely, this technology can save tens of minutes to hours in notifications and workflow activation. Another example is the Stanford study on CheXNet, which screened chest X-rays for 14 pathologies and performed comparably to radiologists across several conditions [42]. In both the US and UK, an AI system developed for mammogram interpretation matched radiologist performance in accuracy [58], and has been validated for use as a standalone reader in double-reading workflows—potentially saving radiologists time and identifying cancers the initial reader may miss.

It is important to note that, in clinical practice, these algorithms serve as mechanical adjunct tools—not stand-alone diagnostic systems. They are embedded within Picture Archiving and Communication Systems (PACS) or scanner software and produce outputs that radiologists consider alongside their interpretations. Moving forward, the integration of human clinical judgment with the pattern recognition power of AI—unfailing and consistent—represents a vision of the future of radiology.

2.2.7 *Challenges and Considerations*

Despite remarkable advancements, the introduction of AI as a reasoned component in the diagnostic imaging workflow in radiology presents many challenges. These include technical issues on the imaging side, data-related biases, ethical questions, and practical considerations.

- **Data bias and generalizability**: AI models are only as good as the data they are trained on. If a training dataset is not representative of the broader patient population or imaging modalities, the model may perform poorly on new data. Typical sources of bias include scanner and protocol differences between hospitals, demographic bias, and prevalence bias. For example, a model trained primarily on adult data may fail to generalize to pediatric cases [59]. Bias can be introduced at every stage—data collection, model training, and evaluation [60–62]. To mitigate this, researchers are working to increase data diversity. Meanwhile, external validation still remains the most important step in assessing generalizability. Many models perform well internally but fail in external settings due to overfitting. Including diverse cases during data collection and analyzing errors across subgroups are recommended practices for reducing bias.
- **Interpretability and trust**: DL models are often complex and lack intuitive explanations for their outputs. The inability of models to explain their decisions undermines clinician trust, especially in high-stakes scenarios. For instance, a CNN may flag an image as abnormal but offer no explanation as to why. Tools like Gradient-weighted Class Activation Mapping (Grad-CAM) and SHapley Additive exPlanations (SHAP) can improve explainability, but they are not perfect. Additionally, radiologists need training to understand both the capabilities and limitations of AI. Some have proposed including an "AI interpretation" section in radiology reports, similar to how radiologists incorporate patient history. Improving interpretability—through better model design and post-hoc explanations—and promoting trust through robust validation are essential to safe AI deployment.
- **Data privacy and availability**: Medical data is highly sensitive, making it difficult to share across institutions due to privacy regulations such as the Health Insurance Portability and Accountability Act (HIPAA) and the General Data Protection Regulation (GDPR), and proprietary concerns. This limits access to the large, diverse datasets needed to train high-performing models. FL algorithms offer one solution by training models across multiple sites without transferring raw data. Still, curating and annotating datasets—particularly with expert labels like pixelwise tumor outlines—is labor-intensive. However, the need for large and well-annotated datasets remains a major challenge. Some areas like pediatric imaging are especially affected by limited data availability [63]. Ensuring consistent labeling and protocol adherence is also crucial to avoid introducing misleading patterns.
- **Regulatory and legal barriers**: AI systems intended for clinical use must demonstrate safety and efficacy and gain regulatory approval (e.g., FDA, CE marking). This is particularly complex for AI because models may evolve over time (e.g., in

continuous learning systems). The FDA has begun issuing guidance for Software as a Medical Device (SaMD) [64]. Legal liability is another unresolved issue: if an AI system fails to detect a cancer and a radiologist also misses it, who is responsible? Similarly, if a physician follows an AI's incorrect recommendation, where does accountability lie? These concerns contribute to medicolegal anxieties—will reliance on AI raise the expected standard of care? Regulatory frameworks must evolve to address these questions.

- **Incorporating into workflow**: AI tools must integrate seamlessly into existing radiology workflows, including PACS. If models are slow or require extra manual steps (e.g., exporting to another system), they may be underused. For triage tasks, near real-time processing is essential, which imposes hardware and computational constraints. A powerful model is of limited use if it takes five minutes per scan in an emergency setting. Most deployed systems rely on GPU-accelerated hardware or hybrid cloud platforms. Efficient model design (e.g., pruning, quantization) is necessary for practical deployment. Some institutions also face IT infrastructure challenges when hosting or maintaining AI systems.
- **Overfitting and spurious feature learning**: AI models can learn the wrong features and still perform well on test data if the test set shares the same spurious correlations. A historical example is a model that associates ink marks on pathology slides with malignancy labels, falsely interpreting the ink as predictive [65]. Similar risks exist in radiology, such as models learning to associate pneumonia with unrelated features like an apical TB scar. These issues require careful experimental validation. Researchers must intentionally manipulate or mask potential confounders to test whether performance degrades. Techniques like data augmentation, adversarial training, and explainability tools can help prevent or detect spurious learning.
- **Human-AI interaction**: Radiologists' interaction with AI affects its success. Studies show that human-AI collaboration can outperform either alone, but only when users understand and trust the system. Poorly presented AI outputs or automation bias (over-reliance on AI even when it is wrong) can harm clinical decision-making. There is concern that routine AI use might erode clinicians' skills. The field is moving towards considering AI to serve as an assistant—for example, auto-generating preliminary reports for normal studies to save time and reduce burnout. Proper training and education in AI usage are key to fostering appropriate trust and understanding.
- **Computational constraints**: Training cutting-edge AI models often requires extensive hardware resources, which are not readily available at all academic institutions. There is a growing digital divide between well-resourced and under-resourced centers. Cloud computing helps but raises concerns about latency and data privacy. On-device AI (e.g., embedded in ultrasound machines) is promising but demands efficient models that can run on limited hardware. As models grow in size, their deployment becomes increasingly limited to well-funded institutions. Model distillation (compressing large models into smaller ones by transferring knowledge from a large "teacher" model to a smaller "student" model) and hardware advancements are needed to make AI broadly accessible.

- **Ethical Issues**: Beyond technical concerns, AI's impact on the workforce is an ethical issue. While most experts believe AI will augment rather than replace radiologists, job security remains a concern. Patient perception is also important—some may be uncomfortable knowing a computer helped interpret their scan. Transparent communication, emphasizing that physicians still oversee AI results, can help with acceptance.

Despite these issues, there is reason for optimism. Radiology has historically embraced digital innovation, and over 75% of FDA-cleared AI medical devices to date are in radiology—underscoring the field's readiness for AI adoption [13]. Research continues to address bias, fairness, and interpretability, and initiatives such as FL are helping build the diverse datasets needed for robust AI development.

The realization of AI's full potential in radiology requires a coordinated effort: strong algorithm design, rigorous validation, collaboration across disciplines (AI researchers, radiologists, clinicians), and a clear regulatory pathway. Addressing these challenges is essential to integrating AI as a standard tool for radiologists—enhancing diagnostic accuracy, efficiency, and patient outcomes while minimizing risks and unintended consequences.

2.3 Early Disease Detection Algorithms

Early detection algorithms utilize AI and data analytics to identify medical conditions at their earliest stages, often before symptoms appear. This shift promotes a preventive approach to healthcare rather than reactive treatment and is already under way. AI systems are processing massive amounts of data—including EHRs, genomic profiles, and wearable sensor data—and monitoring for subtle variances that may signal an emerging pathological condition. In this section, we discuss three aspects of early disease detection, including predictive analytics, genetic analytics, and AI-supported screening programs.

2.3.1 Predictive Analytics

Predictive analytics in healthcare concern the use of AI models to predict risk of disease in an individual before the disease is clinically evident. By using heterogeneous data—such as demographics, medical history, lab testing, imaging, lifestyle factors, and even environmental exposures—AI algorithms can combine inputs to compute risk scores or probability of being diagnosed with multiple diseases, conditions, or health events. These models represent a dramatic shift to more proactive forms of medicine. Ideally, rather than waiting for a patient to become ill, clinicians may be notified that a patient has, for example, a 70% probability of developing diabetes or cancer in the next five years, allowing for interventions (e.g., changes in diet and lifestyle, screening tests, or prophylactic therapies) to prevent or mitigate the disease process.

2.3.1.1 Data and Methods

Predictive analytics systems draw on the enormous amount of health data generated daily in contemporary healthcare and leverage various ML algorithms—from basic regression models to deep NNs—to identify patterns that clinicians may not catch before disease onset. For example, an AI system might detect subtle trends in hospitalization data correlated with routine lab tests, vital signs, and demographic characteristics. Predictive analytics models can use data from EHRs, insurance claims, social determinants of health, and increasingly, wearable devices or remote sensors. Wearables provide a continuous stream of physiological data (heart rate, activity level, sleep), offering real-time signals of physiological changes.

One of the major strengths of predictive analytics is its ability to integrate multiple data sources and uncover complex interactions among risk factors. Through training on large cohorts, AI models learn predictive signatures—often non-intuitive combinations of variables—that can forecast disease with impressive accuracy. DL is especially useful in this context, as NNs can automatically learn high-dimensional features from raw data. For instance, a CNN applied to a chest X-ray might identify an incidental, asymptomatic lung nodule likely to grow [42], while RNNs or LSTMs can analyze time-series data like electrocardiograms (ECGs) to detect early deterioration indicative of sepsis or heart failure. CNNs perform well on image-based predictions, RNNs (especially LSTM variants) on temporal data, and tree-based models (e.g., Random Forests (RF)) on structured tabular data like risk scores for diabetes or heart disease [9, 66]. In practice, ensemble approaches that combine multiple models often achieve the best results when handling diverse inputs.

2.3.1.2 Effects on Early Diagnosis

The ultimate goal of predictive analytics is earlier intervention and improved outcomes. These models have demonstrated success in predicting chronic diseases like diabetes, cardiovascular conditions, and cancers [67, 68]. If high-risk patients are identified well before clinical presentation, clinicians can implement targeted prevention strategies. For instance, an AI model might flag a patient as high risk for stroke based on blood pressure patterns, lifestyle, and genetic risk. The clinician can then initiate early interventions such as antihypertensive therapy or lifestyle counseling. By avoiding hospitalizations because of taking preventive action, healthcare costs can be reduced. This proactive approach can transform outcomes, as catching disease in incipient stages typically makes it more treatable and less debilitating.

A notable example is DeepCare by Pham et al. [69], an AI system built on LSTM networks trained on longitudinal medical records. DeepCare reads medical records, stores previous illness history, infers current illness states and predicts future medical outcomes. It handles irregular intervals between visits and incorporates treatment effects. In cohorts with diabetes and mental health conditions, DeepCare significantly improved prediction accuracy and enabled more timely clinical interventions.

Similarly, predictive models applied to ICU data, such as those from the MIMIC database, have been used to anticipate deterioration hours in advance [70]. Early warning scores powered by AI have been implemented to anticipate sepsis in hospitalized patients, reducing mortality by prompting earlier administration of antibiotics and fluids. One notable system is the Targeted Real-Time Early Warning System (TREWS) developed at Johns Hopkins University, which led to an 18.7% relative decrease in in-hospital mortality when providers confirmed alerts within three hours [71, 72]. Studies comparing automated AI alerts to standard care in sepsis management showed a reduction in sepsis-related mortality, primarily due to earlier administration of antibiotics and fluids [73, 74].

2.3.1.3 Implementation and Limitations

Although predictive analytics is promising, it is not infallible. There is inherent uncertainty in early predictions, and continuous validation is critical. Nevertheless, the tools are advancing rapidly and becoming more reliable. One particularly compelling application is risk stratification—AI models can identify subsets of younger patients who, based on genetic, biometric, or environmental profiles, have the disease risk of someone older. This allows clinicians to offer screening or preventive interventions earlier than standard guidelines recommend. In doing so, predictive analytics supports the transition toward precision public health.

Importantly, many predictive models go beyond risk scoring by identifying the most influential variables contributing to risk. This transparency is beneficial when counseling patients, as they can understand the relevance of specific risk factors (e.g., blood glucose levels, BMI, family history) and make lifestyle changes accordingly. By streamlining complex data analysis, predictive analytics help clinicians empower patients to take proactive roles in their health—often before any symptoms arise.

2.3.2 *Genetic Analysis*

Our DNA is the beginning of a story about the diseases we may eventually develop. AI is becoming a vital component in the study of genetic variability, offering new ways to assess disease predisposition. Genomic technologies now enable rapid sequencing of an individual's genome, or profiling of millions of variants (such as SNPs), generating vast amounts of data. Embedded in this data are early indicators of future disease. Certain mutations (not just common variants) can markedly increase disease risk—for example, BRCA1 and BRCA2 mutations are linked to heightened risk of breast and ovarian cancer [75]. Still, identifying meaningful risk is often complex, as it can involve thousands of variants with small effects that combine to influence disease, forming what are known as polygenic risks. This is where AI excels as ML models can scrutinize through high-dimensional genomic data to identify patterns linked to disease.

2.3.2.1 AI Application in Genomic Data Interpretation

Traditionally, genetic analysis relied on manual, hypothesis-driven inquiry—evaluating individual genes for known mutations linked to disease. AI has reversed this approach. Instead of evaluating one gene at a time, algorithms are trained on genomic and phenotypic data from thousands of individuals, both healthy and affected, and are tasked with identifying distinguishing DNA patterns. This data-driven approach allows AI to uncover subtle or rare associations that may escape human reviewers. For instance, algorithms can scan an entire genome and flag a rare, possibly pathogenic variant—an effort akin to finding a needle in a haystack. These capabilities have already helped identify novel genetic mutations linked to rare disorders that might have been overlooked using conventional methods [76]. By comparing a patient's genome against databases of known variants and predicted gene functions, algorithms can flag anomalies likely to cause disease, expediting diagnosis for conditions that standard genetic tests failed to explain.

AI models also offer value in interpreting more common genetic variants. One of the long-standing dilemmas in clinical genetics has been the interpretation of Variants of Uncertain Significance (VUS). These are changes in the genome that may or may not be clinically relevant, often leaving clinicians and patients in diagnostic limbo. AI models can combine evidence from diverse biological datasets to assess whether a VUS is likely to impact gene function. In effect, AI can provide a probabilistic functional impact assessment for variants. For example, if a patient carries a missense mutation in a tumor suppressor gene, and similar changes have been linked to cancer in variant databases or biochemical simulations, AI might reasonably classify the variant as potentially pathogenic. Such insight enhances clinical decision-making, offering greater clarity on whether intensified screening or preventative treatment should be considered.

Another area where AI is showing promise is in calculating Polygenic Risk Scores (PRS) for complex diseases. Unlike single-gene disorders, most common diseases such as heart disease, type 2 diabetes, and many cancers arise from the combined influence of multiple genetic variants, each contributing a small amount to risk. PRS summarize this influence into a single risk metric. Whereas traditional PRS models were based on statistical models and limited in their integration of other health data, AI models can incorporate nonlinear interactions and contextual information, such as lifestyle, family history, and other clinical parameters. A recent review noted that AI could revolutionize how PRS are applied in clinics by enabling more individualized assessments and better-targeted preventive strategies [77]. For example, AI might identify a young patient who—despite low traditional risk—has a genetic profile indicating high cardiovascular risk, thereby prompting early interventions that could prevent future events.

2.3.2.2 From Prediction to Prevention

Interpreting genetic predisposition through AI has tangible clinical implications. If a person is found to carry high genetic risk for a disease, clinicians can tailor prevention strategies accordingly. A woman at elevated polygenic risk for breast cancer might begin mammography at a younger age or start chemoprevention, even without a BRCA mutation. Similarly, someone with high genetic risk for coronary artery disease could begin aggressive lipid management early in life. In hereditary cancer syndromes, AI can help identify at-risk individuals and trigger cascade testing of family members, potentially preventing serious outcomes through early surveillance or prophylactic surgery.

AI can also contribute to precision medicine by matching patients to specific therapies based on their genetic makeup. In oncology, certain tumor mutations predict sensitivity to particular drugs. AI tools can identify these patterns and support therapeutic decisions. In inherited conditions, AI can point to molecular pathways disrupted by specific mutations, suggesting tailored treatment strategies that may intervene before symptoms begin. Though many of these applications remain in early stages, they offer a future in which AI not only predicts disease but helps prevent or treat it at the molecular level.

2.3.2.3 Challenges in Genomic AI

Despite its promise, AI-guided genetic analysis faces important challenges. First, genomic data is highly sensitive, and privacy must be protected through secure data handling practices, including encryption, consent protocols, and compliance with legal regulations like GDPR [78]. Second, clinicians need proper training to interpret and communicate AI-generated genetic insights. Genetic counselors and physicians must be equipped to understand risk outputs and explain them to patients in meaningful ways [79]. Third, genetic risk is inherently probabilistic—AI predictions do not guarantee outcomes. Careful communication is essential to prevent undue anxiety or overconfidence based on risk scores.

Nevertheless, AI is steadily advancing the field of genetic risk assessment. It allows us to detect health risks before symptoms arise and offers a more comprehensive understanding of disease predisposition. With continued refinement, AI could help reorient medicine around prevention, early action, and personalized care—placing genetics at the heart of a more proactive health strategy.

2.3.3 *AI for Screening Programs*

Screening programs are planned efforts to uncover disease in individuals without symptoms in the population (e.g., mammography for breast cancer, colonoscopies for colon cancer, low-dose CT for lung cancer, blood pressure checks for hypertension). Early detection through screening has a long history of improving outcomes for many conditions. However, expedited access to services remains a challenge for screening programs due to traditional factors including human resources, personal interpretation, and false-positive or false-negative results. Utilization of AI will aid screening programs by providing increased accuracy, consistency, and scalability of screening processes targeting diseases such as cancer and cardiovascular conditions, where early intervention may be lifesaving.

2.3.3.1 Improving Cancer Screening

Cancer screening is often linked to medical imaging, where modern AI (especially DL models) is making tremendous strides in learning patterns. Consider breast cancer screening as an example. A radiologist looks at a mammogram X-ray to try and detect subtle evidence of tumors. AI algorithms could serve as an automated second reader (or even primary reader) for the mammogram, reducing radiologists' workload while standardizing quality. Indeed, deep CNN models have been able to achieve expert-level performance in the detection of breast cancer on mammograms. A recently published landmark study evaluated an AI system on mammography data from both USA and UK datasets and demonstrated improved accuracy over a single radiologist, with 9.4% and 2.7% reductions in false negatives (USA and UK), and 5.7% and 1.2% reductions in false positives, respectively [58]. In an independent study of six radiologists, this AI system outperformed the average radiologist with an absolute margin of 11.5% in the Area Under the Receiver Operating Characteristic Curve (AUC-ROC). This means that while the AI caught cancers that some radiologists missed, it also avoided flagging many benign lesions (which may lead to unnecessary stress and biopsies) (see Fig. 2.10). These improvements can be directly related to better outcomes through fewer missed cancers (patients are promptly treated) and fewer false positives (otherwise healthy people aren't put through invasive procedures or the anxiety of being called back).

Many breast screening programs use double-reading (two radiologists independently read each mammogram) in order to detect as many cancers as possible. A high-quality AI model might be able to replace one human reader (or pre-screen mammograms so that only those with suspicious findings are flagged for radiologists), thus alleviating the radiologist shortage while maintaining quality. An effective AI system could be potentially a solution to radiologist shortages by creating a single-reader model with AI support [80]. This could allow screening programs to increase their capacity and speed of service without jeopardizing overall reading performance.

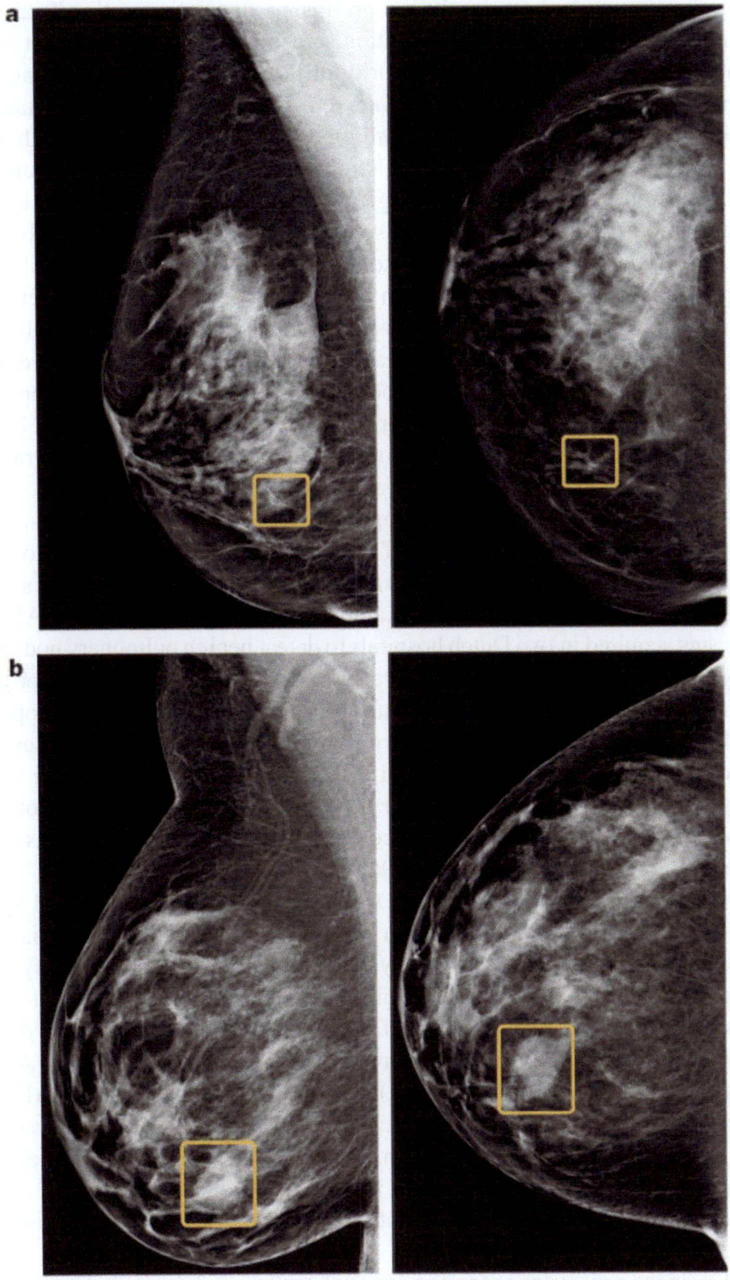

Fig. 2.10 Examples showing discrepancies in identifying cancer cases in the lower inner right breast between the AI system and US readers: **a** a cancer case missed by all six readers but correctly identified by the AI system, and **b** a case detected by all six readers but missed by the AI system. Left, mediolateral oblique view; right, craniocaudal view. Reproduced from McKinney et al. [58], published in Nature 577 (2020) 89–94, © 2020, with permission from Springer Nature

Nevertheless, while these results are promising, experts warn that "real-world" validation is needed before fully entrusting screening to AI. Houssami et al. [80], in their scoping review, noted that majority of the studies published to date on AI performance in breast cancer screening were retrospective, using curated datasets that were not true representations of a screening population. They concluded that while results were promising—with AI models reporting AUC performance from ~0.69 up to 0.98 in some studies—methodological concerns, and evidence gaps exist that limit translation into clinical screening settings. Key gaps included the absence of prospective trials and limited comparisons of AI metrics to radiologists' metrics under real screening conditions. Bias in the training datasets (e.g., datasets highly enriched with cancers or from a singular population) can affect AI's applicability. To demonstrate generalizability and real-world impact, large prospective studies are needed, potentially using AI collaboratively with radiologists. In conclusion, there is significant promise for AI in large-scale cancer screening—from breast to lung cancers and beyond—but actual adoption into national screening programs will require further research and careful consideration.

Apart from breast cancer, AI is being applied to other screening tests. In lung cancer screening, radiologists review CT scans for small nodules, and AI tools have shown similar or higher sensitivity than radiologists, especially when prior scans are unavailable and nodules are small. For example, a study tested a DL -based AI system on CT scans acquired in two Dutch hospitals to detect benign pulmonary nodules and primary lung cancers [81]. This system achieved a sensitivity of 94.3% for benign nodules and 96.9% for primary lung cancers at a clinically acceptable operating point of one false positive per scan—performance equal to or, in some cases, better than radiologists. This could help identify lung cancers at Stage I, when they are much more treatable. In cervical cancer screening, DL algorithms can potentially evaluate cervix images to detect precancerous changes, which may increase access to screening in low-resource settings lacking expert cytologists [82, 83].

For colon cancer, the integration of AI into colonoscopy has enabled systems that assist in real-time polyp detection. These systems use DL analysis during the procedure to highlight potential polyps, aiding endoscopists in identifying and removing precancerous lesions. Randomized clinical trials indicate that AI-assisted colonoscopy improves both Adenoma Detection Rates (ADR) and Polyp Detection Rate (PDR) [84]. In a meta-analysis of 33 trials with 27,404 patients, AI-aided colonoscopy showed a Relative Risk (RR) of 1.24 (95% confidence interval) for ADR compared to standard colonoscopy [85]. This increase suggests more precancerous polyps are detected and removed, which could ultimately reduce colorectal cancer rates. Still, caution is warranted to avoid false positives and overtreatment, ensuring the benefits of improved detection do not lead to unnecessary procedures or patient anxiety.

AI also opens new avenues for non-invasive screening. For example, researchers have used AI to assess retinal photographs—initially designed for diabetic retinopathy screening—to predict systemic conditions like cardiovascular risk. One study demonstrated that a DL model could evaluate retinal images to estimate age, blood pressure, and smoking status, indirectly assessing cardiovascular risk, with results comparable to traditional risk screening [86]. While still preliminary, this demonstrates AI's potential to uncover health markers from common screening data.

An especially interesting application is AI analysis of regular ECGs. In one case, an AI trained on ECGs was able to detect subtle patterns indicating a patient had atrial fibrillation even when the ECG was in normal rhythm [87]. This signal is undetectable by the human eye, but AI identification allows earlier treatment, reducing the risk of serious events like stroke.

2.3.3.2 Expanding Screening with AI

A key advantage of AI in screening programs is scalability. Countries with few specialists could deploy AI to screen images or data and prioritize patients who truly need physician evaluation. For instance, diabetic retinopathy screening often involves yearly fundus photographs. AI is making progress here. Gulshan et al. [88] developed a DL model to detect diabetic retinopathy from retinal photographs, which had high sensitivity and specificity for detecting referable diabetic retinopathy. In simpler terms, the AI could reliably identify patients needing referrals, a major advantage in areas with limited specialist access. Early detection of diabetic retinopathy is crucial, as timely pharmacologic treatment can prevent blindness. Healthcare systems can use AI to automate initial screenings and ensure patients aren't missed due to workforce shortages. Multiple AI-based diabetic retinopathy screening tools have been FDA-approved for use in primary care, providing immediate evaluations of fundus photos and alerting patients when specialist care is needed [89, 90]. This convenience improves adherence and enables earlier detection.

Similarly, AI can support population-level cardiovascular screening. For example, one can imagine mobile apps that use AI to analyze smartwatch data to flag arrhythmia like atrial fibrillation in the general population—the Apple Heart Study showed the feasibility of this approach [91]. For hypertension, AI could analyze blood pressure data and other personal health inputs to identify who is developing sustained hypertension and needs close monitoring. For familial hypercholesterolemia—a genetic cause of early heart disease—AI could search EHRs for patterns (e.g., very high LDL cholesterol plus family history) and alert providers for follow-up.

In short, AI is transforming screening programs by improving accuracy, lessening cognitive load on clinicians, and enabling new forms of screening. AI can serve as a force multiplier, maintaining high standards as screening demand grows. Advancements in AI, particularly in cancer and ophthalmology screening, point toward clinical adoption in the near future. Future success will require strong collaboration among clinicians, researchers, and policy makers to ensure safe, equitable integration of AI tools into screening workflows—enabling AI to be a trusted partner in early disease detection.

2.4 AI Applications in Pathology

Digital pathology—the process of converting glass microscope slides into high-resolution WSIs—has opened a new frontier for AI in medicine. While radiology images are digital by nature and capture organ-level features, pathology images capture cellular-level detail and are orders of magnitude greater in size (often reaching billions of pixels per slide). This section discusses how AI is being applied in pathology, including the digitization of slides, automated disease detection, and the advantages of these tools.

2.4.1 Digital Pathology

Digital pathology refers to scanning conventional histopathology slides to create WSIs that can then be viewed and analyzed on a computer. The emergence of WSIs together with a digital workflow has enabled laboratories worldwide to conduct remote consultations, share slides, and archive slides for teaching, research, and conferences [92]. For example, by 2018, around 60% of pathology departments in the UK were already connected to digital pathology scanners—a number that has likely continued to increase since [93]. The COVID-19 pandemic emphasized the value of digital workflows, enabling pathologists to work and consult remotely on cases when use of a microscope as part of clinical care was not possible [94].

This conversion—from microscope to computer monitor—and the ability to analyze the images with AI is a crucial step toward applying AI in pathology. Once the slide(s) are digitized, AI algorithms can ingest the pixel data to decode patterns and features within the images that might be impossible or time-consuming for a human to recognize. The basic workflow for a pathologist is to microscopically examine sections of tissue; however, this is labor-intensive and subject to interobserver variability. In contrast, a digital workflow combined with AI can mechanize or automate portions of the process. In Fig. 2.11, AI applications are shown across the workflow: performing quality assurance in the pre-analytic stage (e.g., specimen or slide quality), aiding in analytic work (e.g., integrating clinically meaningful data, ordering special studies, flagging important regions), and supporting post-analytic tasks (e.g., report generation, preparation for tumor boards). The transition from glass to data allows pathologists to collaborate with data scientists, enabling the application of "big data" principles in pathology. With large collections of WSIs, DL models can be trained on thousands of examples—a scale not achievable with traditional microscope-based collections—enabling unprecedented exploration of disease patterns.

Importantly, WSIs are very large and complex, presenting a number of technical challenges. A single slide can be 4–5 GB in size, much larger than typical images in radiology [95]. Because of these challenges, early adopters have used high-performance servers and image management systems to store the images and

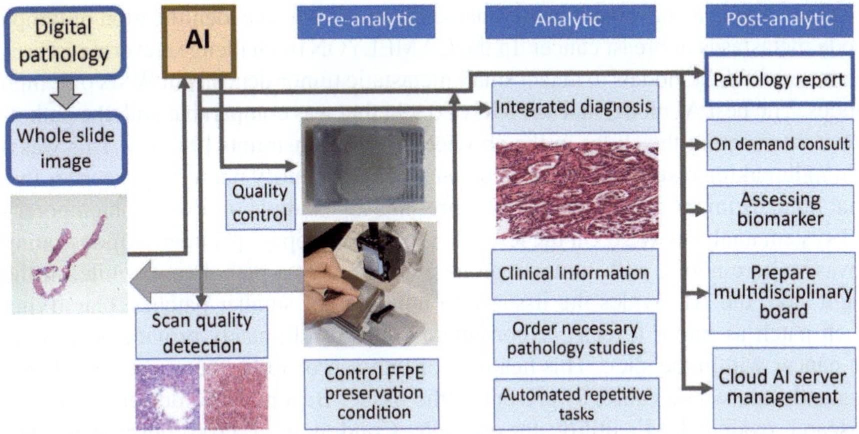

Fig. 2.11 AI integration into the pathology workflow. Reproduced from Kim et al. [95], published in Diagnostics 12 (2022) 2794, under the Creative Commons Attribution 4.0 International License (CC BY), (https://creativecommons.org/licenses/by/4.0/). Font style and text size were adjusted for improved readability; the figure content is unchanged

allow the WSIs to be viewed. AI algorithms must also be able to process these gigapixel images efficiently, which is often done by segmenting the WSI into smaller "tiles" or patches that can be evaluated more quickly. Regardless, digital pathology combined with AI appears to have the potential to ease the workload on pathologists and increase productivity by improving diagnostic accuracy and reducing turnaround times [96]. In summary, the digitization of pathology slides has been a critical enabler for AI, ushering in what is often called "computational pathology"—the application of computational algorithms to analyze digital pathology data.

2.4.2 *Automated Diagnosis with AI*

Now that glass slides can be digitized, AI approaches can be utilized to assist pathologists in the automated detection of disease and recognition of key histologic features at the cellular level. Among these AI approaches, DL within CNNs has emerged as the preferred method. CNNs are effective at recognizing patterns in images and discerning subtle differences in cellular morphology and tissue architecture. Pathology AI models being developed today are capable of a vast array of specific functions, including automated identification of abnormalities, localization of regions of interest (e.g., tumors), quantification of histological features, and diagnosis of disease [97]. In meaningful terms, a CNN algorithm can be presented with an entire WSI of a case and automatically identify and highlight possible cancerous foci, count mitotic figures, measure the distance of tumor invasion, or classify tumor subtype, with the objective of aiding the pathologist's assessment.

One notable achievement in automated diagnosis was the identification of lymph node metastases in breast cancer. In the CAMELYON16 challenge, several research teams created AI models to detect small metastatic tumor deposits in WSIs of lymph nodes. The best AI model had an AUC of 0.994 that was comparable with the pathologist interpreting the slides in the absence of time constraints [98, 99]. This was a groundbreaking result, as it suggested that AI could identify microscopic cancer foci that humans might miss. Figure 2.12 represents an example of how a contemporary AI system analyzes WSI. On the left side is a breast biopsy specimen demonstrating invasive carcinoma, with tumor regions annotated by a pathologist, while on the right side, the AI divides the tissue into hundreds of smaller patches, classifying each patch as tumor (green) or non-tumor (red), to ultimately provide a heatmap of cancer within the slide. This heatmap of tumor probability helps the pathologist instantly see where cancer is present in the tissue. Beyond basic detection, further research extended AI's utility; for example, Coudray et al. [100] developed a DL model which was trained on lungs WSIs and could not only classify lung cancer into subtypes like Lung Adenocarcinoma (LUAD) and Lung Squamous Cell Carcinoma (LUSC) but even predict the mutation status of six genes, including STK11, EGFR, FAT1, SETBP1, KRAS and TP53, directly from the pathology images.

Several commercial AI systems have also been developed to assist in screening and detecting breast lesions in core biopsy specimens [92]. One such example is the Galen Breast algorithm (IBEX Medical Analytics, Israel), which analyzes entire WSIs from breast core needle biopsies to generate heat maps highlighting a range of lesions. These include invasive and in situ carcinomas (both ductal and lobular), atypical hyperplasia, and benign findings such as sclerosing adenosis and fat necrosis. The algorithm uses an ensemble of CNNs trained on over two million annotated image patches derived from more than two thousand Hematoxylin and Eosin (H&E) slides. When evaluated on an independent dataset of 436 breast biopsies, it achieved excellent diagnostic performance, with AUC of 0.99 for invasive carcinoma and 0.98 for Ductal Carcinoma in Situ (DCIS). Moreover, the system demonstrated strong capability in distinguishing between histological subtypes and grades, reaching AUC of 0.97 for invasive ductal vs. invasive lobular carcinoma and 0.92 for high-grade DCIS vs. low-grade DCIS or atypical ductal hyperplasia.

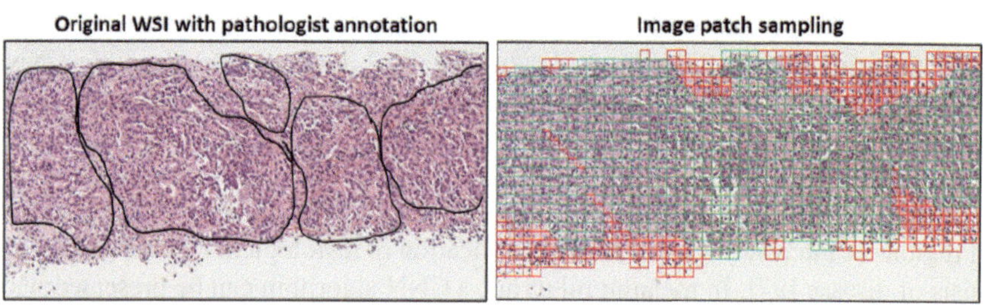

Fig. 2.12 An example of how AI examines a digitized pathology slide by breaking it into many small patches. Reproduced from Kim et al. [95], published in Diagnostics 12 (2022) 2794, under the Creative Commons Attribution 4.0 International License (CC BY), (https://creativecommons.org/licenses/by/4.0/)

It is essential to mention that in the clinical environment, these AI systems are assistive technologies. They are decision-support tools that can flag abnormal areas for the pathologist, pre-screen slides to help prioritize workload, and perform tedious measurements, allowing the expert to focus on interpretation. For instance, Tomita et al. [101] proposed an Attention-Based Deep NNs for distinguishing between low- and high-risk dysplasia samples. This capability can be potentially used for the triage of Barrett's esophagus biopsy specimens, allowing the pathologist to prioritize high-risk cases as a form of automated screening. In real-world use, an AI system might screen all incoming biopsies overnight and mark those slides with probable cancer before the human pathologist reviews and confirms them. Overall, AI assists in improving efficiency while sustaining—or even improving—diagnostic accuracy. In summary, AI is being used to automate diagnosis in pathology: from identifying cancer and other diseases at the microscopic level to grading and measuring disease characteristics and even supporting prognostic and predictive applications—all in aid of helping pathologists deliver timely and accurate diagnoses.

2.4.3 *Advantages of AI in Pathology*

There are some obvious advantages to putting AI into workflow processes for pathology. The largest benefit, undoubtedly, is improved diagnostic accuracy. AI algorithms that are adequately trained can identify minute details or patterns that may be missed by humans, particularly after processing dozens of slides within a busy day. AI can act as a second reader that never gets tired and can help reduce the chance of a missed diagnosis. A recent systematic review of 100 studies demonstrated very high average sensitivity (~96%) and specificity (~93%) for the detection of disease on WSIs by AI algorithms [99]. Our initial understanding is that this shows they can reach the intensity of expert diagnostic performance under research conditions. Some AI systems have a unique ability to identify subtle features, such as tiny metastases or rare single tumor cells, which might have led to missed diagnoses. Studies evaluating Paige Prostate Detect (the first FDA-cleared AI-enabled pathology device for prostate biopsy) have shown that pathologists improve their detection of cancerous features when supported by the AI system [102, 103]. This means that AI, as it develops, can serve as a safety net: at worst, it will help increase cancer detection rates, and at best, it will help users avoid missing critical features in their diagnosis.

Another key advantage is the reduction of workload and, therefore, increases in the efficiency of pathologists. Pathology departments around the globe are inundated with high case volumes but are also experiencing a shortage of specialists. AI can ease some of those squeezes because it can at least automate the most time-consuming tasks. To give an example, when a pathologist performs screening in a batch of lymph node slides for evidence of metastases, this representation of our current practice is very labor-intensive. In contrast, an AI can screen through the entire batch of lymph node slides for a pathologist and either flag a few slides or tell the pathologist which slides were abnormal to some degree. The pathologist still needs to read the slides, but AI-driven triaging means the pathologist spends more time on the slides that are likely to have tumor and significantly less time on the negatives. This means time savings, which can add up. In one breast screening study, an AI triage service was able to safely exclude up to 60% of mammograms from radiologist reviews without missing any screen-detected cancers, thereby substantially reducing workload [104]. The study suggested that using a commercial AI system to triage mammograms into no radiologist assessment and enhanced assessment could potentially cut radiologists' workload by more than half, while also enabling earlier detection of many cancers that would otherwise be found later.

Consistency and reproducibility are additional advantages. Human interpreters can sometimes be subjective—perhaps two pathologists could grade the same tumor differently or count a different number of mitoses. AI algorithms, given the same input, will produce the same output every time and apply a standardized measure. This may lower the inter-observer variability that comes with human interpretation. For instance, an AI-based quantification of immunohistochemical markers, such as estrogen receptor (ER) and progesterone receptor (PR), was found to exhibit excellent agreement with scores provided by experts, as well as significantly improved reproducibility over conventional manual scores [92]. Moreover, researchers have developed an AI-assisted microscope by integrating a human epidermal growth factor receptor 2 (HER2) scoring AI algorithm and an augmented reality module into a conventional microscope. While this system provided pathologists with real-time HER2 assessments for each field of view, it enhanced both the consistency and accuracy of their scoring [105]. By standardizing assessments, AI can establish uniform quality control, and pathology laboratories may increasingly adopt such systems for comprehensive quality assurance.

Ultimately, AI in pathology enhances workflow flexibility. The use of digital slides and AI allows pathologists to conduct work remotely, with the ability for cases to be automatically distributed or prioritized by the AI, making better use of specialist knowledge. The turnaround time can be decreased when AI creates efficiencies in case triaging or case reviews. Overall, the potential benefits to pathology include more accurate and consistent diagnoses, decreased manual burden on pathologists, faster case turnaround, and in some cases, new diagnostic or prognostic information derived from a routine slide. Laboratories using AI tools can potentially achieve greater productivity and clinician satisfaction, as these systems can reduce task load and allow pathologists to be more engaged in higher-level decision-making. Patients will eventually benefit from the changes with more reliable diagnoses and possibly quicker results.

2.5 Conclusion

AI has arrived in the area of medical diagnostics through a variety of means—from AI in radiology and in predictive/ML algorithms for early indications of disease, to its growing role in pathology. As we look toward the future, one can envision a better, faster, and more efficient system to deliver care to patients at scale. In this chapter, we have outlined some exciting AI applications in real-world medical diagnostics.

In radiology, we noted that the latest generation of AI models based on DL can classify and identify abnormalities in medical images with high sensitivity and accuracy, with some models performing comparably to human experts [106]. It is possible that AI will augment radiologists' practice by offering AI-based detection results to highlight areas of interest (e.g., a suspicious lung nodule on a CT scan or a small fracture on an X-ray). In early disease detection, we observed evidence that AI algorithms can evaluate clinical data and patterns, based on routine assessments, to identify diseases earlier than if clinicians were working independently. We provided examples of using AI to review mammographic screening data for early indications of breast cancer; and AI could be used in predictive risk models to forecast events, like stroke or heart disease, before they fully manifest. AI offers new opportunities for clinical engagement and interventions that can improve care delivery.

In pathology, AI-based image analysis is enhancing the diagnostic workflow on digitized tissue slides. These algorithms can identify cancer regions in histopathology images and also extract quantitative features [107]. This not only streamlines the pathologist's workflow—reducing repetitive tasks and turnaround time—but also shifts the diagnostic process toward a more quantitative and data-rich model. Collectively, these advances have substantial clinical impact: patients receive more precise, earlier, and safer treatments, alongside the benefit of AI-based diagnostic comparisons and reduced diagnostic errors or delays.

Beyond these examples, several major themes emerge regarding AI's clinical and technological impact in diagnostics. Clinically, AI acts as a force multiplier for healthcare providers—assisting, not replacing, expert judgment. When properly validated, AI can increase diagnostic throughput, alleviate specialist shortages, reduce inter-observer variability, and uncover patterns related to prognosis or treatment responses that human observers may overlook. Technologically, AI integration drives innovation in health systems, prompting hospitals to adopt new software, build computational infrastructure, and devise new workflows that incorporate AI outputs. Regulatory approvals (e.g., FDA-cleared algorithms for medical image analysis) already demonstrate the feasibility of integrating AI into real-world practice. In the future, we may routinely see diagnostic reports—whether radiologic or pathologic—include AI-generated assessments alongside expert interpretations. This integration supports the vision of personalized medicine, where AI synthesizes imaging, clinical, and genomic data to stratify patients and tailor therapies beyond one-size-fits-all approaches.

That said, several challenges must be addressed to fully realize the potential of AI in diagnostics:

- **Explainability and Trust**: Some AI models—especially deep NNs—function as "black boxes," offering predictions without clear rationale. This lack of transparency can erode trust. Efforts to develop explainable AI (XAI) that clarifies the reasoning behind predictions are essential to maintain confidence among clinicians and patients.
- **Generalization and Clinical Validation**: AI tools must be robust across varied clinical settings and populations. Algorithms that perform well in controlled studies may struggle when exposed to different equipment, demographics, or clinical workflows. External validation, multi-center trials, and standards akin to clinical trials are critical for assessing bias, accuracy, and safety before deployment.
- **Data Privacy and Security**: AI thrives on large datasets, but healthcare data is sensitive. Medical image and record sharing raises concerns around patient privacy and must comply with regulations like HIPAA and GDPR. Emerging solutions like FL enable collaborative model training without exposing raw patient data, balancing access and security.
- **Workflow Integration and Adoption**: Seamless AI adoption requires thoughtful implementation. Clinicians must be educated on how to use AI outputs, and intuitive interfaces must facilitate easy interaction. Legal frameworks also need to clarify accountability—if an AI system contributes to a diagnostic error, responsibility must be clearly defined among developers, vendors, and healthcare providers.

In summary, AI in medical diagnostics offers groundbreaking advantages: higher accuracy, earlier detection, and novel clinical insights across radiology, early disease prediction, and pathology. This chapter has shown how DL and other AI methods process complex medical data with remarkable skill, complementing human expertise. But realizing the full promise of AI will depend on overcoming challenges related to explainability, validation, data governance, and regulatory compliance.

Ongoing R&D is already tackling these challenges—by developing more interpretable models, curating broader training datasets, and creating evaluation standards. As these efforts mature, we can expect AI to become a trusted partner in the diagnostic process. With continued interdisciplinary collaboration between AI researchers, clinicians, and policymakers, AI-based diagnostics will evolve further—ultimately advancing patient care and outcomes in the years to come.

References

1. H. Singh, A.N.D. Meyer, E.J. Thomas, The frequency of diagnostic errors in outpatient care: estimations from three large observational studies involving US adult populations. BMJ Qual. Saf. **23**, 727–731 (2014)
2. J.G. Elmore, C.K. Wells, C.H. Lee, D.H. Howard, A.R. Feinstein, Variability in radiologists' interpretations of mammograms. N. Engl. J. Med. **331**, 1493–1499 (1994)

3. E.A. Ooms, H.M. Zonderland, M.J.C. Eijkemans, M. Kriege, B.M. Delavary, C.W. Burger, A.C. Ansink, Mammography: interobserver variability in breast density assessment. The Breast **16**, 568–576 (2007)
4. B. Acs, M. Rantalainen, J. Hartman, Artificial intelligence as the next step towards precision pathology. J. Intern. Med. **288**, 62–81 (2020)
5. S.L. Kausch, J.R. Moorman, D.E. Lake, J. Keim-Malpass, Physiological machine learning models for prediction of sepsis in hospitalized adults: an integrative review. Intensive Crit. Care Nurs. **65**, 103035 (2021)
6. J. Yang, S. Hao, J. Huang, T. Chen, R. Liu, P. Zhang, M. Feng, Y. He, W. Xiao, Y. Hong, The application of artificial intelligence in the management of sepsis. Med. Rev. **3**, 369–380 (2023)
7. J. Xu, P. Yang, S. Xue, B. Sharma, M. Sanchez-Martin, F. Wang, K.A. Beaty, E. Dehan, B. Parikh, Translating cancer genomics into precision medicine with artificial intelligence: applications, challenges and future perspectives. Hum. Genet. **138**, 109–124 (2019)
8. R. Mishra, B. Li, The application of artificial intelligence in the genetic study of Alzheimer's disease. Aging Dis. **11**, 1567 (2020)
9. M. Li, Y. Jiang, Y. Zhang, H. Zhu, Medical image analysis using deep learning algorithms. Front. Public Health **11**, 1273253 (2023)
10. J. Li, J. Chen, Y. Tang, C. Wang, B.A. Landman, S.K. Zhou, Transforming medical imaging with transformers? A comparative review of key properties, current progresses, and future perspectives. Med. Image Anal. **85**, 102762 (2023)
11. J. Schock, D. Truhn, D. Nürnberger, S. Conrad, M.S. Huppertz, S. Keil, C. Kuhl, D. Merhof, S. Nebelung, Artificial intelligence-based automatic assessment of lower limb torsion on MRI. Sci. Rep. **11**, 23244 (2021)
12. P. Lakhani, B. Sundaram, Deep learning at chest radiography: automated classification of pulmonary tuberculosis by using convolutional neural networks. Radiology **284**, 574–582 (2017)
13. C.P. Langlotz, The future of AI and informatics in radiology: 10 predictions. Radiology **309**, e231114 (2023)
14. M.M. Srikantamurthy, V.P.S. Rallabandi, D.B. Dudekula, S. Natarajan, J. Park, Classification of benign and malignant subtypes of breast cancer histopathology imaging using hybrid CNN-LSTM based transfer learning. BMC Med. Imaging **23**, 19 (2023)
15. A. Dosovitskiy, L. Beyer, A. Kolesnikov, D. Weissenborn, X. Zhai, T. Unterthiner, M. Dehghani, M. Minderer, G. Heigold, S. Gelly, An image is worth 16x16 words: Transformers for image recognition at scale. ArXiv:2010.11929 (2020)
16. J. Wang, L. Wei, L. Wang, Q. Zhou, L. Zhu, J. Qin, Boundary-aware transformers for skin lesion segmentation, in: Medical Image Computing and Computer Assisted Intervention–MICCAI 2021: 24th International Conference, Strasbourg, France, September 27–October 1, 2021, Proceedings, Part i 24, (Springer, 2021), pp. 206–216
17. D.K. Saha, A.M. Joy, A. Majumder, YoTransViT: a transformer and CNN method for predicting and classifying skin diseases using segmentation techniques. Inf. Med Unlocked **47**, 101495 (2024)
18. A. Sriram, M. Muckley, K. Sinha, F. Shamout, J. Pineau, K.J. Geras, L. Azour, Y. Aphinyanaphongs, N. Yakubova, W. Moore, Covid-19 prognosis via self-supervised representation learning and multi-image prediction. ArXiv:2101.04909 (2021)
19. S. Park, G. Kim, Y. Oh, J.B. Seo, S.M. Lee, J.H. Kim, S. Moon, J.-K. Lim, J.C. Ye, Vision transformer for covid-19 cxr diagnosis using chest x-ray feature corpus, ArXiv:2103.07055 (2021)
20. S. Park, G. Kim, Y. Oh, J.B. Seo, S.M. Lee, J.H. Kim, S. Moon, J.-K. Lim, J.C. Ye, Multi-task vision transformer using low-level chest X-ray feature corpus for COVID-19 diagnosis and severity quantification. Med. Image Anal. **75**, 102299 (2022)
21. J. Jiang, N. Tyagi, K. Tringale, C. Crane, H. Veeraraghavan, Self-supervised 3D anatomy segmentation using self-distilled masked image transformer (SMIT), in: International Conference on Medical Image Computing and Computer-Assisted Intervention, (Springer, 2022), pp. 556–566

22. J. Chen, Y. Lu, Q. Yu, X. Luo, E. Adeli, Y. Wang, L. Lu, A.L. Yuille, Y. Zhou, Transunet: Transformers make strong encoders for medical image segmentation. ArXiv:2102.04306 (2021)
23. I. Vaccari, V. Orani, A. Paglialonga, E. Cambiaso, M. Mongelli, A generative adversarial network (GAN) technique for internet of medical things data. Sensors **21**, 3726 (2021)
24. J. Hussain, M. Båth, J. Ivarsson, Generative adversarial networks in medical image reconstruction: a systematic literature review. Comput. Biol. Med. **191**, 110094 (2025)
25. Z. Huang, J. Zhang, Y. Zhang, H. Shan, DU-GAN: generative adversarial networks with dual-domain U-Net-based discriminators for low-dose CT denoising. IEEE Trans. Instrum. Meas. **71**, 1–12 (2021)
26. X. Gu, Y. Zhang, W. Zeng, S. Zhong, H. Wang, D. Liang, Z. Li, Z. Hu, Cross-modality image translation: CT image synthesis of MR brain images using multi generative network with perceptual supervision. Comput. Methods Programs Biomed. **237**, 107571 (2023)
27. Y. Liu, A. Chen, H. Shi, S. Huang, W. Zheng, Z. Liu, Q. Zhang, X. Yang, CT synthesis from MRI using multi-cycle GAN for head-and-neck radiation therapy. Comput. Med. Imaging Graph. **91**, 101953 (2021)
28. W. Li, Y. Li, W. Qin, X. Liang, J. Xu, J. Xiong, Y. Xie, Magnetic resonance image (MRI) synthesis from brain computed tomography (CT) images based on deep learning methods for magnetic resonance (MR)-guided radiotherapy. Quant. Imaging Med. Surg. **10**, 1223 (2020)
29. H. Zhang, W. Guo, S. Zhang, H. Lu, X. Zhao, Unsupervised deep anomaly detection for medical images using an improved adversarial autoencoder. J. Digit. Imaging **35**, 153–161 (2022)
30. F. Kadri, A. Dairi, F. Harrou, Y. Sun, Towards accurate prediction of patient length of stay at emergency department: a GAN-driven deep learning framework. J. Ambient. Intell. Humaniz. Comput. **14**, 11481–11495 (2023)
31. Y. Yang, F. Nan, P. Yang, Q. Meng, Y. Xie, D. Zhang, K. Muhammad, GAN-based semi-supervised learning approach for clinical decision support in health-IoT platform. IEEE Access **7**, 8048–8057 (2019)
32. M. Kohli, L.M. Prevedello, R.W. Filice, J.R. Geis, Implementing machine learning in radiology practice and research. Am. J. Roentgenol. **208**, 754–760 (2017)
33. R.S. Olson, W. La Cava, Z. Mustahsan, A. Varik, J.H. Moore, Data-driven advice for applying machine learning to bioinformatics problems, in: Pacific Symposium on Biocomputing 2018: Proceedings of the Pacific Symposium, World Scientific (2018), pp. 192–203
34. B. Kocak, E.A. Kus, O. Kilickesmez, How to read and review papers on machine learning and artificial intelligence in radiology: a survival guide to key methodological concepts. Eur. Radiol. **31**, 1819–1830 (2021)
35. S. Faghani, B. Khosravi, K. Zhang, M. Moassefi, J.M. Jagtap, F. Nugen, S. Vahdati, S.P. Kuanar, S.M. Rassoulinejad-Mousavi, Y. Singh, Mitigating bias in radiology machine learning: 3. Performance metrics. Radiol. Artif. Intell. **4**, e220061 (2022)
36. F. Schwarzhans, G. George, L.E. Sanchez, O. Zaric, J.E. Abraham, R. Woitek, S. Hatamikia, Image normalization techniques and their effect on the robustness and predictive power of breast MRI radiomics. Eur. J. Radiol. **187**, 112086 (2025)
37. H. He, E.A. Garcia, Learning from imbalanced data. IEEE Trans. Knowl. Data Eng. **21**, 1263–1284 (2009)
38. M.A. Mazurowski, P.A. Habas, J.M. Zurada, J.Y. Lo, J.A. Baker, G.D. Tourassi, Training neural network classifiers for medical decision making: the effects of imbalanced datasets on classification performance. Neural Netw. **21**, 427–436 (2008)
39. C. Hu, N. Cao, H. Zhou, B. Guo, Medical Image classification with a hybrid SSM model based on CNN and transformer. Electronics (Basel) **13**, 3094 (2024)
40. A. Zeynali, M.A. Tinati, B.M. Tazehkand, Hybrid CNN-transformer architecture with Xception-based feature enhancement for accurate breast cancer classification. IEEE Access (2024)
41. G. Wang, M. Zhou, X. Ning, P. Tiwari, H. Zhu, G. Yang, C.H. Yap, US2Mask: image-to-mask generation learning via a conditional GAN for cardiac ultrasound image segmentation. Comput. Biol. Med. **172**, 108282 (2024)

42. P. Rajpurkar, J. Irvin, K. Zhu, B. Yang, H. Mehta, T. Duan, D. Ding, A. Bagul, C. Langlotz, K. Shpanskaya, Chexnet: radiologist-level pneumonia detection on chest x-rays with deep learning. ArXiv:1711.05225 (2017)
43. J. Tang, R.M. Rangayyan, J. Xu, I. El Naqa, Y. Yang, Computer-aided detection and diagnosis of breast cancer with mammography: recent advances. IEEE Trans. Inf Technol. Biomed. **13**, 236–251 (2009)
44. F.J. Dorfner, J.B. Patel, J. Kalpathy-Cramer, E.R. Gerstner, C.P. Bridge, A review of deep learning for brain tumor analysis in MRI. NPJ. Precis. Oncol. **9**, 2 (2025)
45. T. Prodanovic, S. Petrovic Savic, N. Prodanovic, A. Simovic, S. Zivojinovic, J.C. Djordjevic, D. Savic, Advanced diagnostics of respiratory distress syndrome in premature infants treated with surfactant and budesonide through computer-assisted chest x-ray analysis. Diagnostics **14**, 214 (2024)
46. L. Topff, S. Steltenpool, E.R. Ranschaert, N. Ramanauskas, R. Menezes, J.J. Visser, R.G.H. Beets-Tan, N.S. Hartkamp, Artificial intelligence-assisted double reading of chest radiographs to detect clinically relevant missed findings: a two-centre evaluation. Eur. Radiol. **34**, 5876–5885 (2024)
47. İÖ. Koska, Ç. Koska, Deep learning classification of MGMT status of glioblastomas using multiparametric MRI with a novel domain knowledge augmented mask fusion approach. Sci. Rep. **15**, 3273 (2025)
48. K. Ben Ahmed, L.O. Hall, D.B. Goldgof, R. Gatenby, Ensembles of convolutional neural networks for survival time estimation of high-grade glioma patients from multimodal MRI. Diagnostics 12:345 (2022)
49. J. Tromp, D. Bauer, B.L. Claggett, M. Frost, M.B. Iversen, N. Prasad, M.C. Petrie, M.G. Larson, J.A. Ezekowitz, S.D. Solomon, A formal validation of a deep learning-based automated workflow for the interpretation of the echocardiogram. Nat. Commun. **13**, 6776 (2022)
50. S. Kumar, S. Sharma, K.T. Megra, Transformer enabled multi-modal medical diagnosis for tuberculosis classification. J. Big Data **12**, 5 (2025)
51. M. Sirshar, M.F.K. Paracha, M.U. Akram, N.S. Alghamdi, S.Z.Y. Zaidi, T. Fatima, Attention based automated radiology report generation using CNN and LSTM. PLoS ONE **17**, e0262209 (2022)
52. R. Noor, A. Wahid, S.U. Bazai, A. Khan, M. Fang, U.A. Bhatti, Y.Y. Ghadi, DLGAN: undersampled MRI reconstruction using deep learning based generative adversarial network. Biomed. Signal Process. Control **93**, 106218 (2024)
53. Denoised ultra-low dose CT offers safe pneumonia diagnosis for immunocompromised patients, (n.d.). https://www.news-medical.net/news/20250313/Denoised-ultra-low-dose-CT-offers-safe-pneumonia-diagnosis-for-immunocompromised-patients.aspx. Accessed 18 Mar 2025
54. A. Zayed, G. Cloutier, H. Rivaz, Automatic frame selection using CNN in ultrasound elastography, in: 2020 42nd Annual International Conference of the IEEE Engineering in Medicine & Biology Society (EMBC) (IEEE, 2020), pp. 2027–2030
55. V. Kumar, There is no substitute for human intelligence. Indian J. Crit. Care Med. **25**, 486 (2021)
56. C.A. Vitellas, N.C. Mannix, S.M. Nimjee, M.T. Shujaat, S. Heaton, V.H. Lee, Abstract 130: real world experience with Viz.AI automated large vessel occlusion detection. Stroke 53 (2022). https://doi.org/10.1161/STR.53.SUPPL_1.130.
57. Viz LVO - Viz.ai, (n.d.). https://healthairegister.com/products/vizai-lvo/. Accessed 18 Mar 2025
58. S.M. McKinney, M. Sieniek, V. Godbole, J. Godwin, N. Antropova, H. Ashrafian, T. Back, M. Chesus, G.S. Corrado, A. Darzi, International evaluation of an AI system for breast cancer screening. Nature **577**, 89–94 (2020)
59. A. Chen, J. Huang, Y. Liao, Z. Liu, D. Chen, C. Yang, R. Yang, X. Wei, Differences in clinical and imaging presentation of pediatric patients with COVID-19 in comparison with adults. Radiol. Cardiothorac. Imaging **2**, e200117 (2020)

60. I.Y. Chen, S. Joshi, M. Ghassemi, Treating health disparities with artificial intelligence. Nat. Med. **26**, 16–17 (2020)
61. J. Wiens, S. Saria, M. Sendak, M. Ghassemi, V.X. Liu, F. Doshi-Velez, K. Jung, K. Heller, D. Kale, M. Saeed, Do no harm: a roadmap for responsible machine learning for health care. Nat. Med. **25**, 1337–1340 (2019)
62. Z. Obermeyer, B. Powers, C. Vogeli, S. Mullainathan, Dissecting racial bias in an algorithm used to manage the health of populations. Science **366**(2019), 447–453 (1979)
63. M.M. Moore, E. Slonimsky, A.D. Long, R.W. Sze, R.S. Iyer, Machine learning concepts, concerns and opportunities for a pediatric radiologist. Pediatr. Radiol. **49**, 509–516 (2019)
64. A. Ceross, J. Bergmann, Tracking the presence of software as a medical device in US food and drug administration databases: retrospective data analysis. JMIR Biomed. Eng. **6**, e20652 (2021)
65. J.D. Ianni, R.E. Soans, S. Sankarapandian, R.V. Chamarthi, D. Ayyagari, T.G. Olsen, M.J. Bonham, C.C. Stavish, K. Motaparthi, C.J. Cockerell, Tailored for real-world: a whole slide image classification system validated on uncurated multi-site data emulating the prospective pathology workload. Sci. Rep. **10**, 3217 (2020)
66. K.K. Napa, R. Govindarajan, S. Sathya, J.S. Murugan, B.K.P. Vijayammal, Comparative analysis of explainable machine learning models for cardiovascular risk stratification using clinical data and Shapley additive explanations. Intell. Based Med. 100286 (2025)
67. E. Afrifa-Yamoah, E. Adua, E. Peprah-Yamoah, E.O. Anto, V. Opoku-Yamoah, E. Acheampong, M.J. Macartney, R. Hashmi, Pathways to chronic disease detection and prediction: mapping the potential of machine learning to the pathophysiological processes while navigating ethical challenges. Chronic. Dis. Transl. Med. **11**, 1–21 (2025)
68. D. Dixon, H. Sattar, N. Moros, S.R. Kesireddy, H. Ahsan, M. Lakkimsetti, M. Fatima, D. Doshi, K. Sadhu, M.J. Hassan, Unveiling the influence of AI predictive analytics on patient outcomes: a comprehensive narrative review. Cureus 16 (2024)
69. T. Pham, T. Tran, D. Phung, S. Venkatesh, Predicting healthcare trajectories from medical records: a deep learning approach. J. Biomed. Inform. **69**, 218–229 (2017)
70. S. Yang, L. Cao, Y. Zhou, C. Hu, A retrospective cohort study: predicting 90-day mortality for ICU trauma patients with a machine learning algorithm using XGBoost using MIMIC-III database. J. Multidiscip. Healthc. 2625–2640 (2023)
71. Using AI to Predict the Onset of Sepsis - Mayo Clinic Platform, (n.d.). https://www.mayoclinicplatform.org/2024/05/02/using-ai-to-predict-the-onset-of-sepsis/. Accessed 18 Mar 2025
72. R. Adams, K.E. Henry, A. Sridharan, H. Soleimani, A. Zhan, N. Rawat, L. Johnson, D.N. Hager, S.E. Cosgrove, A. Markowski, Prospective, multi-site study of patient outcomes after implementation of the TREWS machine learning-based early warning system for sepsis. Nat. Med. **28**, 1455–1460 (2022)
73. F. Li, S. Wang, Z. Gao, M. Qing, S. Pan, Y. Liu, C. Hu, Harnessing artificial intelligence in sepsis care: advances in early detection, personalized treatment, and real-time monitoring. Front. Med. (Lausanne) **11**, 1510792 (2025)
74. Z. Zhang, L. Chen, P. Xu, Q. Wang, J. Zhang, K. Chen, C.M. Clements, L.A. Celi, V. Herasevich, Y. Hong, Effectiveness of automated alerting system compared to usual care for the management of sepsis. NPJ Digit. Med. **5**, 101 (2022)
75. What Causes Hereditary Breast and Ovarian Cancers | Hereditary Breast and Ovarian Cancer | CDC, (n.d.). https://www.cdc.gov/breast-ovarian-cancer-hereditary/causes/index.html. Accessed 19 Mar 2025
76. O.S.M. El Nahhas, C.M.L. Loeffler, Z.I. Carrero, M. van Treeck, F.R. Kolbinger, K.J. Hewitt, H.S. Muti, M. Graziani, Q. Zeng, J. Calderaro, Regression-based deep-learning predicts molecular biomarkers from pathology slides. Nat. Commun. **15**, 1253 (2024)
77. N.N. Khanna, M. Singh, M. Maindarkar, A. Kumar, A.M. Johri, L. Mentella, J.R. Laird, K.I. Paraskevas, Z. Ruzsa, N. Singh, Polygenic risk score for cardiovascular diseases in artificial intelligence paradigm: a review. J. Korean Med. Sci. **38** (2023)
78. L. Bonomi, Y. Huang, L. Ohno-Machado, Privacy challenges and research opportunities for genomic data sharing. Nat. Genet. **52**, 646–654 (2020)

79. D. Duong, B.D. Solomon, Artificial intelligence in clinical genetics. Eur. J. Hum. Genet. 1–8 (2025)
80. N. Houssami, G. Kirkpatrick-Jones, N. Noguchi, C.I. Lee, Artificial Intelligence (AI) for the early detection of breast cancer: a scoping review to assess AI's potential in breast screening practice. Expert Rev. Med. Devices **16**, 351–362 (2019)
81. W. Hendrix, N. Hendrix, E.T. Scholten, M. Mourits, J. Trap-de Jong, S. Schale-kamp, M. Korst, M. van Leuken, B. van Ginneken, M. Prokop, Deep learning for the detection of benign and malignant pulmonary nodules in non-screening chest CT scans. Com-mun Med. (Lond) **3**(1), 156 (2023)
82. Researchers create AI approach for cervical cancer screening - NCI, (n.d.). https://www.cancer.gov/news-events/press-releases/2019/deep-learning-cervical-cancer-screening. Accessed 19 Mar 2025
83. L. Hu, D. Bell, S. Antani, Z. Xue, K. Yu, M.P. Horning, N. Gachuhi, B. Wilson, M.S. Jaiswal, B. Befano, An observational study of deep learning and automated evaluation of cervical images for cancer screening. JNCI: J. Nat. Cancer Inst. **111**, 923–932 (2019)
84. D. Huang, J. Shen, J. Hong, Y. Zhang, S. Dai, N. Du, M. Zhang, D. Guo, Effect of artificial intelligence-aided colonoscopy for adenoma and polyp detection: a meta-analysis of randomized clinical trials. Int. J. Colorectal. Dis. 1–12 (2022)
85. S. Lou, F. Du, W. Song, Y. Xia, X. Yue, D. Yang, B. Cui, Y. Liu, P. Han, Artificial intelligence for colorectal neoplasia detection during colonoscopy: a systematic review and meta-analysis of randomized clinical trials. EClinicalMedicine **66** (2023)
86. R. Poplin, A.V. Varadarajan, K. Blumer, Y. Liu, M.V. McConnell, G.S. Corrado, L. Peng, D.R. Webster, Prediction of cardiovascular risk factors from retinal fundus photographs via deep learning. Nat. Biomed. Eng. **2**, 158–164 (2018)
87. Z.I. Attia, P.A. Noseworthy, F. Lopez-Jimenez, S.J. Asirvatham, A.J. Deshmukh, B.J. Gersh, R.E. Carter, X. Yao, A.A. Rabinstein, B.J. Erickson, An artificial intelligence-enabled ECG algorithm for the identification of patients with atrial fibrillation during sinus rhythm: a retrospective analysis of outcome prediction. The Lancet **394**, 861–867 (2019)
88. V. Gulshan, L. Peng, M. Coram, M.C. Stumpe, D. Wu, A. Narayanaswamy, S. Venugopalan, K. Widner, T. Madams, J. Cuadros, Development and validation of a deep learning algorithm for detection of diabetic retinopathy in retinal fundus photographs. JAMA **316**, 2402–2410 (2016)
89. X. Xu, M. Zhang, S. Huang, X. Li, X. Kui, J. Liu, The application of artificial intelligence in diabetic retinopathy: progress and prospects. Front. Cell Dev. Biol. **12**, 1473176 (2024)
90. FDA clears fully autonomous AI for portable diabetic retinopathy screening, (n.d.). https://www.healio.com/news/optometry/20240430/fda-clears-fully-autonomous-ai-for-portable-diabetic-retinopathy-screening. Accessed 19 Mar 2025
91. M.P. Turakhia, M. Desai, H. Hedlin, A. Rajmane, N. Talati, T. Ferris, S. Desai, D. Nag, M. Patel, P. Kowey, Rationale and design of a large-scale, app-based study to identify cardiac arrhythmias using a smartwatch: the apple heart study. Am. Heart J. **207**, 66–75 (2019)
92. Y. Liu, D. Han, A.V. Parwani, Z. Li, Applications of artificial intelligence in breast pathology. Arch. Pathol. Lab. Med. **147**, 1003–1013 (2023)
93. B.J. Williams, J. Lee, K.A. Oien, D. Treanor, Digital pathology access and usage in the UK: results from a national survey on behalf of the National Cancer Research Institute's CM-Path initiative. J. Clin. Pathol. **71**, 463–466 (2018)
94. M.G. Hanna, V.E. Reuter, O. Ardon, D. Kim, S.J. Sirintrapun, P.J. Schüffler, K.J. Busam, J.L. Sauter, E. Brogi, L.K. Tan, Validation of a digital pathology system including remote review during the COVID-19 pandemic. Mod. Pathol. **33**, 2115–2127 (2020)
95. I. Kim, K. Kang, Y. Song, T.-J. Kim, Application of artificial intelligence in pathology: trends and challenges. Diagnostics **12**, 2794 (2022)
96. S. Morales, K. Engan, V. Naranjo, Artificial intelligence in computational pathology–challenges and future directions. Digit. Signal Process **119**, 103196 (2021)
97. A. Janowczyk, A. Madabhushi, Deep learning for digital pathology image analysis: a comprehensive tutorial with selected use cases. J. Pathol. Inform **7**, 29 (2016)

98. B.E. Bejnordi, M. Veta, P.J. Van Diest, B. Van Ginneken, N. Karssemeijer, G. Litjens, J.A.W.M. Van Der Laak, M. Hermsen, Q.F. Manson, M. Balkenhol, Diagnostic assessment of deep learning algorithms for detection of lymph node metastases in women with breast cancer. JAMA **318**, 2199–2210 (2017)
99. C. McGenity, E.L. Clarke, C. Jennings, G. Matthews, C. Cartlidge, H. Freduah-Agyemang, D.D. Stocken, D. Treanor, Artificial intelligence in digital pathology: a systematic review and meta-analysis of diagnostic test accuracy. NPJ Digit. Med. **7**, 114 (2024)
100. N. Coudray, P.S. Ocampo, T. Sakellaropoulos, N. Narula, M. Snuderl, D. Fenyö, A.L. Moreira, N. Razavian, A. Tsirigos, Classification and mutation prediction from non–small cell lung cancer histopathology images using deep learning. Nat. Med. **24**, 1559–1567 (2018)
101. N. Tomita, B. Abdollahi, J. Wei, B. Ren, A. Suriawinata, S. Hassanpour, Attention-based deep neural networks for detection of cancerous and precancerous esophagus tissue on histopathological slides. JAMA Netw. Open **2**, e1914645 (2019)
102. The Paige Prostate Suite: Assistive Artificial Intelligence for Prostate Cancer Diagnosis, The Paige Prostate Suite: Assistive Artificial Intelligence for Prostate Cancer Diagnosis: Emerging Health Technologies (2024). https://www.ncbi.nlm.nih.gov/books/NBK608438/. Accessed 21 Mar 2025
103. P. Raciti, J. Sue, J.A. Retamero, R. Ceballos, R. Godrich, J.D. Kunz, A. Casson, D. Thiagarajan, Z. Ebrahimzadeh, J. Viret, Clinical validation of artificial intelligence–augmented pathology diagnosis demonstrates significant gains in diagnostic accuracy in prostate cancer detection. Arch. Pathol. Lab. Med. **147**, 1178–1185 (2023)
104. K. Dembrower, E. Wåhlin, Y. Liu, M. Salim, K. Smith, P. Lindholm, M. Eklund, F. Strand, Effect of artificial intelligence-based triaging of breast cancer screening mammograms on cancer detection and radiologist workload: a retrospective simulation study, Lancet Digit. Health **2**, e468–e474 (2020)
105. M. Yue, J. Zhang, X. Wang, K. Yan, L. Cai, K. Tian, S. Niu, X. Han, Y. Yu, J. Huang, Can AI-assisted microscope facilitate breast HER2 interpretation? A multi-institutional ring study. Virchows Archiv. **479**, 443–449 (2021)
106. R. Aggarwal, V. Sounderajah, G. Martin, D.S.W. Ting, A. Karthikesalingam, D. King, H. Ashrafian, A. Darzi, Diagnostic accuracy of deep learning in medical imaging: a systematic review and meta-analysis. NPJ Digit. Med. **4**, 65 (2021)
107. A. Echle, N.T. Rindtorff, T.J. Brinker, T. Luedde, A.T. Pearson, J.N. Kather, Deep learning in cancer pathology: a new generation of clinical biomarkers. Br. J. Cancer **124**, 686–696 (2021)

Chapter 3
AI in Treatment and Patient Care

In this chapter, we explore the evolving field of Artificial Intelligence (AI) for inpatient treatment and treatment planning. This chapter looks at how AI's role in medicine has progressed from being a highly advanced diagnostic tool to now being a significant player in therapeutic decision-making and the management of long-term healthcare. AI can now provide technology-assisted decision-making to clinicians, aiding principles of care that personalize care and guide treatment outcomes based on a person's clinical history, genomic profile and real-world data. In essence, this advancement shifts medicine from a series of fixed protocols to a more adaptive approach. This chapter explores how AI may enhance precision medicine by providing individualized treatment recommendations based on complex biological and clinical data. The chapter also discusses the potential of AI in improving outcomes in clinical surgical environments through pre-operative procedure planning, risk assessment, and outcome evaluation. In addition, the chapter examines AI in the form of telehealth and telemedicine, including intelligent triage, remote patient monitoring, and other forms of applied virtual health support systems. Finally, the chapter discusses the importance of ethical, regulatory, and equity considerations, as well as the importance of responsible integration of AI systems in the current healthcare practices.

3.1 Introduction

AI is rapidly outgrowing its diagnostic capabilities and is beginning to extend into therapy planning and patient care. In previous chapter, we have demonstrated how well AI can identify diseases in medical images and data. Nonetheless, diagnosis is only the first step in the overall process; the end goal is to improve patient outcomes through effective therapy and care. AI is changing treatment paradigms by helping

L. Tayebi et al., *Artificial Intelligence in Medicine and Dentistry*,
https://doi.org/10.1007/978-3-032-15977-9_3

clinicians select the right interventions for individual patients and enabling continuous and proactive management of patients' health conditions. AI fundamentally shifts care away from the "one-size-fits-all" model toward providing individualized, data-driven care. Physicians can make medical decisions based more on a person's own genomic, clinical, and lifestyle profile rather than on the average characteristics of a population. Care can extend beyond episodic visits in clinics to continuous attention and monitoring in people's day-to-day lives.

One significant shift is the emergence of precision, or personalized, medicine, where AI algorithms analyze and integrate extensive genomic and clinical data in selecting the best treatment appropriate for a patient. Current treatment guidelines are based on the "average" patient, which fails to account for real patients who differ widely in genetics, environment, and behaviors. AI is able to leverage that variability—e.g., identifying which cancer therapy a tumor is most likely to respond to base on specific genetic mutations, or which drug dosage would provide the appropriate therapeutic effect without causing side effects [1]. These tools give clinicians the additional capability to harmonize treatment from generic protocols to individualized therapy plans, with better efficiency and safety outcomes. Meanwhile, AI systems can summarize the data from Electronic Health Records (EHRs), data from clinical trials, and real-world evidence to facilitate decision-making in complex cases. This may mean a recommendation for preferred drug combinations for complex diseases or a recommendation to adjust treatment based on a patient's particular risk factors. In each instance, AI is there not to replace clinicians; rather, it is meant to enhance their own competence with integrated "augmented intelligence" [1].

A second important transition is the application of AI for chronic disease management and patient engagement. Many chronic conditions (like diabetes, heart failure, or hypertension) require steady monitoring and adjustments (even sometimes minor) to the treatment plan. Here AI facilitates a shift from reactive care (when a crisis occurs) to proactive care (the environment is set to reduce complications). Wearable biosensors, mobile health applications, and the Internet of Things (IoT) allow for continuous gathering of patient data—from blood glucose levels, blood pressure readings, and even activity and sleep. AI processes this streaming data in real-time and identifies changes that could signal a problem missed by a human provider. An example is when AI informs clinicians when a patient's weight and blood pressure trends show signs of an issue in a chronic heart failure patient, allowing for intervention before the patient returns to the hospital. Essentially AI is providing an extra layer of monitoring capability for patients throughout the entirety of their day, where clinicians would manually, and reactively, respond to acute events or issues. AI-enabled reminders and conversational agents on smartphones can also encourage patients to follow their treatment recommendations—whether it is taking medications on time or following dietary recommendations. This way of providing care continuously to patients through AI-assisted decrease unnecessary visits and gives patients a chance to stay healthy at home, where they prefer [2].

AI's incorporation into treatment and patient care is shaping a new paradigm of more personalized, preventive, and participatory medicine. By using AI tools, doctors can consider unique biology and situational context to provide personalized treatment, and patients can enjoy increased support for their experience in between visits. In the following, this primary shift across medicine will be discussed in several domains. Section 3.2 discusses how AI assists in the analysis of genomic data and patient-specific data for treatment personalization. Section 3.3 explores AI transforming role in the management of chronic disease, with the use of continuous monitoring, predictive analytics, and greater patient participation in their own ongoing long-term care. The application of AI in surgery design and robot-assisted surgery is presented in Sects. 3.4 and 3.5. Finally, in Sect. 3.6, we discuss how AI can change telemedicine and enable enhanced healthcare access through real-time monitoring, advance assessment of symptoms in advance, and enhanced access to care in disadvantaged locations. Collectively, each of these areas illustrates how AI is transitioning medicine away from reactive, generic, episodic care, and toward predictive, personalized, and continuous care.

3.2 Personalized Medicine and Genomics

3.2.1 Definition and Benefits of Personalized Medicine

Personalized medicine refers to specific medical treatment of an individual based on the characteristics of that patient. It is a different notion from what the medical community has historically relied on, which has been to extrapolate findings from clinical trials and generalize them to the average individual in a population. In personalized medicine, clinicians can account for a person's unique genetic profile, environmental influences, and lifestyle when preventing, diagnosing, and treating a disease. Much of personalized medicine has been made possible by advances in the area of high-throughput genomics, as these studies have demonstrated the variability among patients based on genetic differences. A patient may respond differently to a drug than another patient depending on their gene variants; what might be a therapeutic dose for one patient could be a toxic dose or even ineffective for another. The concept behind personalized medicine is to collect this information ahead of time and select the best possible therapy or dosage for that patient. There are quite a few advantages. For example, treatments can be more effective by reducing cycles of trial-and-error and adverse effects can be minimized by avoiding therapies that are unlikely to have any positive impact [1]. This ultimately leads to a higher cure rate, longer life expectancy, and continued health and quality of life by situating medical care around the needs of each individual patient.

AI functions as the enabling technology for personalized medicine because it can make sense of all the "big data" of human variability [3]. The human genome is vast, and billions of variants (mutations) exist across individuals. Traditional analytical approaches do not cope well with this staggering amount of genomic information, especially when integrated with other data types like clinical records. AI algorithms, especially Machine Learning (ML) and Deep Learning (DL), have been successful in finding patterns in large, complicated datasets. In genomics, AI is able to rapidly scan a patient's DNA sequence to distill pathogenic mutations or disease-relevant variants from the millions of benign differences [1]. ML models are even able to merge genomic data with clinical information to help predict outcomes or treatment responses. For example, in oncology, AI models use a tumor's genomic profile (mutated gene's expression levels, etc.) to predict which targeted therapy the tumor is most likely to respond to [4]. Similarly, in pharmacogenomics (the study of how genes affect drug responses), AI can predict the best medication and dose for a patient based on that patient's genetic variants in their drug-metabolizing enzymes [5]. Genotype-guided dosing has been employed to select warfarin dosages and other therapies to prevent adverse reactions [6]. In summary, AI allows clinicians to utilize genomic and other personal data to guide their decision-making, transforming medical care from a reactive, one-size-fits-all approach to predictive, personalized medical care.

3.2.2 AI in Genomic Data Analysis for Tailored Treatments

The steps to convert genomic data into clinical insights are a complex process, and this is where AI-based tools are irreplaceable. A standard example in precision medicine may involve sequencing a patient's tumor DNA or whole genome; in this example, calling variants in the extracted sequence generates a huge list of thousands of variants. The challenge is to find clinically actionable insights, for example, if there is a mutation suggesting that a certain drug will work or not work. AI algorithms, particularly those using DL techniques, have been shown to be effective in variant interpretation. One example is when applied to variant calling—identifying true genetic variants from raw sequencing data—where older algorithms (relied on hand-crafted filtering) still missed some variants or falsely flagged others. AI-based variant calling systems use deep Neural Networks (NNs) trained on known genomes to provide much more accurate identification of mutations that can greatly improve the foundation for downstream analysis [7, 8]. Once the variants are identified, other ML models can assess which problems were likely disease-causing by recognizing specific patterns that human experts might miss, subtle combinations of mutations or effects on protein structure, thus allowing for much faster variant interpretation for an individual genome than could ever be done manually.

AI can also be key in synthesizing many forms of data (multi-omics) to personalize treatment. In addition to DNA sequences, a patient may also have data from RNA expression profiles, proteomic studies, microbiome studies, and clinical phenotyping. Each form of information provides a part of the whole, and AI can synthesize this information to develop a more comprehensive representation of the health of a patient. An example of this is in oncology, where a precision medicine AI platform could take genomics (for the detection of targetable mutations), transcriptomics (for the identification of active pathways), and digital pathology images (to characterize tumor morphology) and recommend a therapy. This ability to make sense of a holistic system is one area where advanced AI systems perform particularly well, making connections between heterogeneous data sources. Another rapidly developing area is predicting drug responses using AI. Researchers have begun training algorithms on databases of cancer cell lines to learn the patterns of genomic features that predict sensitivity or resistance to therapies. Those models can then be applied to a new patient to predict which drug is most likely to provide a clinical response [1]. Such approaches may bring us closer to in silico trials, where computations simulate how a patient will respond to different treatments, creating personalized choices for therapy without exposing the patient to ineffective treatments.

Importantly, these AI genomics approaches can have significant potential for deployment into clinical care systems [9, 10]. Many of these tools are currently in pilot projects, but their role in precision medicine would allow for a more evidence-based foundation for clinical decisions. In both academic medical centers and healthcare organizations, there is a growing interest in developing AI-based genomic decision support tools to help interprofessional teams provide personalized care. Consider referring a patient, with a known medical history and current medications, to an AI-based pharmacogenomics clinic. The system would pull together different types of data from the patient. An AI platform could then be utilized to analyze the combination of these data and help discover gene-drug interactions or genetic risks. The final product would be a personalized medication management plan, which would be sent to the physician to review and act upon. The flow from data collection from the patient (genetic test, lab tests, history) into an AI analytical core and out to a personalized treatment recommendation (like altered drug treatment regimens) for that individual patient is demonstrated in Fig. 3.1. The AI system will analyze the complexities of drug-drug interactions based on a particular patient's genetics or biology and then suggest personalized therapy.

3.2.3 Real-World Applications of AI-Powered Personalized Medicine

Personalized medicine is advancing beyond the theoretical domain and has realistic potential to change clinical practice, and AI will likely be a driving force in that change. One of the best places to see that potential is oncology (cancer care). Cancer treatment is evolving over time from toxic chemotherapies geared toward the broadest categories of cancer to targeted therapies aimed at specific genetic mutations in tumors. AI systems can assist oncologists in matching tumor genomic data to the most likely effective drugs. For example, in non-small cell lung cancer cases, AI-driven platforms may analyze DNA sequencing results to ascertain available mutations in genes such as EGFR or ALK that may be targetable by therapies, such as EGFR inhibitors [12]. Instead of relying on trial-and-error methodology, these systems could generate AI-curated reports that highlight "actionable" mutations and document the specific treatments across trials that have worked for similar tumors with matching

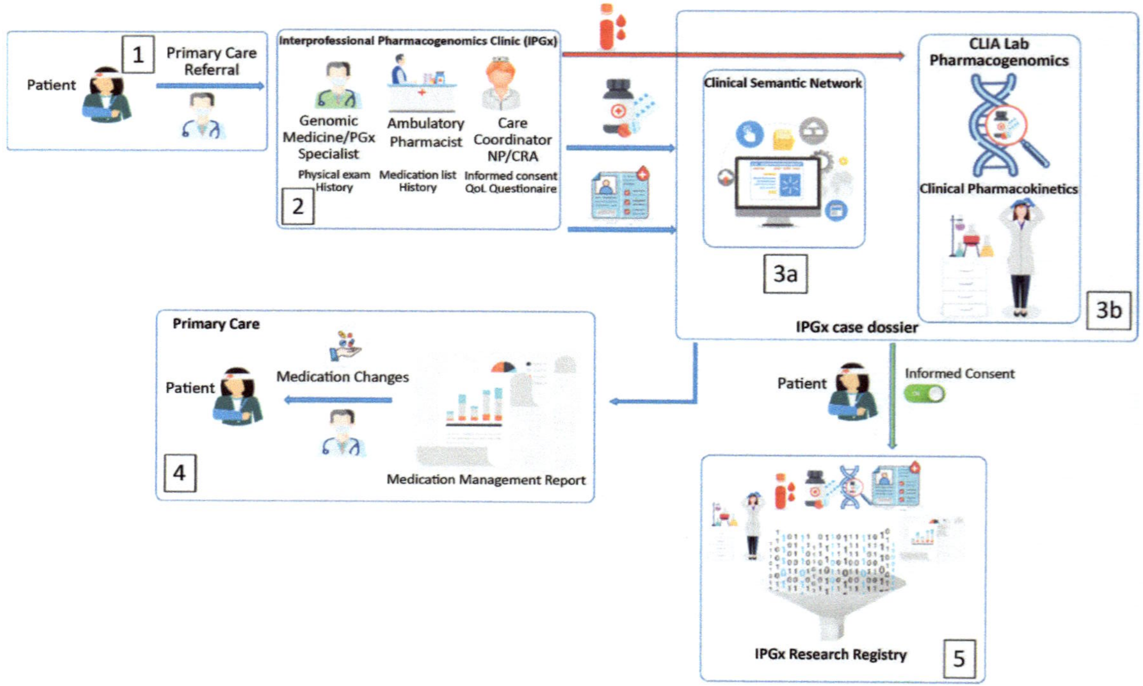

Fig. 3.1 Interprofessional Pharmacogenomics (IPGx) Model integrating AI. In this workflow, a patient with polypharmacy (multiple medications) undergoes genomic testing and clinical data review. An AI-driven system (central "Clinical Semantic Network" and analytics engine) processes the patient's medical history, identifies symptoms that may have pharmacological root causes, and when appropriate, triggers pharmacogenomic analysis (step 3a) or pharmacokinetic profiling (step 3b). The AI then generates a medication management report with recommendations tailored to the patient's genetic profile and clinical status (step 4), which is reviewed by clinicians to optimize the treatment plan. If the patient consents, their data also contributes to a growing clinical-genomic registry for further learning (step 5). This figure exemplifies how AI and genomics combine to personalize treatment in practice, ensuring therapy decisions account for each patient's unique genetic makeup. Reproduced from Silva et al. [11], published in Journal of Personalized Medicine 11 (2021) 443, under the Creative Commons Attribution 4.0 International License (CC BY), (https://creativecommons.org/licenses/by/4.0/). Font style and text size were adjusted for improved readability; the figure content is unchanged

molecular characteristics. In the case of breast cancer, predictive algorithms may use genomic and clinical information to determine whether the patient will benefit from adjuvant chemotherapy or whether it can be safely avoided, reducing overtreatment [13]. A number of AI-powered platforms (e.g., IBM Watson for Oncology) have been piloted and deployed to help doctors' teams to integrate and analyze the vast amounts of genomic and clinical data and recommend individualized therapy. However, these tools have shown limited success in real practice, with reports of poor adoption by clinicians [14]. Thus, the future application of AI in oncology will require not just additional validation and transparency of models but also integration into workflows and acceptance by health care providers.

AI is also empowering personalized medicine through population-scale initiatives. Large biobank projects, for instance the UK Biobank and the U.S. All of Us Research Program, are utilizing AI to identify findings from genomic and health record data collected from hundreds of thousands of people which may in turn be relevant for individual patients [15, 16]. ML models trained on these enormous datasets may be able to identify an individual's risk for certain diseases (such as type 2 diabetes or coronary artery disease) based on their specific individual's combination of genetic variants—known as Polygenic Risk Scores (PRSs). Even as these are currently still under development, such AI derived scores may soon allow for true individualized prevention strategies. For example, an individual determined at high genetic risk for diabetes might utilize early lifestyle coaching and interventions years before having symptoms of disease, while a low genetic risk individual would avoid potentially unnecessary interventions. In effect, these kinds of efforts consider each patient's data as a part of a big learning network, working to benefit all patients. In this network, AI discovers the "clusters" of similarity that relate one patient experience to another patient experience. This networked learning reduces the time it takes to discover treatment rules.

While there have been many successes, challenges still exist in delivering AI-based personalized medicine. Models need to be rigorously validated before health professionals can trust them to provide reliable recommendations. Clinicians require training to use and integrate AI-generated reports into their clinical judgement. There is always a concern about bias and equity, as there might be populations that have not been adequately represented in the training of AI models. We should ensure that advances in personalized medicine do not only benefit those individuals whose data are well represented in the databases. There are some ethical dilemmas we will examine next.

3.2.4 *Ethical and Privacy Considerations*

The integration of AI and personalized genomic medicine presents numerous ethical and privacy challenges that need to be managed effectively. First, dealing with genomic data requires ensuring privacy and security; genomic data is the ultimate Personally Identifiable Information (PII) that may reveal a person's predisposition to disease, ancestry information, and even unknown familial relationships. If genomic data is to be used at scale for AI algorithms, it must be stored securely and protected with safeguards for processing to prevent unauthorized use or access to an individual's genomic data. Patients may fear that their DNA information could be used by third parties (e.g., insurers, employers) to discriminate against them, so it is important to ensure that genomic databases are encrypted, anonymized, and governed. Relatedly, AI developers and healthcare sectors are expected to comply with Health Insurance Portability and Accountability Act (HIPAA) and General Data Protection Regulation (GDPR) regulations and often have to obtain additional consent for the use of genomic data. By making use of Federated Learning (FL), researchers are starting to develop AI models based on genomic data across institutions at scale, without the need to transfer the data across institutions [16]. The use of FL can thus lower the risks associated with privacy while still harnessing the strength of larger datasets.

Another issue is the ethical use of AI and minimizing bias in personalized medicine. AI systems are trained on existing data, which may lack representation of some groups (e.g., ethnic minorities or women) or reflect disparities in previous healthcare. For example, if a precision medicine AI algorithm is mainly trained on a dataset consisting of genomic information from people with European ancestry (a noted bias in genomics), then it is likely that it will be less reliable in generating recommendations for people from under-represented groups. In fact, this AI algorithm could literally add to health access inequities, rather than diminish them. Equity in AI-driven health care is now an important focus area, with calls for the field to address the sources of bias, improve transparency of algorithms, and to validate prediction performance across all subgroups. Clinicians using these AI-driven recommendations in practice should be completely aware of this kind of bias. They should dive deeper into the recommendation when an AI recommendation pathway seems out-of-context for a patient.

Consent and patient autonomy also come into play. Physicians must be able to clarify (to the greatest extent possible) why a recommendation is made. Providing the rationale for a recommendation is part of building trust. In addition, researchers are exploring explainable AI techniques that make ML models less of a "black box," which is important when the stakes are life and death. Moreover, patients typically have to consent to the use of their data (i.e., DNA) in AI training.

Finally, there is the overarching issue of clinical responsibility. These AI programs and decision-support tools can help rationalize clinical problems and help make treatment decisions. However, the ultimate responsibility for treatment decisions lies with the human clinician. If the AI recommends a therapy that is inappropriate for the patient, and that patient is harmed, the question of who is liable becomes very complicated. That being said, it is important to think about AI as a tool for decision-making purposes in the realm of personalized medicine and not as a decision-maker or authority. Clinicians will need to engage with AI in conjunction with their own assessment of the patient. Regulatory agencies, particularly in the United States the FDA, should become more engaged in evaluating AI systems—including those used for genomic decision support—to ensure they align with rigorous safety and efficacy criteria and ethical use prior to clinical adoption.

In summary, AI is ready to serve as a powerful adjunct in personalized medicine and genomics. It is starting to reveal usable information from the vast amounts of genetic and clinical data we have now, enabling a fundamentally different approach to health care for patients—from selecting the most effective cancer therapy to considering disease risk and customized prevention. As we see these possibilities grow, it is essential that we remain cognizant of privacy, bias, and transparency in order to ensure that the personalized medicine revolution is held accountable. With these things in mind, AI-guided precision medicine could make healthcare much more effective, safer, and more patient-centered than it has ever been before.

3.3 AI in Managing Chronic Diseases

3.3.1 Transforming Chronic Disease Management with AI

Chronic diseases—such as heart disease, diabetes, chronic respiratory disease, and cancer—are the world's leading causes of morbidity and mortality, accounting for an estimated 41 million deaths annually (around 74% of all deaths globally) [17]. Chronic diseases tend to be persistent, long-term conditions that are controlled, not cured. The management of chronic diseases has historically been quite complex because they are multifactorial and require ongoing engagement from the patient. Patients must stick to medication, stay on top of lifestyle changes, and constantly monitor their health indicators (such as blood pressure, weight, or glucose levels). Clinicians must regularly adjust the treatment plan and are also charged with early intervention when potential complications arise. Hospitals also feel the burden of chronic illnesses. Outpatient care for chronic patients is one of the most common sources of hospitalization. The use of AI in healthcare is an emerging area that could change the game by enhancing chronic disease management through continuous monitoring, early prediction of issues, custom care strategies/interventions, and patient self-management support. The goal is to push care from the clinic and hospital into the natural day-to-day lives of patients, seeking to minimize crises in favor of maintaining stability instead of reacting to deteriorating health.

One key aspect of AI's impact on chronic disease care is remote monitoring and early warning systems. Traditionally, physicians could only track the status of a chronic disease patient between visits using patient-reported information. Now, we can continuously collect data about vital signs, symptoms, and behavior through connected devices and wearable sensors. Using AI algorithms, this real-time data can be processed to detect trends or acute changes that might indicate issues for the patient. This approach has been described as a transition from reactive to proactive health care. For example, when managing patients with heart failure, patients can weigh themselves daily using Bluetooth-connected scales, wear blood-pressure cuffs, or even receive daily readings from implanted hemodynamic monitors. The AI systems then continuously analyze the daily readings and identify a pattern of weight gain, rising blood pressure, and lower activity to tell us, for example, there is a very high likelihood of fluid retention, which is an early sign of an exacerbation of heart failure. Clinicians can then intervene early in the process, before the patient may reach the point of hospitalization. Similarly, patients with atrial fibrillation (an irregular heart rhythm disorder) can use wearables, such as smartwatches, that continuously record their pulse or Electrocardiogram (ECG) information. AI algorithms that can analyze those data in real time, will see even very early signs of irregularities or patterns of atrial fibrillation episodes and can recommend patients seek clinical evaluation and early intervention [18]. Further evidence shows these types of AI-supported remote monitoring systems are safe and effective and can significantly reduce hospitalizations for heart-failure-related issues through earlier interventions [2].

In Chronic Obstructive Pulmonary Disease (COPD) management, AI-systems can analyze data obtained from remote monitoring of blood oxygen and respiratory rate and provide warnings of approaching exacerbation, so that early therapy can be initiated at home to prevent further complications [19]. In diabetes, researchers developed AI predictive models that use data from Continuous Glucose Monitors (CGMs) to accurately forecast glucose levels 30-min, or even 2 h, ahead, which permits early intervention and optimizes glycemic control [20–22]. When a system recognizes the probability of a steep drop in glucose (hypoglycemia) overnight, it can automatically decrease insulin delivery from an insulin pump or instruct the patient to eat a snack to prevent actual hypoglycemia. Preventive suggestions by the system help avoid emergencies and keep patients safe. Indeed, advances in hybrid closed-loop insulin pumps (the "artificial pancreas") have demonstrated improvements in glycemic control in type 1 diabetes [23]. AI has the ability to observe patients' data 24 h a day and apply feedback control to chronic diseases on an intelligent level, something that human providers by themselves can never practically achieve. From the perspective of the patient, continuous monitoring by AI offers a safety net of sorts. Knowing that their condition is being monitored in real-time may make patients feel more secure.

One of the strengths of AI is the ability to collate numerous parameters of data for chronic disease management. Consider hypertension (high blood pressure): management is not only related to blood pressure readings, but also to diet, stress levels, compliance with the prescribed medications, and other perpetually evolving factors. An AI application may obtain data from a patient's smart blood pressure cuff or smartwatch activity readings and, additionally, lab results at periodic intervals, and aggregate all of them. The app may build models showing that, for instance, a patient's blood pressure spikes two hours before taking their medication (potentially due to the waning levels of the drug), or that a patient's blood pressure improves on days when they have more sleep. The AI may then be able to send that individual targeted coaching messages or reminders about their medications and develop personalized plans. These plans could lead to better control of the disease condition.

AI's predictive analytics are more than just improvements in tracking, as they are changing how the near- and long-term management of chronic disease patients is adjusted. Risk stratification is one area where AI has made a big impact. When providing ongoing care for chronic patients, clinicians must consider which ones are at greater risk for potential complications such as stroke, heart attack, or hospitalization, so they can direct resources to the patients most in need. In healthcare, traditional risk scores typically combine two to three individual variables with a static algorithm. However, AI risk models can consider multiple variables, including patient demographics, comorbidity lists, past laboratory or testing data, and even whether the patient is adherent to medication therapy. AI risk models, unlike traditional risk scores, can also be updated in near real-time when new data becomes available. AI predictive models have shown that they can improve accuracy over traditional prediction models for numerous clinical outcomes [24]. Some hospitals are already using AI-driven "early warning systems" in their EHR databases to identify chronic disease patients at risk of deterioration, which allows for early intervention [25, 26].

AI-based systems for chronic disease management can also be used as decision support systems for clinicians. For example, an AI-based system may offer guidelines on the individualized target blood pressure and the combination of antihypertensive drugs that are likely to work best for that individual patient after analyzing the results of care from a large number of similar patients. This kind of analysis that utilizes findings of past patients is known as "predictive analytics" because it identifies the best care for an individual patient as a function of the care given to past patients. Predictive analytics does not merely dip into a population of past patients but rather learns who is at high risk of complications and for whom the potential intervention will likely reduce risk. The idea is to anticipate which patients need which interventions in a cost-effective way, so that resources can be optimally used across a population of chronic disease patients [24].

One specific example of AI-enabled decision support is the creation of knowledge-graph-based systems for chronic disease management. Knowledge graphs are networked representations of biomedical knowledge. For instance, in a study on pediatric asthma management, researchers constructed a knowledge graph from thousands of clinical notes and then added AI to reason with the knowledge contained in the graph [27]. AI could track the graph using an individual child's data (e.g., symptoms, tests) to suggest the best steps for management, some of which may not be obvious from existing guidelines. Figure 3.2 provides an example of how such an AI-enabled chronic disease management system can be conceptualized. In the example system, patient data streams are collected from wearables and home monitoring devices, and the patient data streams are aggregated with hospital patient data and medical knowledge into a central AI platform that performs assessment and risk analysis and uses that data to communicate with patients (through a smartphone app or chatbot) and to their healthcare providers (through alerts, dashboards, and EHR alerts). This approach exemplifies what the future of chronic disease management looks like, that is data-driven, personalized, and anticipatory.

AI does far more in chronic disease management than provide analytics behind the scenes; it engages and empowers patients in their own care. Patient self-management is at the heart of chronic care, with daily decisions and behaviors having a significant

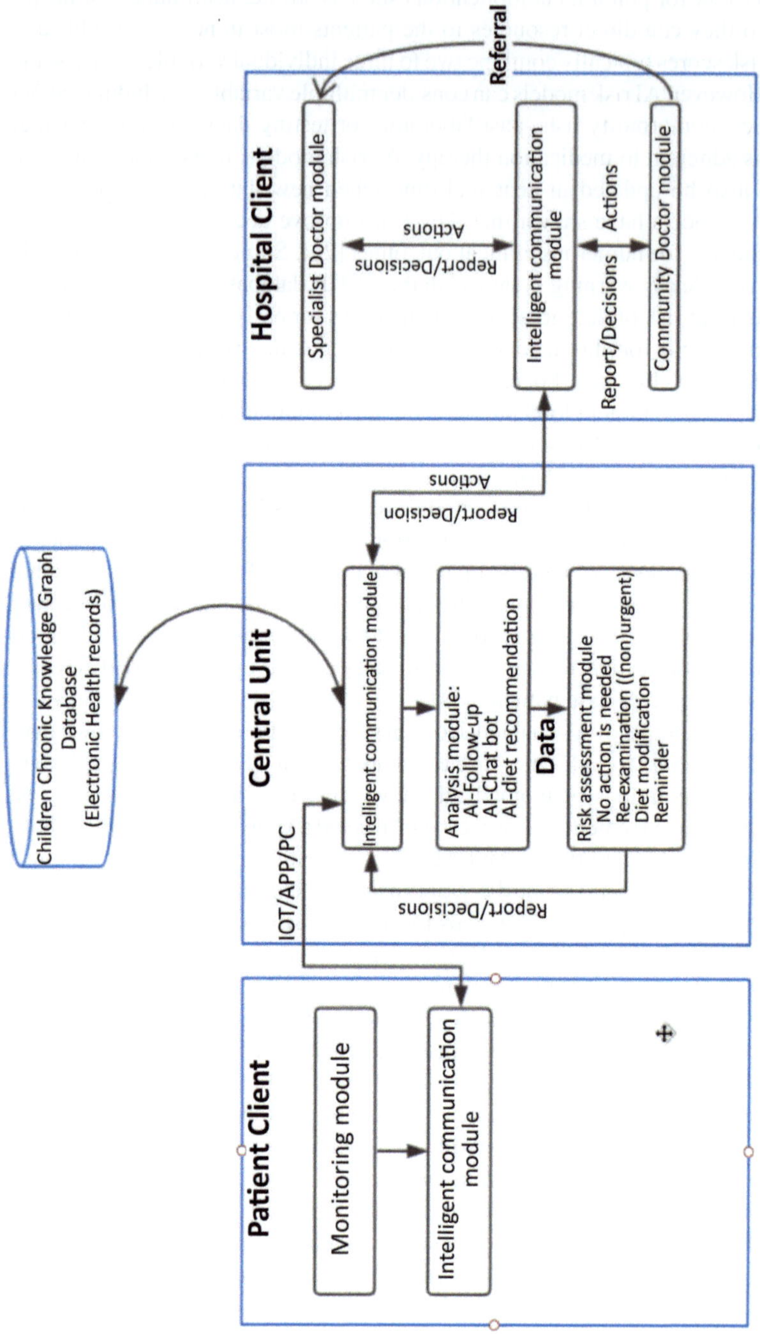

Fig. 3.2 The structure of the AI chronic disease management system. Reproduced from Yu et al. [27], published in Expert Systems With Applications 201 (2022) 117,026, under the Creative Commons Attribution 4.0 International License (CC BY), (https://creativecommons.org/licenses/by/4.0/). Font style and text size were adjusted for improved readability; the figure content is unchanged

impact on outcomes. AI tools, such as chatbots and virtual coaches, provide continuous support—answering questions, offering reminders, and delivering personalized feedback based on a patient's behavior or health data. As the AI coach learns the nuances of a particular patient's behavior, it can use this information to be more personal in its engagement. For example, if the AI learns that a patient is likely to forget their evening medications, it can center its reminders and problem-solving around that area. Research shows that these at-home, AI-facilitated interventions increase patient engagement and accountability, leading to benefits in medication adherence and lifestyle changes [2]. Because patients view AI tools as non-judgmental partners, this can be especially beneficial for challenging subjects (like dietary indiscretions or smoking relapses), which they may feel comfortable sharing with an AI before a clinician. Continuous engagement through AI support helps bridge the time gaps between clinic visits, allowing patients to assume a co-partner role in managing their own health.

Lastly, it's important to consider the impact on a patient's quality of life. Chronic diseases typically have a psychological burden too, as patients feel anxious about changes in their health or distressed by the level of involvement required to self-manage their condition. AI technology can help improve the patient's feeling of being supported and not being alone in managing their condition. For instance, if something goes wrong in the middle of the night, a patient may be able to get an answer or get some action from an AI-enabled platform instantly, instead of worrying until 8 am when they can reach their doctor. Secondly, as AI contributes to stabilizing disease control (i.e., timely intervention and adherence support), patients are more able to enjoy well days and physical activity and have fewer days suffering from complications. Even a few extra well days can make a big difference over months and years—helping patients work, enjoy activities, and manage their condition more effectively. In addition, family members and caregivers have the comfort of knowing an intelligent system is observing and managing their loved one. All these improvements in health and life participation are the central goal of chronic disease management, and AI is emerging as a strong tool to attain those goals.

3.3.2 System-Level Impact

Treatment of chronic disease also has implications for the healthcare system. If AI can reduce hospitalizations and emergency visits through timely engagement, it could be a great help. Prevention of hospitalization and emergency visits leads to reduced costs and burden. Avoided hospitalization for heart failure, or avoided episodes of diabetic ketoacidosis, provides the patient with better outcomes and healthcare savings of tens of thousands of dollars. As an example, the Livongo® diabetes management program (which uses AI and utilizes data from clients' self-service blood glucose levels and other clinical data to provide tailored coaching and monitoring) achieved a medical spending reduction of 21.9% for program participants over a one year period, which translates to about $88 per patient per month reduction in spending (most of which was due to reductions in hospital and office visits) [28, 29]. As the number of patients multiplies to hundreds or thousands, the economic impact becomes very large. AI can also improve efficiency of clinical workflows by employing remote monitoring programs. Meanwhile, by stratifying risk, healthcare teams are able to deliver their efforts more efficiently, for example, prioritizing nurses and care managers for patients with the highest-risk status, while lower-risk patients may be safely supported with an automated system that maximizes human effort. This improves the productivity of the healthcare workforce in the context of a global shortage of healthcare professionals.

In addition, AI can support population health management and a continuous quality improvement cycle. Beyond anticipatory analytics that support the clinical care of individuals or groups of patients, health systems can analyze the aggregate data of AI-monitored patients to highlight trends. For example, if health systems notice a spike in the number of asthma exacerbations in a certain population or geographic area, they may want to explore the issue, and the results may correlate with environmental conditions. Having this kind of population health measurement and continuous quality improvement feedback mechanism allows organizations to rapidly improve the quality of care in their chronic care programs.

In conclusion, AI is introducing a new paradigm in chronic disease management. It provides the ability to continuously monitor patients, and in the worst cases, to prevent catastrophic events. AI's predictive analytics and decision support systems empower clinicians to evolve long-term therapy plans tailored to patients' needs. It engages patients as participants while reducing stress on the healthcare system. Early implementation of these technologies in diabetes, heart disease, and chronic respiratory illness has shown improvements in control, decreased hospitalizations, and cost savings [2, 28, 29]. There are challenges that will need to be overcome, such as data sharing, patient privacy, and seamless integration into clinical practice, but the path is clear. As AI for chronic disease management evolves and matures, we can create healthcare delivery environments that focus on prevention, personalization, and participation, ultimately improving outcomes and quality of life for the millions of people living with chronic disease. The intersection of constant data and intelligent analysis transforms chronic disease management from a historical, periodic, reactive process into a continuous, proactive partnership of patients, machines, and healthcare providers.

3.4 AI in Surgery Design

AI is now beginning to shape the way in which the surgery is organized and performed, even before the first incision, and this field is evolving rapidly. A number of new, advanced AI algorithms are emerging that can aggregate and analyze large pools of patient data, including imaging data, genomic data, and more, to help surgeons optimize unique surgical approaches for each patient. For surgery, this design includes preoperative planning, realistic simulation of the procedure and potential outcomes, risk assessment for complications, and iterative processes that ensure surgical techniques improve with results. AI technologies are now involved in most of these components, providing surgeons with data to guide their decision-making. In this section, we will discuss how AI models can assist in preoperative planning, simulation and modeling through virtual surgeries, risk assessment for potential complications, and provide assistance in improving surgical outcomes.

3.4.1 Preoperative Planning: AI Models in Surgical Strategy

Preoperative planning is an important stage of surgery where careful strategy and preparation occurs. The emergence of AI as a tool of preoperative planning has made it a powerful collaborator in this phase, as it can analyze complicated medical images, anatomical information, and past surgical cases to create a potential surgical plan or optimize a surgical plan. For instance, algorithms using AI can segment medical imaging (CT, MRI) for surgeons to create 3D models of the patient's anatomy and help identify important structures such as blood vessels or tumors [30]. This functionality allows surgeons to experience the operative field in 3D before the operation. In plastic and reconstructive surgery, researchers have combined Reinforcement Learning (RL) with image enhancement AI to facilitate surgeons to make decisions, such as mapping the blood vessels (perforators) in flap surgery. This technique can save surgeons significant time in analyzing sites for critical blood vessels while maintaining accuracy [30]. In the field of orthopedic or spine surgery, AI software can help surgeons improve their accuracy in screw placement [31].

AI has also improved the planning aspects of dental surgery. A noteworthy illustration of the effectiveness of AI is the interaction between AI and Augmented Reality (AR) in a surgical planning program for dental implants. In one research example, the authors developed a protocol for the use of AI in conjunction with AR, where a patient underwent Cone-Beam Computed Tomography (CBCT) scanning and the AI algorithm automatically segmented the scan to create a 3D model of the jaw that could be visualized and manipulated into the operative field, displayed as an overlay through AR goggles [32]. The surgeon wore goggles that allowed visualization of the anatomic structures through holographic images aligned with the patient's anatomy. The surgeon could also plan virtual 3D placement of the implants in the surgical field through AR. Initial trials demonstrated that the AI + AR approach was a feasible and effective method that allowed efficient surgical planning of implants without requiring conventional surgical guide software. The deviations of implant placements using the AI + AR software were clinically acceptable and fell within minor margins, indicating that AI-assisted surgical planning can be as effective as conventional planning approaches.

AI-driven planning tools are also helping surgeons predict variations and complexities in patient anatomy. For example, AI algorithms can evaluate CT scans to show the identifiable branches of blood vessels or tumor margins, so the surgical team can make decisions about how much tissue to resect while preserving normal tissue

[33, 34]. In neurosurgery, ML algorithms help surgeons determine the locations of brain tumors relative to important functional brain areas and potentially create safer access points [35, 36]. These pre-operative AI programs serve as augmented intelligence, providing objective analysis and suggestions for the surgical team to add to their plan. The surgeon is ultimately in charge, while AI provides a second opinion supported by data. This helps the surgeon potentially better individualize the surgical plan to the anatomy and pathology of the patient, while also increasing the chances of success and minimizing intraoperative surprises.

3.4.2 Simulation and Modeling: Virtual Surgeries and Outcome Prediction

Another significant addition of AI in surgical design is the potential for virtual surgery capability and predictive understanding. Advanced Computer Vision (CV) and physics-based modeling, along with AI, enable us to develop virtual surgery simulators that behave like the real procedures. In this scenario, surgeons could rehearse a complex procedure on a patient-specific virtual model multiple times to improve their approach before doing it on their patient. Such simulations are often augmented with AI so that it provides feedback and guidance—effectively serving as a "virtual coach". For example, the Virtual Operative Assistant (VOA), an AI-based simulator, was developed as a training tool for neurosurgeons and other surgical specialties [37]. As demonstrated in Figs. 3.3 and 3.4, in this scenario, trainees were performing a virtual surgery (e.g., brain tumor removal in VR), while the VOA's use of ML was analyzing the trainee's performance—such as instrument movements, safety, precision—and compared that data against expert benchmarks. The unique features of the VOA allow it to classify a trainee's skill level (novice versus expert) with over 90% accuracy. The trainee received immediate feedback on specific metrics. The explainable AI simulator not only predicts likely outcomes (e.g., whether a novice's technique presents a complication risk) but also teaches the user how to improve performance on identified errors.

Aside from training, simulation via AI may be valuable in assisting practitioners in predicting outcomes prior to surgery. AI can be utilized to predict surgical difficulty or related outcomes by virtually undertaking the planned surgery on a patient's digital twin. In orthopedic surgery, for instance, preoperative imaging can inform implant allocation, and implant simulations can be used to predict outcomes such as range of motion or impingement risk based on surgical navigation expectations. In these cases, based on simulation outcomes, the implant size or position may be adjusted to improve postoperative results. Recent trials have shown that AI-assisted planning significantly improves surgical workflow and technical precision in orthopedic procedures [38]. In the context of cancer surgery, AI-based simulation may compute whether an anticipated resection approach would provide clear margins, or if not, advise how margins should be extended in the surgical plan.

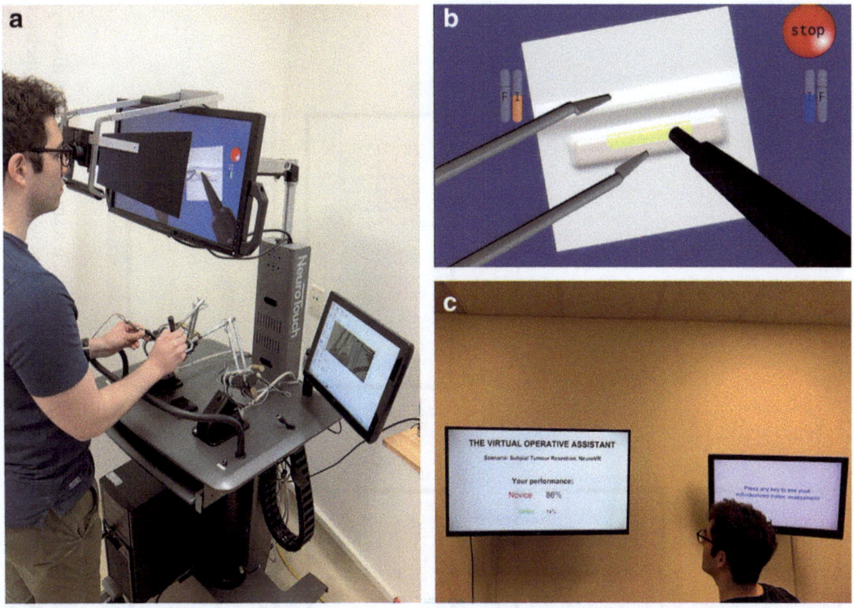

Fig. 3.3 AI-enabled surgical simulation system in use: **a** trainee using a VR surgical simulator, **b** simulation of cortical tumor (yellow) removal with preservation of healthy brain tissue (white), and **c** simulation data automatically uploaded to VOA for real-time feedback. Reproduced from Mirchi et al. [37], published in PLoS One 15 (2020) e0229596, under the Creative Commons Attribution 4.0 International License (CC BY), (https://creativecommons.org/licenses/by/4.0/)

Simulation enhanced by AI accounts not only for the logistics of surgery, such as maneuvers and processes, but also for patient counselling and expectation management. AI models can produce realistic visual representations of potential outcomes following surgery, especially in plastic or aesthetic procedures. In cosmetic surgery, AI models can be used to generate "after" images directly from a patient's "before" photo, illustrating possible changes from procedures such as rhinoplasty or breast reconstruction. Alongside more traditional educational methods, AI simulation can provide patients with virtual possibilities while ensuring their expectations are aligned with what can feasibly be achieved surgically [30]. By using multiple simulated outcomes, surgeons and patients can negotiate the best possible plan for the operating room (for example, how much tissue to remove or reshape).

In summary, AI-based simulation and modeling has added an important ingredient to surgical design: rehearsal and foresight. Emotional strain and difficulty in communicating the surgical plan often exist in the operative suite, and AI helps mitigate this by allowing the surgeon to iterate a plan in silico repeatedly until the system indicates a high likelihood of achieving the desired outcome or a low risk of failure, making the process both safer and more efficient than relying solely on the operation itself. Furthermore, once improved theoretical surgical sequences are tested virtually, AI performance can be validated by completing fewer real surgeries, while the data

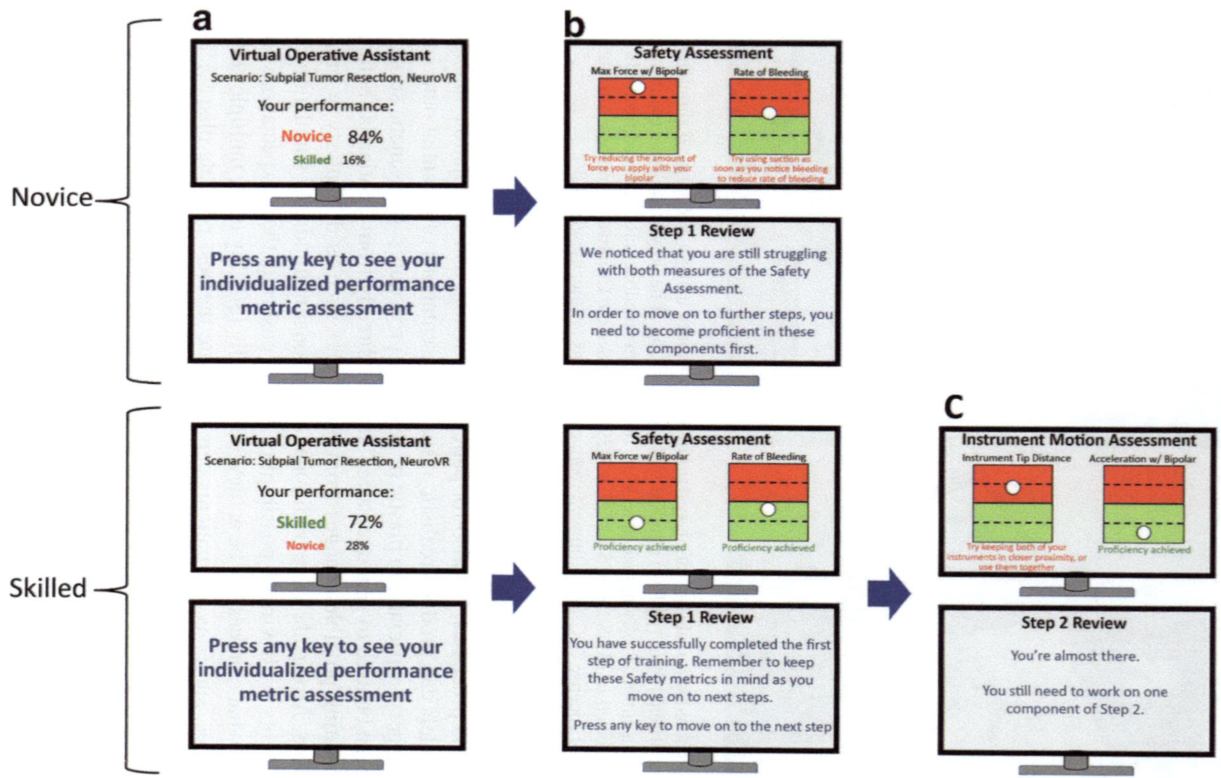

Fig. 3.4 Example of performance feedback from the VOA. The VOA provides trainees with real-time feedback on two monitors: **a** a summary screen displays the trainee's skill classification (e.g., novice, intermediate, expert) along with associated probabilities, **b** a feedback screen reports two safety-related metrics, with positive reinforcement or improvement instructions depending on performance. If competency in all safety metrics is not achieved, the trainee must repeat the scenario, and **c** a third screen (optional) provides feedback on two instrument motion metrics with performance-specific comments. Reproduced from Mirchi et al. [37], published in PLoS One 15 (2020) e0229596, under the Creative Commons Attribution 4.0 International License (CC BY), (https://creativecommons.

from these simulations help refine and improve predictive accuracy. This creates a positive feedback loop in which more surgeries generate better simulations for the future. As these systematic and powerful capabilities of virtual tools advance, we can envision a future where every complex surgery is rehearsed on a patient's digital twin with AI assistance to identify uncertainties, reduce risks, and develop optimal strategies before the real patient is ever put under general anesthesia.

3.4.3 Risk Assessment: AI's Role in Identifying Complications

It's important for every surgical design to consider risks, both general ones (e.g., infection, bleeding) and specific patient ones (e.g., a patient having anatomical variant that increases risk of injury). Historically, risk assessment relies on the surgeon's experience as well as standard risk scores. AI is revolutionizing risk assessment by mining large datasets that include surgical patients with known outcomes. AI can create individualized risk profiles with much greater precision and accuracy than human surgeons. For instance, MySurgeryRisk is an ML algorithm designed to predict major complications or death from surgery [39]. MySurgeryRisk was trained in tens of thousands of surgical cases with known outcomes and has detected very complex patterns in preoperative variables (lab values, comorbidities, medications) that might not be obvious to human surgeons. The model showed high accuracy, with Area Under a Curve (AUC) values above 0.8 for complications and 0.77–0.83 for mortality, and outperformed traditional surgical risk scores.

Aside from general complications, there are some AI models aimed at specific prediction tasks, such as prediction of risk of surgical site infection, risk of tumor recurrence, or risk of requiring blood transfusion, among others. These models usually use DL algorithms on heterogeneous data, which includes both structured health records and unstructured data, such as free-text notes and imaging. For example, there have been recent examples of using Natural Language Processing (NLP) on clinical or operative notes, in combination with ML, to improve prediction of postoperative outcomes such as complications or hospital readmissions by capturing subtle patterns and contextual details that are not apparent in structured data alone [40–42]. Thus, AI can be used to inform care teams about high-risk patients earlier and push the team to make an intervention (perhaps with closer postoperative observation, prophylactic measures, or discussing with a specialist) to mitigate the risk.

In the operating room itself, AI assesses risk in real time, as illustrated in Fig. 3.5. The area of anesthesia can use AI models that assess key vital sign trends to predict hypotension or hypoxemia before they occur, allowing the anesthesiologist to intervene proactively and prevent a medical emergency. In the example of an AI monitoring a patient during cardiac surgery, an AI system could analyze live vital sign data to proactively warn the surgical team of impending arrhythmia or ischemia, effectively combining multiple data points while patients are in the operating room. Surgical robots are also being equipped with smart sensors powered by AI. These systems are capable of, for example, continuous monitoring of organ movements in real time, resulting in enhanced precision and accuracy [43]. By detecting these small nuances, AI acts as a sentinel of safety in the surgical suite.

It is important to emphasize that AI risk assessment is augmentative and does not replace clinical judgement. It provides evidence-based risk analysis for clinicians to use when making care decisions and planning subsequent treatment. Surgeons can also share AI-generated risk scores to guide discussions around informed consent (for example: "Based on your patient profile, the AI estimates a 30% chance of complication X; here's how we would mitigate or reduce that risk for you"). Also, the third-order predictions has an effect on surgical planning. For example, if a patient is rated high risk for cardiac stress and the surgical team agrees to proceed, they may consider developing a plan for a less invasive procedure or potentially staging surgery over multiple individual surgical operations to reduce physiological strain.

A key hurdle that we have to overcome is to make sure that these AI risk models are generalizable and unbiased. Because they learn from historical data, they need

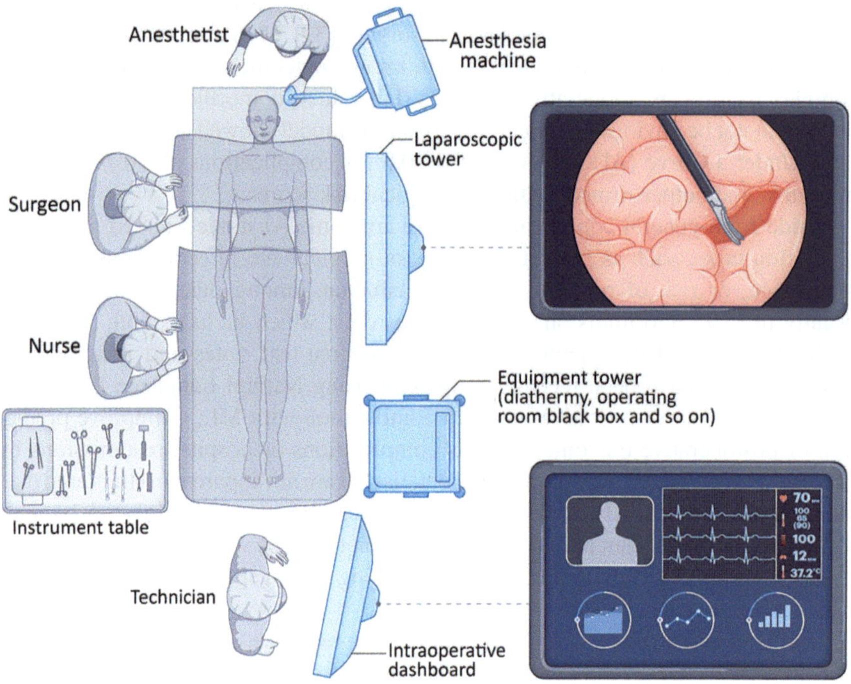

Fig. 3.5 Integration of novel AI-powered digital interventions in the intraoperative setting. Reproduced from Varghese et al. [38], published in Nature Medicine 30 (2024) 1257–1268, © 2024, with permission from Springer Nature. Font style and text size were adjusted for improved readability; the figure content is unchanged

to be well validated across patient populations and maintained with regular updates. Nevertheless, the results to date have been encouraging. In several studies across a range of surgical specialties, ML algorithms showed superior performance compared to traditional risk indices, such as American Society of Anesthesiologists (ASA) score or Surgical Apgar Score (SAS), in predicting outcomes such as complications, length of stay, or recovery time [44–46]. By more accurately identifying who is at risk for specific outcomes, surgeons can customize perioperative care, for example, by adjusting the level of postoperative monitoring required, or choosing one surgical plan over another to effectively plan the surgical journey of patients around possible pitfalls.

3.4.4 Improving Outcomes: Evidence of Enhanced Surgical Success

The overall aim of using AI in surgical design is to enhance patient outcomes. AI in surgery is an area that is still developing; however, there is growing evidence that its applications are correlated with better surgical outcomes. A documented area for improvement is surgical precision and the extent of tumor resection. As we mentioned earlier, the use of patient-specific 3D models in prostate cancer surgery resulted in an observable decrease in positive surgical margins [47]—that is, more patients were cancer-free after surgery and required less need for adjuvant treatments.

Another outcome benefit is decreased operative time and complications for complex cases. If AI planning tools can order surgical steps more efficiently, then operative time may decrease further. For example, in liver surgery, AI-assisted systems that integrate AR and 3D models can guide the surgeon in navigating vascular structures [48]. By helping determine the optimal sequence of vessel management, these tools can potentially reduce intraoperative blood loss and shorten operative time, ultimately enhancing surgical efficiency. Clinical studies on orthopedic surgeries using AI and other supported methods of pre-operative planning, including image-based patient-specific guides, have reported decreased surgical times and improved technical accuracy [38]. In general, a shorter surgical procedure will likely lead to less time under anesthesia and a reduction of complications as patients' risk of infection diminishes.

AI's influence on intraoperative decision support also provides benefits for outcomes. Take, for instance, a laparoscopic case where an AI vision system indicates anatomic landmarks in real time through the video feed. Early studies of intraoperative AI systems have shown that when surgeons work with the AI overlays, they make fewer inadvertent injuries as the critical structures are explicitly pointed out by the computer (even if buried in fat or bleeding) [38, 49, 50]. Fewer injurious actions lead to fewer adverse outcomes and reoperations. In neurosurgery, AI-based image guidance that distinguishes tumor tissue from normal brain tissue facilitates more complete resection and treatment while preserving function, leading to enhanced oncologic and neurologic outcomes for patients [35].

Outcomes in robotic surgery will also potentially improve with AI (see Sect. 3.5 for more). Indeed, an autonomous surgical robot has been developed that demonstrated better performance than human surgeons performing the suturing of bowel tissue in experiments [51]. The Smart Tissue Autonomous Robot (STAR) has been more consistent with evenly spaced sutures than surgeons with several years of experience. Although not yet demonstrated in a clinical setting, the consistent precision of STAR may result in fewer leaks and complications following surgery. This illustrates the principle that certain routine aspects of surgery could exceed human performance when automated via AI, thereby enhancing outcomes such as healing and recovery.

It's important to see these improvements in context, since AI is a tool that must be incorporated into surgical practice properly. Best outcomes occur when surgeons and AI are working together, with the surgeon providing oversight, ethical decision-making, and creativity while the AI does data analysis, pattern recognition, and mechanical precision—day and night—indefatigably. When that occurs—early data indicates—patients might benefit from safer surgeries, more effective disease treatment, or faster recovery. Eventually, as more prospective trials and longitudinal studies take place, we may begin to have better quantification of AI's effects, such as lower rates of complications, better survival after cancer surgery, or better functional outcomes.

As previously discussed, AI is rapidly changing surgical design from planning through postoperative outcomes analysis. Using AI to help with planning in a thorough manner, providing realistic simulations, anticipating and mitigating risk, and learning from previous surgical interventions, the surgical field is closer to the surgical ideal of precision surgical interventions that are individually and optimally defined, performed without error, and that produce the optimal outcome for each patient.

3.5 AI in Robot-Assisted Surgery

Robot-assisted surgery is being pursued more aggressively in operating rooms, and procedures such as episiotomies are now possible with robotic arms and systems like the da Vinci Surgical System, which surgeons employ for minimally invasive procedures. Historically, these surgical robots operated on a master–slave paradigm, where hand movements at a console performed by the surgeon were converted into precise movements of instruments inside of the patient [51]. When a surgeon is at the console, in its most basic sense, the robot extends the surgeon's hand, eliminates tremor, and scales motion. However, the robot does not make any decisions. The introduction of AI into robot-assisted surgery now exceeds the master–slave paradigm by adding machine autonomy and machine intelligence in a myriad of complex degrees to surgical robots. Ultimately, the goal of AI in robot-assisted surgery is to improve performance in achieving surgical precision, provide decision support during surgery, and incrementally automate surgical tasks under the direct supervision of a surgeon.

3.5.1 *From Assistance to Autonomy: Evolution of Robotic Surgery with AI*

The most commonly used surgical robots approved by the FDA today provide robotic assistance only and are not capable of decision-making. The surgeon always maintains control of all movements and actions [52]. However, advancements in AI are enabling increased levels of autonomy in both research prototypes and specialized systems. Autonomy in surgical robotics is categorized into different levels (Fig. 3.6, Level 0 = No Autonomy, Level 5 = Full Autonomy) [52].

The majority of clinical robots currently function at Level 1 autonomy, providing instrument holding and other assistance with basic tasks under surgeon control. Level 2 and Level 3 systems are currently under development due to advancements in AI. A Level 2 system can perform specific sub-tasks, for instance, suturing or drilling along a pre-defined pattern, autonomously once initiated by the surgeon. Level 3 systems are designed to make conditional decisions and adapt to the surgical field (such as defining a cutting path in relation to patient details) while acting under supervision [52].

Approximately 86% of regulator-cleared surgical robots to date operate at Level 1 autonomy, with a few operating at Level 2—such as orthopedic robots that can autonomously perform pre-planned bone cuts [52]. A very small number of systems have already achieved Level 3 conditional autonomy, meaning that they can plan or change their actions after taking in environmental inputs, such as a patient's anatomy or imaging, under the supervision of a surgeon. However, to our knowledge, no surgical robots have been licensed at Level 4 or 5 autonomy, and they are yet to be developed for fully autonomous surgery without the surgeon's oversight. Nevertheless, it is possible, as shown in advances such as the STAR project, that achieving Level 4 or 5 autonomy is close to possible for specific tasks. In experimental models, STAR was able to perform small bowel anastomosis, demonstrating comparable efficacy—and in terms of suture consistency, superior performance—relative to expert surgeons using both manual laparoscopy and the da Vinci robot-assisted system [51]. The STAR system used CV to guide its suturing and made adjustments to its approach if the tissue was moved or changed shape, illustrating AI decision-making during a surgical task.

One way that AI is contributing to the realm of robot-assisted surgery is via intraoperative guidance. Although not fully autonomous, an AI algorithm is still useful in surgery by interpreting data from the robotic system cameras and sensors, and providing real-time feedback, thereby assisting the surgeon. For example, in robotic laparoscopic surgery, a CV module with AI can identify organs, blood vessels, and/or tumors in the endoscope view and paint an outline around them for the surgeon. Advanced initial work was conducted by Madani et al. [53] using semantic segmentation AI to label structures during laparoscopic cholecystectomy (gallbladder removal) in real time. In the framework of an AI-based robotic system, this could help avert accidents, like cutting the incorrect duct, by effectively making the AI warn or—in the worst-case scenario—prevent the robot from performing a dangerous action

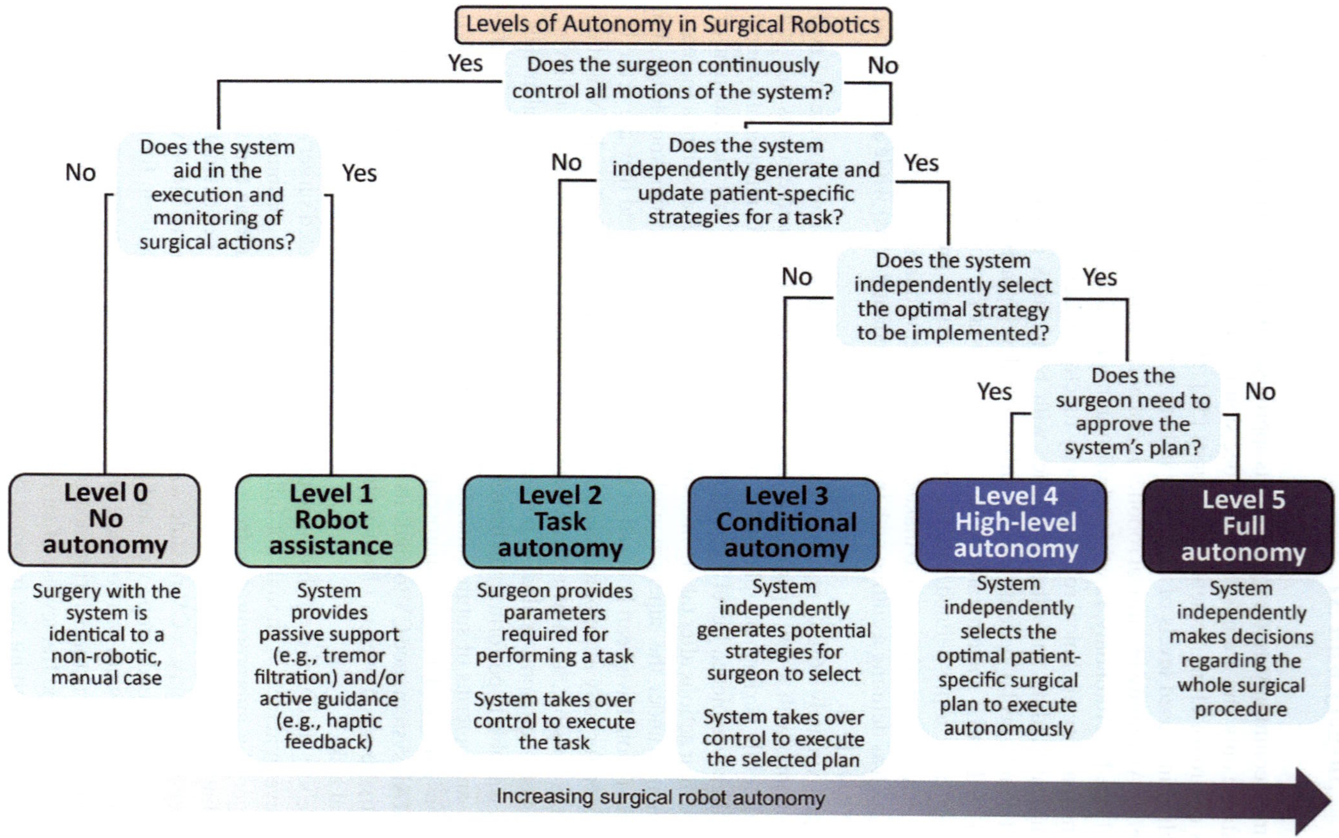

Fig. 3.6 Levels of Autonomy in Surgical Robotics (LASR) taxonomy. Reproduced from Lee et al. [52], published in NPJ Digital Medicine 7 (2024) 103, under the Creative Commons Attribution 4.0 International License (CC BY), (https://creativecommons.org/licenses/by/4.0/). Font style and text size were adjusted for improved readability; the figure content is unchanged

in proximity to a labeled structure. Moreover, AI can monitor robotic instruments movements with force feedback to the robot's sensors and keep a watchful eye on how much force is being applied to delicate structures, tissues, or organs, or if a surgical instrument is existing the defined safe zone in the surgical plan.

Another example of AI guidance in robotics is AR overlays in the robotic surgeon's console. With AR, preoperative imaging (annotated by AI) can be overlaid on the surgeon's view of the operative field. In robot-assisted surgery, AI-generated 3D models of organs and their internal structures can be displayed within the real-time endoscopic video feed. For instance, in the case of a procedure on the kidney, the surgeon could see tumor margins or blood vessels highlighted below the surface in real-time through AI-driven segmentation and automatic registration with the operative field [43]. This improves situational awareness. Some experimental robotic systems have incorporated AR with force feedback sensors—the idea is not just to see critical structures, but to feel engagement when the instrument element of the robot encounters resistance, recognizing that this resistance directly corresponds to that same critical structure [43]. This is in part a vision of compensating for the haptic feedback that surgeons are missing in today's robotic surgical systems, and also a motivation to improve precision (i.e., stopping dissection when a threshold of tension is achieved to avoid tearing a vessel).

The application of AI to improve the safety and efficacy of robot-assisted surgeries is already being realized. AI, by reviewing the vast amount of data generated from robotic systems (all instrument motion, camera views, etc.), can identify patterns associated with poor outcomes. For example, ML analysis of thousands of robotic surgery videos has developed an "AI surgical coach" that can inform a surgeon when they are departing from a known best technique at a particular step [43]. In essence, the AI is observing the actual surgical procedure and prompting suggestions (or warnings) to the surgeon. This is similar to a driving assistant in vehicles—it is not driving for you, but it helps you drive better.

The shift in autonomy also creates challenges. As robots act independently, we have to start thinking about permissions, legal liability, and ethical limits [52]. Right now, everyone (including surgeons and regulators) believe AI-driven robots should work as assistive devices in surgery, not as independent operators, except in very limited situations. The surgeon of record accepts the duty for the patient's safety, which means that the autonomy of the AI is supervised by the surgeon. The community is actively working on frameworks like the LASR to delineate what a robot can do on its own, and what requires formal human confirmation [52]. For example, a Level 2 task-autonomous robot may be able to place a row of sutures after the surgeon says "go", but the surgeon can interrupt, interfere, or abort the task at their discretion if something is incorrect. All of these frameworks help to ensure we adopt autonomy in a systematic and safety-tested way as we transition to AI.

3.5.2 *Evidence of Improved Surgical Performance with Robotics and AI*

Robot-assisted surgery is already associated with advantages, like smaller incisions, less blood loss, and quicker recovery for many procedures, but the impact of AI is expected to enhance these advantages and help solve some outstanding issues. Preliminary evidence suggests that AI can assist robotic surgeons in achieving proficiency more quickly and potentially exceed human-only benchmarks for certain measures. A systematic review published in 2025 reported on recent studies of AI-enabled robotic surgery [54]. It found that AI-enabled robotic systems nearly always improved surgical accuracy, decreased risks and errors in the intraoperative phase of surgery, and improved clinical outcomes. While many studies were observational or still at an early stage, there were multiple reports of improved efficiency and patient outcomes across many surgical specialties when AI assistance was present.

The fully autonomous STAR system described earlier still shows the vision for improvement of outcomes. In comparative studies, STAR-sutured tissues had more uniform suture spacing and tension, thereby showing improved healing outcomes [51]. When suturing blood vessels, human beings showed vast variability from stitch to stitch, whereas STAR consistently achieved the same result. It is consistency that ML was designed for, taking away variability and helping to raise the baseline for surgical quality (despite the fact that humans are likely still the best performers in unpredictable situations based on our ingenuity). With that said, it is conceivable that the robot consistently performs the routine portion of surgery perfectly every time while the surgeon handles the less predictable portion, leading to a better overall outcome.

To conclude, AI is improving robot-assisted surgery in numerous ways, including improving the surgeon's vision and precision, offering a degree of partial automation for efficiency, and laying the foundation for increased autonomy. Current evidence suggests that all of this can bring about safer surgeries, better consistency, and even increased capabilities (e.g., performing a task in a tighter space or making a more precise movement than a human hand). Robot-assisted surgery was already a step into the future for minimally invasive surgery, and now with AI, it is stepping into what we could call intelligent surgery—wherein surgical robots will not just be robotic hands executing commands but will have awareness of the goal and context of the surgery and actively assist in achieving the best result. The movement towards fully autonomous surgery will be slow and deliberate, and rightly so, but each step that AI introduces is making surgery more precise and patient-specific.

3.6 AI in Telemedicine and Remote Patient Care

Telemedicine, the delivery of care through communication technologies in remote spaces, has become a hot topic, particularly in light of COVID-19, as it supports alternatives to in-person services [55]. Telemedicine supports important needs beyond pandemic settings by establishing connection points between patients and providers (in many cases across geographic distances), enabling consultations, diagnosis, and monitoring without requiring travel. In this evolving context, there are opportunities to harness advances in AI to enhance remote care delivery. While virtual spaces inherently lack physical presence, AI decision-support tools could support remote patient care by providing intelligent analysis of digital data and creating personalized remote care solutions that expand access to specialists. Here, we discuss how AI enhances telehealth in two general areas of telemedicine (i.e., tele-consultation and diagnosis) and remote patient monitoring. We also discuss the opportunities and challenges associated with this incorporation.

3.6.1 AI-Enhanced Tele-Consultations and Diagnosis

The beginning of telemedicine's journey often starts with a virtual consultation, a remote meeting between a patient and clinician connecting via video, phone, or chat. AI can be increasingly integrated into these interactions, oftentimes behind the scenes. AI-driven diagnostic tools can also support physicians during video consultations by analyzing patient information in real time. For instance, when a patient is explaining their symptoms via video call, an AI symptom checker (like a virtual triage nurse) is likely gathering data and parsing the patient's conversation and medical history to provide possible diagnoses or questions to ask [56]. Telehealth platforms can start off the process with an AI chatbot engaging the patient directly, gathering structured information about symptoms and medical history through NLP. These AI systems triage the cases, identifying the highest-risk patients so that they can be prioritized, while channeling direct care to lower-acuity cases [55]. By the time the physician joins the video call, the AI has already conducted an initial review and informed the physician of possible diagnoses with some level of confidence, or it flagged the patient's speech for increased risk based on ill-defined symptoms that could suggest a stroke needing emergency management.

The use of telemedicine and AI is particularly exciting in dermatology and radiology. In dermatology, tele-consults usually involve patients capturing and uploading images of their skin lesions. An AI image classification algorithm can analyze the uploaded images, identifying features of malignancy—for example, identifying suspicious moles—and assist the remote dermatologist in prioritizing skin lesions for urgent biopsy. Similarly, AI can facilitate the addition of other medical specialties. At a rural clinic, a CT or MRI scan can be uploaded to a cloud-based AI system, which can then screen for urgent and critical findings (like a brain hemorrhage) and alert the tele-radiologist or local providers directly. In this form, even when specialists do not occupy a site, their expertise is enhanced by additional digital "eyes", reducing the chance of missed diagnoses. In fact, studies have demonstrated that AI-based teleradiology can significantly decrease the interpretation time for urgent, time-sensitive scans—from hours to one or two minutes—by disregarding normal scans and highlighting areas of interest on abnormal scans [57].

AI can also improve telemedicine and address barriers related to language and accessibility. AI language models can facilitate real-time translation services between patients and doctors who speak different languages [58, 59]. These services increase access to care opportunities. AI can reduce medical jargon [60, 61]. AI could function in different ways as an intermediary. For example, it could create a presentation or visual aid so that when the doctor is explaining the health issue at a complex level, AI can distill that into a simpler explanation or text graphic for the patient, which is helpful to promote understanding and adherence to treatments. In remote telemedicine, where establishing rapport can be difficult through a screen, AI can help meditate understanding and adherence to patient instructions.

Security and verification are another layer. AI-based facial recognition, with the right privacy precautions, could verify a patient's identity for telemedicine appointments. Emotion recognition algorithms could also measure if the patient looks distressed or confused and could alert the provider to slow down or clarify communication. Although this emotional AI is still experimental, it could offer some insights into mental health tele-consults by identifying indicators of anxiety or even depression that may not have been expressed verbally.

In short, AI's function in tele-consultations is to enhance the delivery of high-quality virtual care to match the level of an in-person visit. AI can offer decision support, process large amounts of data, and help remote clinicians make accurate diagnoses and decisions. It is as if the telemedicine doctor has a virtual helper whispering in their ear with the best pertinent information based on hundreds of thousands of records from medical databases and the patient's digital footprint. Most importantly, AI can serve to reduce the disparities associated with telemedicine being seen as a "lower-tier" interaction; aided by AI, remote care can now be delivered with the understanding that in certain instances it can be as effective and data-saturated as bedside care.

3.6.2 Remote Patient Monitoring and Management with AI

AI may have the greatest impact in remote patient care through Remote Patient Monitoring (RPM), which is using connected devices/sensors to monitor patients' health outside of the hospital. Devices such as wearables, smart implants, and smartphone applications can continuously collect vital signs (heart rate, blood pressure, oxygen saturation), blood glucose, activity level, and more. This constant stream of patient data greatly benefits from AI, which has the ability to make sense of and transform high-volume, big-data and high-velocity data, and determine what patterns and behaviors warrant intervention.

There are multiple functions that AI algorithms can serve in RPM. One function is to identify the presence of abnormal patient metrics. AI uses ML models to create a baseline for each individual patient and can generate alerts when a patient's metrics are drastically outside of what it has learned. For example, a heart failure patient may have a weight-sensing scale and a blood pressure cuff in their home. The learning algorithm may determine that a patient's daily weight does not typically vary by more than 1 kg. If it detects a 3 kg daily increase over the course of a couple of days, along with rising blood pressure, it would preemptively flag a potential heart failure exacerbation. The care team would be alerted through the RPM dashboard and would be able to initiate an intervention, like adjusting the patient's diuretics or performing a telemedicine visit to intervene before the patient became critically ill. Proactive interventions based on AI pattern recognition have been demonstrated to reduce hospital readmissions related to chronic disease management [2].

Predictive analytics in remote monitoring is more than just a reaction to real-time data; this type of monitoring leverages AI models that not only identify a patient's current status but also project their health path into the future. For instance, an RPM AI system monitoring the glucose readings of a diabetic patient, as well as their diet logs and fitness tracker, might predict the likelihood that this patient will have persistently elevated blood glucose over the next week (i.e., an upward trend in glucose readings while patient activity is decreasing). The RPM AI could suggest preemptive actions by notifying the patient with a tailored notification—"Your activity has decreased during a time where your glucose levels are creeping up; how about going for a 30-min walk today?"—or alerting clinical staff to address possible medication needs. This patient management approach switches care from event-driven (i.e., when patient health is already at risk) to preventive care. This new technique of using AI and RPM to manage an individual patient's health has the potential to move from reactive care to continuous health maintenance. It shifts the focus from episodic care to continuous healthcare.

Importantly, AI doesn't just alert but can also provide interventions or suggestions. In chronic disease management, AI chatbots or virtual coaches can engage with patients to orient their day. Picture a patient with hypertension logging their diet and blood pressure: it is possible for an AI coach (via a smartphone app) to talk to them, congratulating them on days with healthy eating and gently guiding them when salt was higher. It is continual care at a personal level. AI-based coaching could improve taking medications and support significant lifestyle changes by providing more proactive, personalized, real-time support, versus continued reliance on infrequent medical appointments.

The ability of AI to utilize multi-modal data will play an important role in providing remote care. AI can combine sensor data, the patient's EHR, and even social determinants (when available) into a comprehensive representation of the patient. In a rural health telemonitoring environment, for example, AI could recognize that a drop in physical activity on weekends may simply reflect a lack of access to safe walking spaces, and therefore, despite a drop in step count, a health issue was not presented. Based on the knowledge it gains of individual patterns and context, AI has the potential for limiting false alarms and making alerts more relevant.

The use of AI for remote monitoring is already providing benefits. Recent studies have reported reductions in emergency visits among telemonitoring COPD patients through AI-enhanced processes, improved glycemic control in diabetic patients using AI-based coaching, and even the detection of asymptomatic atrial fibrillation in ECG wearers [62]. Collectively, these findings translate into better patient outcomes and reduced utilization of healthcare resources.

3.6.3 Challenges and Considerations in AI-Integrated Telemedicine

AI has the potential to greatly enhance telemedicine, but careful thought must be given to the challenges and factors involved in developing and employing it in an effective and ethical manner. The most pressing challenges in a remote setting will be related to data quality and safety. AI models are only as good as the data the model can see; therefore, if devices used in the home produce poor-quality data—for example, if a patient has a blood pressure cuff that is out of calibration or their smartwatch isn't worn properly—the patient may provide data that is misinterpreted by AI. While device quality is critical, AI design is equally important. Models must be able to detect implausible data points (and, ideally, verify them with the patient) to ensure accuracy.

Privacy concerns are an even greater challenge. Health data streamed from a patient's home must be protected against breaches, which could otherwise violate regulatory standards. AI systems must be compliant with health data protection legislation, and organizations implementing AI must invest in robust cybersecurity measures to prevent unauthorized access. There is also a set of privacy techniques, like FL, that allow AI algorithms to learn from data on individual devices or local networks to continuously update and improve algorithms without requiring the transfer of raw data.

Another important consideration is clinical integration and acceptability. Providers must be able to trust AI in telehealth just as they do in direct clinician–patient interactions. If an AI system indicates that a patient is at high risk, providers need to understand why (explainability), as the lack of rationality can create doubts in the clinician's mind which can dissuade proactive action on the AI's recommendation. Therefore, telehealth AI tools should be developed with explainable outputs. For example: "Mrs. Jones has a 70% risk of a flare of heart failure because her weight increased by 5% in the past week and her resting heart rate changed by 10%." This type of rationale is easy for a clinician to comprehend and validate.

Additionally, other stakeholders, such as regulatory authorities, are developing policies for AI in telehealth to address effectiveness and safety. Just like medications that need to be rigorously proven with trials, AI analytics ideally should be demonstrating their processes benefit with a prospective study (e.g., trialing standard care vs. AI-augmented remote care and reporting more favorable outcomes) prior to market release and end user availability.

Ethical issues arise as well, particularly relating to reliance on AI and less human interaction. In healthcare, patients tend to appreciate human connection and empathy, which are harder to convey from a distance. If patients get responses to most of their questions via an AI (e.g., patients chat with a bot), the therapeutic relationship could be jeopardized. The goal should be to use AI to improve the connection between people, rather than replace that connection. For example, if an AI can handle routine follow-up questions, then when a human clinician speaks with the patient, they can engage in more nuanced conversations.

Furthermore, this comes with the possibility of bias and access issues. An AI model trained on one population may not perform as well on another. For example, a model may succeed in an urban environment with good internet but not in rural communities with limited connectivity or different lifestyle habits. It is important that the training data is inclusive and that researchers continually check how their AI is performing across demographics to ensure there are no gaps. Also, it is ironic that while telemedicine using AI may improve access (for example, bringing specialty care to more remote locations), if everyone does not have suitable devices and access to the internet, this could widen gaps even more. Accessible options for patients must be ensured, along with patient education or tools that are user-friendly for older patients or those less familiar with technology. In locations where smart phones may not be available, "low-tech" options, such as using AI interaction via phone or SMS, can be explored, even if they are not as rich in data.

In sum, AI acts as the invisible hand elevating telemedicine from a simple video consultation to a comprehensive care platform. AI will pull together data from wearables, EHRs, and clinical video/audio of the consultation to provide care-informed perspective and insight that enhances remote care. Four key areas arise where AI significantly impacts remote care in telemedicine:

- **Remote monitoring:** Human surveillance of patient health data to detect issues earlier (e.g., AI monitoring the patient's vitals and using algorithms to determine early warning signs of sepsis in homecare).
- **IT and automation:** Use of IT (and maybe AI) to manage the flow of data from telehealth services or telehealth consultations, automate documentation, and display follow-up recommendations (e.g., AI would transcribe the clinical visit and summarize the tele-visit information into a medical record).
- **Intelligent assistance and diagnosis:** AI assisting clinicians during tele-consults with diagnostic suggestions or decision support related to treatment (e.g., reading images or EHR data in real-time).

- **Collaborative analysis and education:** Bringing multiple remote patients' data together to identify population-level trends and provide decision support or some educational resources to the remote providers and patients.

Together, telehealth and AI are changing the trajectory of healthcare toward a more proactive and continuous-care paradigm, breaking down the physical barriers of space and time between patient and provider. This could lead us to a point where geography becomes far less of an influential factor in accessing and providing high-value healthcare, as AI-augmented telemedicine has the potential to democratize top-tier care to people in any setting—whether in a busy urban center or a remote rural village—and at scale. The main challenge is to achieve this in a way that is equitable, ethical, and still prioritizes providing compassionate, person-centered care, even as the care delivery space increasingly resembles the digital space.

3.7 Conclusion

AI is quickly changing the field of healthcare from a system focused mostly on diagnosing patients to one that actively helps treat and manage conditions while delivering personalized care. In this discussed the evolution of AI in detail and how it adds value to patient care throughout the continuum of care, from precision genomics to robotic surgery and telemedicine. In this conclusion, we present a synthesized overview of these changes, highlighting both the opportunities associated with advancements in AI and the challenges it continues to face.

AI's progress in healthcare has primarily been observed in its ability to customize therapies for individual patients. In personalized medicine, AI systems can combine genomic and patient health record data, along with environmental exposure, to identify the right therapy from many potential options. Oncology provides a clear example of these capabilities, where AI models help clinicians determine the most appropriate drug for patients with mutations like EGFR or ALK [12]. Although personalized medicine has not yet become routine practice in most clinical settings, we are beginning to see how AI can improve outcomes and reduce the trial-and-error process of determining the best drug for patients, especially when AI systems are deployed in research and demonstration projects.

Importantly, the possibilities for personalization using AI extend far beyond acute disease. Among patients with complex or chronic diseases, AI-enabled pharmacogenomic tools can assess drug-gene interactions to promote safer and more effective medication regimens. These tools offer clinicians supportive data to make informed decisions that reflect a patient's biological characteristics, past treatments, and comorbidities. Even though adoption is still in its nascent stages, these systems represent an acceleration of AI's role in becoming a relevant part of treatment workflows.

AI's predictive capability is also evident in the management of chronic diseases. Chronic diseases such as heart disease and diabetes often require lifelong management, and these conditions have begun to be transformed using AI-enabled technologies. For example, wearable sensors, implantable monitors, and other technologies collect and provide real-time data to AI algorithms that detect subtle yet clinically relevant abnormalities in patients' health. Such analyses can sometimes lead to pre-symptomatic intervention [63].

These capabilities are being embedded into telehealth platforms, allowing clinicians to manage chronic diseases remotely. It has been reported that the combination of virtualization technology and AI in telemonitoring can reduce hospital admissions and increase survival rates in heart failure patients [63]. In another transformational capacity, mobile applications with AI are improving patient activation through reminders, educational content, and personalized recommendations. When applied appropriately, these technologies improve health outcomes and reduce costs while advancing a model of care that is more continuum-based.

AI is having a meaningful impact for clinicians in surgical planning and in performing procedures. By leveraging existing large surgical datasets and patient-relevant imaging, ML models can recommend a surgical plan and help assess the risk of harm [32]. AI also has a profound impact in the area of pre-operative planning, particularly with respect to surgical simulation and predicting complications in certain surgical fields, such as orthopedic and craniofacial surgery.

Robot-assisted surgery takes that precision a step further. Surgical robots, integrated with AI, can provide real-time feedback, stabilize instruments, and improve visualization. This allows for an even more accurate, minimally invasive approach with faster recovery times, ultimately leading to better patient safety. While these systems are under the supervision of human operators today, technology is advancing toward the semi-autonomous assistant. A surgeon's role has expanded to partnering with AI as a "co-pilot," allowing it to recommend suggestions to the surgeon but never replace their judgment.

AI-enhanced telemedicine may be one of the most meaningful developments in equitable global health. Access to virtual consultations, symptom checkers, and automatic triage systems easily improve healthcare access around the world, particularly for those living in rural areas, minority populations, and patients with decreased mobility. With the help of AI, these technologies can help patients in real time interpret their symptoms and identify the most appropriate next steps (urgent care, telehealth, or home monitoring).

In addition to triage, AI systems can facilitate ongoing remote monitoring of biometric data obtained from patients in their home environment. AI-generated alerts can help avert emergencies in patients with conditions such as hypertension, diabetes, or respiratory illnesses. These technologies are facilitating a shift towards proactive and inclusive healthcare, as well as relieving pressure on overcrowded hospitals. However, to unlock the full potential of these developments, it is important that concurrent efforts are made to close the digital divide and provide access to all groups across the socioeconomic continuum [64].

Even with the transformative possibilities that AI offers in clinical care, its incorporation raises ethical, regulatory, and operational questions. Systems must be rigorously validated prior to any use to ensure that they are safe and accurate. Transparency in the algorithms' development and decision-making process is essential so that clinicians and patients can trust the output provided by AI. Furthermore, algorithms must be trained using varied datasets to mitigate bias and promote equitable care among populations. Privacy is also a major consideration; AI systems leveraging genomic data or continuous monitoring must employ stringent data security protocols. Patients must also be notified if AI has been involved in their care, and there should always be human oversight of AI, especially when an AI system contributes to a decision associated with treatment, surgery, or medication modifications.

Patient care likely will look like a future where AI is an impactful collaborator—helping clinicians make decisions, supporting patients, and improving their outcomes. The real challenge lies ahead in how we shoulder this opportunity responsibly—building AI that is attuned to safety and inclusion and aligned with the values of medical ethics. Interdisciplinary collaboration between AI designers, clinicians, and policymakers will be critical for using AI to maximize its utility in the future of patient care.

In conclusion, Chapter 3 has shown that the use of AI to inform treatment and care is not limited to one aspect of healthcare—it is a continuum. From personalized prescriptions, individualized by understanding the genome, to national telehealth networks, AI helps rethink healthcare in a more personalized, predictive, and inclusive manner. With careful execution, AI could become one of the most powerful pieces of modern medicine—not replacing any clinician but maximizing their potential by bringing about a change that was previously not possible.

References

1. K.B. Johnson, W. Wei, D. Weeraratne, M.E. Frisse, K. Misulis, K. Rhee, J. Zhao, J.L. Snowdon, Precision medicine, AI, and the future of personalized health care. Clin. Transl. Sci. **14**, 86–93 (2021)
2. P.M. Patel, M. Green, J. Tram, E. Wang, M.Z. Murphy, A. Abd-Elsayed, K. Chakravarthy, Beyond the Pain Management Clinic: The Role of AI-Integrated Remote Patient Monitoring in Chronic Disease Management–A Narrative Review, J. Pain Res. (2024) 4223–4237
3. N.J. Schork, Artificial intelligence and personalized medicine, Precision Medicine in Cancer Therapy (2019), 265–283
4. R.J. Hartmaier, L.A. Albacker, J. Chmielecki, M. Bailey, J. He, M.E. Goldberg, S. Ramkissoon, J. Suh, J.A. Elvin, S. Chiacchia, High-throughput genomic profiling of adult solid tumors reveals novel insights into cancer pathogenesis. Cancer Res. **77**, 2464–2475 (2017)
5. K.E. Caudle, T.E. Klein, J.M. Hoffman, D.J. Muller, M. Whirl-Carrillo, L. Gong, E.M. McDonagh, K. Sangkuhl, C.F. Thorn, M. Schwab, Incorporation of pharmacogenomics into routine clinical practice: the Clinical Pharmacogenetics Implementation Consortium (CPIC) guideline development process. Curr. Drug Metab. **15**, 209–217 (2014)

6. A.L. Jorgensen, C. Prince, G. Fitzgerald, A. Hanson, J. Downing, J. Reynolds, J.E. Zhang, A. Alfirevic, M. Pirmohamed, Implementation of genotype-guided dosing of warfarin with point-of-care genetic testing in three UK clinics: a matched cohort study. BMC Med. **17**, 1–11 (2019)
7. R. Poplin, P.-C. Chang, D. Alexander, S. Schwartz, T. Colthurst, A. Ku, D. Newburger, J. Dijamco, N. Nguyen, P.T. Afshar, A universal SNP and small-indel variant caller using deep neural networks. Nat. Biotechnol. **36**, 983–987 (2018)
8. R. Dias, A. Torkamani, Artificial intelligence in clinical and genomic diagnostics. Genome Med **11**, 70 (2019)
9. H. Taherdoost, A. Ghofrani, Ai's role in revolutionizing personalized medicine by reshaping pharmacogenomics and drug therapy. Intelligent Pharmacy **2**, 643–650 (2024)
10. M. Elhaddad, S. Hamam, AI-driven clinical decision support systems: an ongoing pursuit of potential, Cureus **16** (2024)
11. P. Silva, D. Jacobs, J. Kriak, A. Abu-Baker, G. Udeani, G. Neal, K. Ramos, Implementation of pharmacogenomics and artificial intelligence tools for chronic disease management in primary care setting. J Pers Med **11**, 443 (2021)
12. X. Tan, Y. Li, S. Wang, H. Xia, R. Meng, J. Xu, Y. Duan, Y. Li, G. Yang, Y. Ma, Predicting EGFR mutation, ALK rearrangement, and uncommon EGFR mutation in NSCLC patients by driverless artificial intelligence: a cohort study. Respir. Res. **23**, 132 (2022)
13. S.-J. Sammut, M. Crispin-Ortuzar, S.-F. Chin, E. Provenzano, H.A. Bardwell, W. Ma, W. Cope, A. Dariush, S.-J. Dawson, J.E. Abraham, Multi-omic machine learning predictor of breast cancer therapy response. Nature **601**, 623–629 (2022)
14. E. Loh, Medicine and the rise of the robots: a qualitative review of recent advances of artificial intelligence in health, BMJ Leader (2018) leader-2018.
15. M. Bracher-Smith, E. Rees, G. Menzies, J.T.R. Walters, M.C. O'Donovan, M.J. Owen, G. Kirov, V. Escott-Price, Machine learning for prediction of schizophrenia using genetic and demographic factors in the UK biobank. Schizophr. Res. **246**, 156–164 (2022)
16. D. Kolobkov, S. Mishra Sharma, A. Medvedev, M. Lebedev, E. Kosaretskiy, R. Vakhitov, Efficacy of federated learning on genomic data: a study on the UK Biobank and the 1000 Genomes Project, Front Big. Data **7** (2024) 1266031
17. C. Dong, Y. Ji, Z. Fu, Y. Qi, T. Yi, Y. Yang, Y. Sun, H. Sun, Precision management in chronic disease: An AI empowered perspective on medicine-engineering crossover, I Sci. **28** (2025)
18. Z. Papalamprakopoulou, D. Stavropoulos, S. Moustakidis, D. Avgerinos, M. Efremidis, P.N. Kampaktsis, Artificial intelligence-enabled atrial fibrillation detection using smartwatches: current status and future perspectives. Front Cardiovasc Med **11**, 1432876 (2024)
19. X. Li, H.-P. Zhou, Z.-J. Zhou, N. Du, E.-H. Zhong, K. Zhai, N. Liu, L. Zhou, Artificial intelligence-powered remote monitoring of patients with chronic obstructive pulmonary disease. Chin Med J (Engl) **134**, 1546–1548 (2021)
20. Q. Bian, A. As' arry, X. Cong, K.A. bin M. Rezali, R.M.K. bin Raja Ahmad, A hybrid Transformer-LSTM model apply to glucose prediction, PLoS One **19** (2024) e0310084
21. P. Herrero, M. Andorrà, N. Babion, H. Bos, M. Koehler, Y. Klopfenstein, E. Leppäaho, P. Lustenberger, A. Peak, C. Ringemann, Enhancing the capabilities of continuous glucose monitoring with a predictive App, (2024)
22. M. Iftikhar, M. Saqib, S.N. Qayyum, R. Asmat, H. Mumtaz, M. Rehan, I. Ullah, I. Ud-Din, S. Noori, M. Khan, Artificial intelligence-driven transformations in diabetes care: a comprehensive literature review. Annals of Medicine and Surgery **86**, 5334–5342 (2024)
23. R.P. Wadwa, Z.W. Reed, B.A. Buckingham, M.D. DeBoer, L. Ekhlaspour, G.P. Forlenza, M. Schoelwer, J. Lum, C. Kollman, R.W. Beck, Trial of hybrid closed-loop control in young children with type 1 diabetes. N. Engl. J. Med. **388**, 991–1001 (2023)
24. F. Farid, A. Bello, F. Ahamed, F. Hossain, The roles of ai technologies in reducing hospital readmission for chronic diseases: a comprehensive analysis, Preprints. Org). Doi **10** (2023) 1–19

25. J.K. Ribeiro, H.D.P. dos Santos, F. Barletta, M.C. da Silva, R. Vieira, H.M.P. Morales, C. da Costa Rocha, A machine learning early warning system: multicenter validation in Brazilian hospitals, in: *2020 IEEE 33rd International Symposium on Computer-Based Medical Systems (CBMS)*, IEEE, (2020), pp. 321–326
26. D.P. Edelson, M.M. Churpek, K.A. Carey, Z. Lin, C. Huang, J.M. Siner, J. Johnson, H.M. Krumholz, D.J. Rhodes, Early warning scores with and without artificial intelligence. JAMA Netw. Open **7**, e2438986–e2438986 (2024)
27. G. Yu, M. Tabatabaei, J. Mezei, Q. Zhong, S. Chen, Z. Li, J. Li, L. Shu, Q. Shu, Improving chronic disease management for children with knowledge graphs and artificial intelligence. Expert Syst. Appl. **201**, 117026 (2022)
28. Study Demonstrates Livongo Members More Empowered, Less Distressed in Diabetes Self-Management – Livongo, (n.d.). https://www.mylivongo.com/Study-Demonstrates-Livongo-Members-More-Empowered-and-Less-Distressed/ (Accessed September 27, 2025)
29. C.M. Whaley, J.B. Bollyky, W. Lu, S. Painter, J. Schneider, Z. Zhao, X. He, J. Johnson, E.S. Meadows, Reduced medical spending associated with increased use of a remote diabetes management program and lower mean blood glucose values. J. Med. Econ. **22**, 869–877 (2019)
30. A.K. Kapila, L. De Vleminck, M. Hamdi, Three key domains for optimizing preoperative preparedness in plastic surgery with AI, Plast Aesthet Res **12** (2025) N-A
31. S. Jia, Y. Weng, K. Wang, H. Qi, Y. Yang, C. Ma, W.W. Lu, H. Wu, Performance evaluation of an AI-based preoperative planning software application for automatic selection of pedicle screws based on computed tomography images. Front Surg **10**, 1247527 (2023)
32. F.G. Mangano, O. Admakin, H. Lerner, C. Mangano, Artificial intelligence and augmented reality for guided implant surgery planning: a proof of concept. J. Dent. **133**, 104485 (2023)
33. X. Meng, X. Zhang, G. Wang, Y. Zhang, X. Shi, H. Dai, Z. Wang, X. Wang, Exploiting full resolution feature context for liver tumor and vessel segmentation via integrate framework: Application to liver tumor and vessel 3d reconstruction under embedded microprocessor, ArXiv Preprint ArXiv:2111.13299 (2021)
34. M. Moghbel, S. Mashohor, R. Mahmud, M.I. Bin Saripan, Automatic liver tumor segmentation on computed tomography for patient treatment planning and monitoring, EXCLI J **15** (2016) 406
35. T.T. Dundar, I. Yurtsever, M.K. Pehlivanoglu, U. Yildiz, A. Eker, M.A. Demir, A.S. Mutluer, R. Tektaş, M.S. Kazan, S. Kitis, Machine learning-based surgical planning for neurosurgery: artificial intelligent approaches to the cranium. Front Surg **9**, 863633 (2022)
36. N. Nandakumar, N.S. D'Souza, K. Manzoor, J.J. Pillai, S.K. Gujar, H.I. Sair, A. Venkataraman, A multi-task deep learning framework to localize the eloquent cortex in brain tumor patients using dynamic functional connectivity, in: Machine Learning in Clinical Neuroimaging and Radiogenomics in Neuro-Oncology: Third International Workshop, MLCN 2020, and Second International Workshop, RNO-AI 2020, Held in Conjunction with MICCAI 2020, Lima, Peru, October 4–8, 2020, Proceedings 3, Springer, (2020), pp. 34–44
37. N. Mirchi, V. Bissonnette, R. Yilmaz, N. Ledwos, A. Winkler-Schwartz, R.F. Del Maestro, The Virtual Operative Assistant: An explainable artificial intelligence tool for simulation-based training in surgery and medicine. PLoS ONE **15**, e0229596 (2020)
38. C. Varghese, E.M. Harrison, G. O'Grady, E.J. Topol, Artificial intelligence in surgery. Nat. Med. **30**, 1257–1268 (2024)
39. A. Bihorac, T. Ozrazgat-Baslanti, A. Ebadi, A. Motaei, M. Madkour, P.M. Pardalos, G. Lipori, W.R. Hogan, P.A. Efron, F. Moore, MySurgeryRisk: development and validation of a machine-learning risk algorithm for major complications and death after surgery. Ann. Surg. **269**, 652–662 (2019)
40. L. Matondora, M. Mutandavari, B. Mupini, Nlp based prediction of hospital readmission using clinicalbert and clinician notes, International Journal of Innovative Science and Research Technology (IJISRT) (2024).
41. C. Alba, B. Xue, J. Abraham, T. Kannampallil, C. Lu, The foundational capabilities of large language models in predicting postoperative risks using clinical notes. NPJ Digit Med **8**, 95 (2025)

42. E.L. Barber, R. Garg, C. Persenaire, M. Simon, Natural language processing with machine learning to predict outcomes after ovarian cancer surgery. Gynecol. Oncol. **160**, 182–186 (2021)
43. T. Bellos, I. Manolitsis, S. Katsimperis, P. Juliebø-Jones, G. Feretzakis, I. Mitsogiannis, I. Varkarakis, B.K. Somani, L. Tzelves, Artificial intelligence in urologic robotic oncologic surgery: a narrative review. Cancers (Basel) **16**, 1775 (2024)
44. O. Elfanagely, Y. Toyoda, S. Othman, J.A. Mellia, M. Basta, T. Liu, K. Kording, L. Ungar, J.P. Fischer, Machine learning and surgical outcomes prediction: a systematic review. J. Surg. Res. **264**, 346–361 (2021)
45. K. Merath, J.M. Hyer, R. Mehta, A. Farooq, F. Bagante, K. Sahara, D.I. Tsilimigras, E. Beal, A.Z. Paredes, L. Wu, Use of machine learning for prediction of patient risk of postoperative complications after liver, pancreatic, and colorectal surgery. J. Gastrointest. Surg. **24**, 1843–1851 (2020)
46. M. Graeßner, B. Jungwirth, E. Frank, S.J. Schaller, E. Kochs, K. Ulm, M. Blobner, B. Ulm, A.H. Podtschaske, S.M. Kagerbauer, Enabling personalized perioperative risk prediction by using a machine-learning model based on preoperative data. Sci. Rep. **13**, 7128 (2023)
47. E. Checcucci, A. Pecoraro, D. Amparore, S. De Cillis, S. Granato, G. Volpi, M. Sica, P. Verri, A. Piana, P. Piazzolla, The impact of 3D models on positive surgical margins after robot-assisted radical prostatectomy. World J. Urol. **40**, 2221–2229 (2022)
48. P. Chatzikomnitsa, A.D. Gkaitatzi, M. Papakonstantinou, E. Louri, D. Giakoustidis, V.N. Papadopoulos, A. Giakoustidis, The role of artificial intelligence and 3D printing in minimally invasive liver surgery, Mini-Invasive Surgery 9 (2025) N-A
49. H. Orimoto, T. Hirashita, S. Ikeda, S. Amano, M. Kawamura, Y. Kawano, H. Takayama, T. Masuda, Y. Endo, Y. Matsunobu, Development of an artificial intelligence system to indicate intraoperative findings of scarring in laparoscopic cholecystectomy for cholecystitis, Surg. Endosc. (2025) 1–9.
50. D. Corallino, A. Balla, D. Coletta, D. Pacella, M. Podda, A. Pronio, M. Ortenzi, F. Ratti, S. Morales-Conde, P. Sileri, Systematic review on the use of artificial intelligence to identify anatomical structures during laparoscopic cholecystectomy: a tool towards the future. Langenbecks Arch. Surg. **410**, 1–16 (2025)
51. H. Saeidi, J.D. Opfermann, M. Kam, S. Wei, S. Léonard, M.H. Hsieh, J.U. Kang, A. Krieger, Autonomous robotic laparoscopic surgery for intestinal anastomosis, Sci. Robot. **7** (2022) eabj2908
52. A. Lee, T.S. Baker, J.B. Bederson, B.I. Rapoport, Levels of autonomy in FDA-cleared surgical robots: a systematic review. NPJ Digit Med **7**, 103 (2024)
53. A. Madani, B. Namazi, M.S. Altieri, D.A. Hashimoto, A.M. Rivera, P.H. Pucher, A. Navarrete-Welton, G. Sankaranarayanan, L.M. Brunt, A. Okrainec, Artificial intelligence for intraoperative guidance: using semantic segmentation to identify surgical anatomy during laparoscopic cholecystectomy. Ann. Surg. **276**, 363–369 (2022)
54. J.N.K. Wah, Revolutionizing surgery: AI and robotics for precision, risk reduction, and innovation. J. Robot. Surg. **19**, 1–15 (2025)
55. S. Sharma, R. Rawal, D. Shah, Addressing the challenges of AI-based telemedicine: Best practices and lessons learned, J. Educ. Health Promot (2023) 338
56. E.I. Nwankwo, E.V. Emeihe, M.D. Ajegbile, J.A. Olaboye, C.C. Maha, Integrating telemedicine and AI to improve healthcare access in rural settings. Int. J. Life. Sci. Res. Arch. **7**, 59–77 (2024)
57. A.M. Seetharamapura, D.V. Varadarajan, Framework for Integrating AI-Based Teleradiology Solutions into Modern Healthcare Ecosystem for Predictable Response Time, Enhanced Connectivity, Patient Empowerment, Flexibility and Innovation. Int. J. Commun. Netw. Inf. Secur (IJCNIS) **16**, 514–535 (2024)
58. A.K. Barwise, S. Curtis, D.A. Diedrich, B.W. Pickering, Using artificial intelligence to promote equitable care for inpatients with language barriers and complex medical needs: clinical stakeholder perspectives. J. Am. Med. Inform. Assoc. **31**, 611–621 (2024)
59. H.- www.ushealthconnect.com, The Potential of AI Language Translation Tools for Addressing Healthcare Inequities - ReachMD, (n.d.). https://reachmd.com/programs/clinicians-roundtable/the-potential-of-ai-language-translation-tools-for-addressing-healthcare-inequities/29858/ (Accessed May 12, 2025)

60. J. Zaretsky, J.M. Kim, S. Baskharoun, Y. Zhao, J. Austrian, Y. Aphinyanaphongs, R. Gupta, S.B. Blecker, J. Feldman, Generative artificial intelligence to transform inpatient discharge summaries to patient-friendly language and format. JAMA Netw. Open **7**, e240357–e240357 (2024)
61. A. Phatak, D.W. Savage, R. Ohle, J. Smith, V. Mago, Medical text simplification using reinforcement learning (teslea): Deep learning–based text simplification approach. JMIR Med. Inform. **10**, e38095 (2022)
62. O.J. Mbanugo, AI-Enhanced telemedicine: a common-sense approach to chronic disease management and a tool to bridging the gap in healthcare disparities, department of healthcare management & informatics, coles college of business, Kennesaw State University, Georgia, USA (2025)
63. D. D'Amario, F. Canonico, D. Rodolico, J.A. Borovac, R. Vergallo, R.A. Montone, M. Galli, S. Migliaro, A. Restivo, M. Massetti, Telemedicine, artificial intelligence and humanisation of clinical pathways in heart failure management: back to the future and beyond. Card. Fail. Rev. **6**, e16 (2020)
64. S. Arefin, Chronic disease management through an ai-powered application. J. Serv. Sci. Manag. **17**, 305–320 (2024)

Chapter 4
AI in Medical Education and Healthcare Management

This chapter examines how Artificial Intelligence (AI) changes medical education and the management of health care. It discusses that AI is fundamentally changing the learning of health care professionals, as well as improving the productivity of health care organizations. AI-enabled systems involving intelligent learning platforms, adaptive learning environments, virtual patients, AI-enabled assessments, and curriculum design tools are changing how students learn knowledge and clinical skills in medical education. These technologies can provide personalized learning, real-time feedback, and data-informed adjustments to the curriculum that enhance readiness for clinical practice. In terms of health care management, AI is improving hospital administration solutions, predictive analytics for resource allocation, strategic governance, and regulatory compliance monitoring. Examples of applications include staff scheduling, billing, patient flow forecasting, and fraud detection, among others. These technologies improve productivity and cost efficiency in health care. The chapter highlights that AI affords us tremendous chances for efficiency, personalization, and equity, but barriers related to data privacy, bias, and human decisions will continue to be important. The conclusion reinforces that to be successful, AI will need to balance between technology and human capacity to guarantee care that is ethical, transparent and patient-centered.

4.1 Introduction

AI has transitioned from a specialty technology to an impactful transformational force across domains of health care fields. In previous chapters we considered how AI supports clinical diagnosis (Chap. 2) and treatment (Chap. 3) and how it is revolutionizing clinical practices in medicine. In this chapter we shift our considerations from medicine as it relates to education and management systems in health care. Upon first glance, the learning and managing health systems may be unrelated, however, the

L. Tayebi et al., *Artificial Intelligence in Medicine and Dentistry*,
https://doi.org/10.1007/978-3-032-15977-9_4

two themes highlight a common element, the capacity for AI to add value to human decision-making and efficiencies outside of direct practice with patients. With AI, medical education is transforming the way health care professionals are able to learn and develop skills. In health care management, AI-enabled systems will efficiently manage operational functions, from managing hospital administrative systems to strategic decision-making. By considering them simultaneously, we emphasize how AI spans throughout the entire continuum of the "learner-to-leader" concept, from training an individual clinician to aiding decision-making in a health organization, thus creating a cohesive improvement in healthcare delivery.

AI methods, such as Machine Learning (ML) and data-driven decision support, are now present in academic environments and health care systems. For instance, intelligent tutoring systems can provide personalized responsiveness to medical students, while predictive algorithms can assist hospital administrators in resourcing health care [1, 2]. The implications of these applications are substantial. In education, AI facilitates potentially greater efficiency, very personalized pathways to learning, and greater access to information. In management, AI will help improve operational efficiency, take some of the administrative burden off from health care professionals, and promote equitable care by flagging deficiencies and distributing resources in an equitable way. Educators and managers alike will also face similar challenges, from privacy of data to need for interpretability, and the need to prevent bias, which we will summarize in context.

This chapter provides a thorough overview of the advancements AI is bringing to education in medicine (Sect. 4.2), and management of health care (Sect. 4.3). In the medical education part of this chapter, we will look at intelligent learning platforms, adaptive and personalized educational systems, immersive simulations with virtual patients, AI-assisted assessments, and data-informed curriculum design. In health care management, we review AI-enabled hospital administration, intelligent resource distribution and predictive analytics for capacity planning, AI in health system governance and policy decisions, and AI in regulatory compliance and fraud detection. The chapter connects how AI is integrated "from the Ward to the Boardroom" and the classroom to the clinic, to achieve a more adaptive, responsive, and efficient health care ecosystem.

4.2 AI in Medical Education

Advancements in AI are changing the landscape of medical training and education. Intelligent systems are introducing novel, effective ways of learning, practicing, and assessing competencies across the educational spectrum, from the lecture hall through the bedside. Traditionally, medical education balanced knowledge acquisition with the development of skills for clinical practice; AI is enhancing both domains. The educational applications of AI can be in the form of customized educational content, on-demand tutoring, simulated clinical scenarios, or even online assessment and evaluation tools of assessment. In this section, we discuss how AI-powered applications and platforms can provide support to medical educators and learners.

4.2.1 Intelligent Learning Platforms

There is a growing trend within medical education to embed AI directly into Learning Management Systems (LMS) and educational platforms to produce "intelligent" learning environments. An intelligent learning platform used in education is an LMS that uses AI algorithms to categorize content, provide tutorial support, and monitor student learning as opposed to a traditional LMS. One example is educational material tagging and recommendation. The LMS can support autonomous tagging of educational materials—lectures, articles, clinical cases—by subject and level of difficulty and then make that tagged educational material available for the right learner at the right time [3]. For example, if a medical student struggles with interpreting an electrocardiogram (ECG), the LMS recognizes this based on quiz performance or a pattern of student interaction and will recommend specific modules or practice clinical cases on cardiology based on the student's performance.

AI-driven chatbot tutors that provide on-demand instruction are another development. These chatbots are able to answer students' questions, clarify complex concepts, and quiz learners in an interactive format, all while providing access as needed, 24/7. They can act as virtual teaching assistants to help students when human faculty are not available. Early implementations demonstrate that chatbot tutors can answer questions such as anatomy or pharmacology questions to help students clarify doubts by sharing immediate and contextualized responses [4–6].

Intelligent platforms simplify administrative tasks in education. With automatic scheduling and personalized learning experiences, students may follow along with slightly different sequences of learning. For example, an AI system could schedule a student who needs support in pathology with additional quizzes, while allowing for faster pacing in the content for a student who has already demonstrated competency. This continuous pacing occurs because the system continuously monitors learning performance and lowers or raises an individual's difficulty [7, 8]. Over time, the system grows to understand the student's learning preferences and knowledge gaps, similar to the way Netflix usually learns an audience's viewing preferences, except now in the context of life-or-death educational content of medicine.

One of the most impactful features of intelligent learning platforms is their ability to use predictive analytics to identify students at risk. Using data about students' performance and engagement (e.g., videos watched, quizzes attempted), AI-based systems can identify those learners that are underperforming for large student populations. Martinez et al. [9] applied supervised ML algorithms to identify risk using engagement, performance, and demographic data. Their findings showed that all tested ML algorithms could generate acceptable prediction outcomes with more than 78% overall accuracy. Tsekhmister et al. [10] conducted an empirical study with Ukrainian medical program students to apply predictive analytics for risk identification and for motivation enhancement purposes. Their work integrated statistical modeling and Decision Trees (DTs) to find a motivation index. Following the implementation of a multi-component intervention strategy which altered content, methods, assessments, and pedagogy, the number of students facing risk of dropout declined by 4.27%, while the number of students facing potential risks declined by 9.4%. This suggested that predictive modeling, when tied to tailored pedagogical strategies, could favorably influence engagement and learning outcomes in a medical education context. At a broader educational level, a systematic review of 124 studies by Almalawi et al. [11] reported that ML models consistently outperformed traditional statistical tools to identify at-risk learners. Importantly, they reported that behavioral measures, such as class attendance, LMS participation, and study habits were particularly effective for identifying at-risk students and accurately predicting short-term outcomes, such as course completion rates.

These developments are all intended to advance aspects of efficiency and individualization in the education of physicians. By freeing educators from the tasks of content curation and basic level tutoring work to AI, educators can devote more attention toward higher order mentorship, while engaging in experiential (or hands-on) training with learners. It should be noted that AI and the intelligent learning systems are meant to support but not replace the needs of faculty. The role of educators evolves to guiding AI's use, by investigating AI output, determining whether it meets curricular objectives and is consistent with professional competence standards. As medical schools and medical education programs engage with intelligent learning systems, there are research studies underway to evaluate its impact. Initial reports of student engagement and satisfaction have been reported, since students receive assistance tailored to their own interests and contexts [12]. Educators will need to keep an eye out for potential issues that may arise, such as over-dependence on AI suggestions or pre-existing algorithmic biases in the learning material presented to learners. Used in responsible ways, newly developed intelligent platforms mark a shift toward a more responsive and ultimately more effective education system for physicians.

4.2.2 Adaptive Learning and Personalized Education

Of all AI's potential contributions to medical education, the most significant is its ability to enable adaptive learning, which provides learning experiences that continually adapt to the individual learner's needs. Traditionally, medical curricula have maintained a fixed pace, but with AI, adaptive systems personalize the difficulty, modality, and pace in real time—just as a qualified tutor may adjust the difficulty of their instruction based on the student's understanding. Adaptive systems rely on algorithms that create a learner model for each student based on various data, such as quiz results, errors, and speed of learning. By interpreting multiple streams of this data, the system estimates the learner's knowledge in various domains and determines what the learner is ready to learn next.

Research suggests that adaptive learning promotes knowledge retention and reduces the time to competence. By directing study time toward individual needs, students avoid spending excessive time on material they have already learned. One example from nursing education suggested a benefit to adaptive quizzing in terms of course performance and completion rates [13]. The Adaptive Quizzing System (AQS) used algorithms to modify the learning process and present questions tailored to each student's ability. Thus, concepts that were difficult would continue to trigger practice until mastery was achieved, while students did not practice material they had already mastered. The system also evaluated each student's level and provided feedback that increased student confidence. Particularly, increased mastery levels through the use of the AQS had a significant impact on students' success in both course grades and performance on standardized predictors such as HESI. Students using the program had the highest on-time graduation rates compared to other cohorts in previous years. Simon-Campbell and Phelan [14] examined the effectiveness of an AQS as a self-regulated study tool for nursing students. Their study showed that students voluntarily used the AQS (without any grades incentives), benefited from improved mastery of course content, with a strong correlation between the number of questions answered and the achieved mastery level. Importantly, students who engaged in the AQS outperformed their peers on ATI standardized tests and all passed the NCLEX-RN on either the first or second attempt, highlighting the efficacy of adaptive learning environments as an important adjunct to virtual patient training. Another benefit is engagement; students consistently report that personalized challenges are more inspiring than standardized practice assignments because the content feels more relevant to their learning journey, focusing on their progress.

Adaptive learning has unique opportunities to aid learners in complex decision-making training scenarios where the learner must iteratively reason through dynamically evolving clinical decisions, for example, differential diagnosis or treatment planning [15, 16]. In these types of training contexts, adaptive learning systems can mimic branching clinical scenarios with the ability to adjust the complexity of the case and provide personalized feedback based on the learner's clinical reasoning performance. A notable example of such an approach is the e-MedLearn system implemented by Xu et al. [17]. The authors incorporate adaptive learning into a problem-based learning (PBL) framework to improve differential diagnosis training from the learner's perspective. The sequence and steps of their system are shown in Fig. 4.1. The platform is designed to enhance structured clinical reasoning by directing students through evidence chains and logical diagnostic pathways. Enhanced support for students' clinical reasoning skills and engagement was reported, particularly in clinical decision analysis and justification of diagnostic rationale. Socratic AI, developed by Golchini et al. [16], is an Large Language Model (LLM)-based adaptive tutor that transforms clinical cases from passive learning into engaging, active-learning Socratic dialogues between a student and an AI tutor. The tutor engages students with Socratic questioning and provides real-time feedback on their diagnostic logic throughout the case. When used with the NEJM clinical pathological case series, students demonstrated more transparency in their reasoning and were more cognizant of their diagnostic bias. The authors demonstrated the potential for AI-based tutors in personalized case-based learning. Hicke et al. [18] developed MedSimAI, an AI-based simulation platform to improve educational training for clinical decision-making. The system uses realistic virtual patient cases and provides

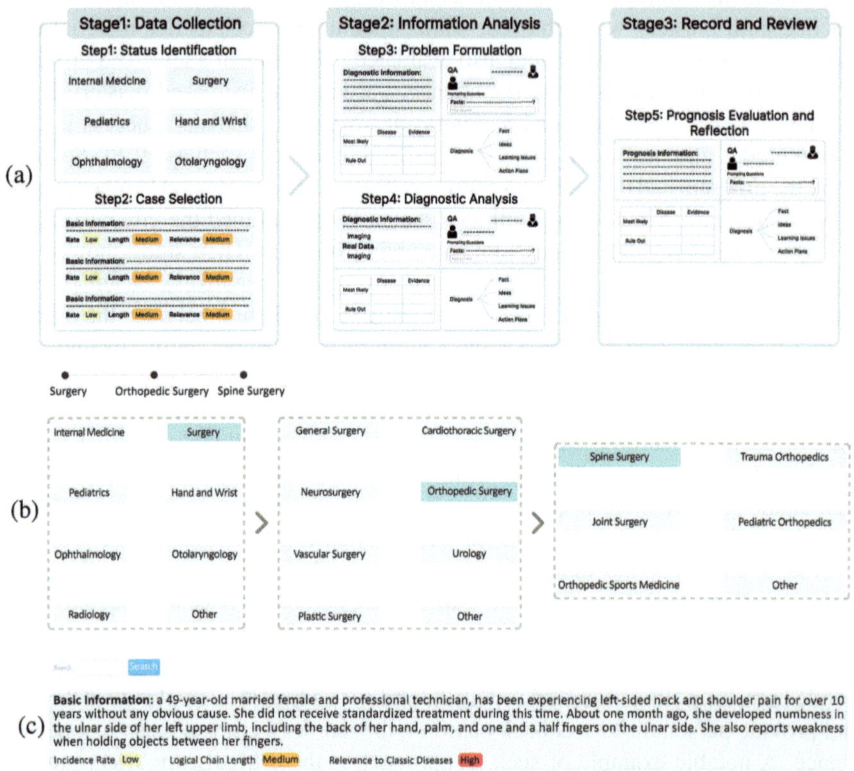

Fig. 4.1 Overview of the e-MedLearn system's workflow for clinical reasoning and differential diagnosis: **a** The main stages of the e-MedLearn platform guiding learners through a structured diagnostic process. **b** In Step 1 (Status Identification), a top-down, multi-level interface helps users define their learning objectives. **c** In Step 2 (Case Selection), learners browse case cards enriched with difficulty scores and search functionality for targeted selection. **d** In Step 3 (Problem Formulation), the interface includes (A) a case summary card, (B) a question-prompting module to support reasoning, and (C) a mind map template to structure and record analyzed information. **e** In Step 4 (Diagnostic Analysis), multimodal clinical data—imaging (visuals), physical exam findings (text), and lab results (indicators)—are provided in an interactive, collapsible format. Reproduced from Xu et al. [17], published in Proceedings of the 2025 CHI Conference on Human Factors in Computing Systems, 2025: pp. 1–32, under the Creative Commons Attribution 4.0 International License (CC BY), (https://creativecommons.org/licenses/by/4.0/). Font style and text size were adjusted for improved readability; the figure content is unchanged

(d)

(e)

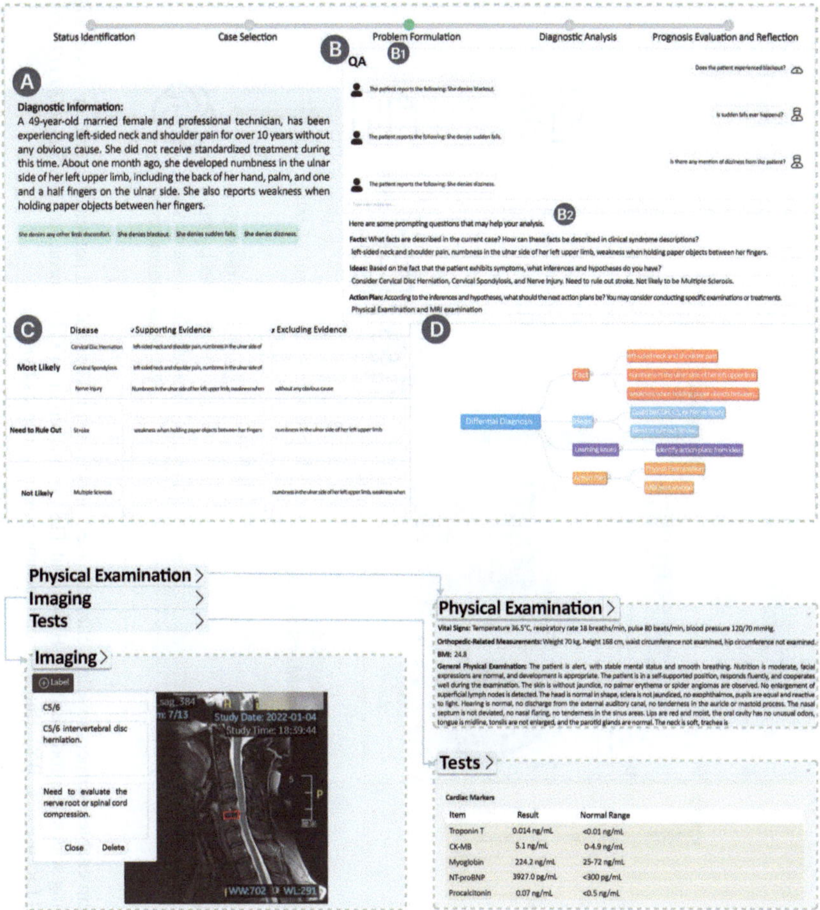

Fig. 4.1 (continued)

immediate, systematic, and tailored feedback. In a pilot study with medical students, it was found that MedSimAI significantly improved learners' ability to engage in systematic diagnostic interviews. MedSimAI's workflow is illustrated in Fig. 4.2 and provides insight into the adaptive learning loop from clinical case selection to real-time feedback generation.

AI-driven personalization is also concerned with the preferred learning modality. Not every learner will learn most effectively through text-based narratives or a lecture, as some learners will prefer visual diagrams, and other learners will thrive in interactive experiments. Adaptive platforms can determine which modality produces the best performance or fastest learning for a learner [19, 20]. For example, if a learner can repeatedly answer ECG questions correctly after watching an animation but struggles with textbook material on the same ECG content, the system can subsequently show more animations for cardiology-based content. Biometric measurements, such

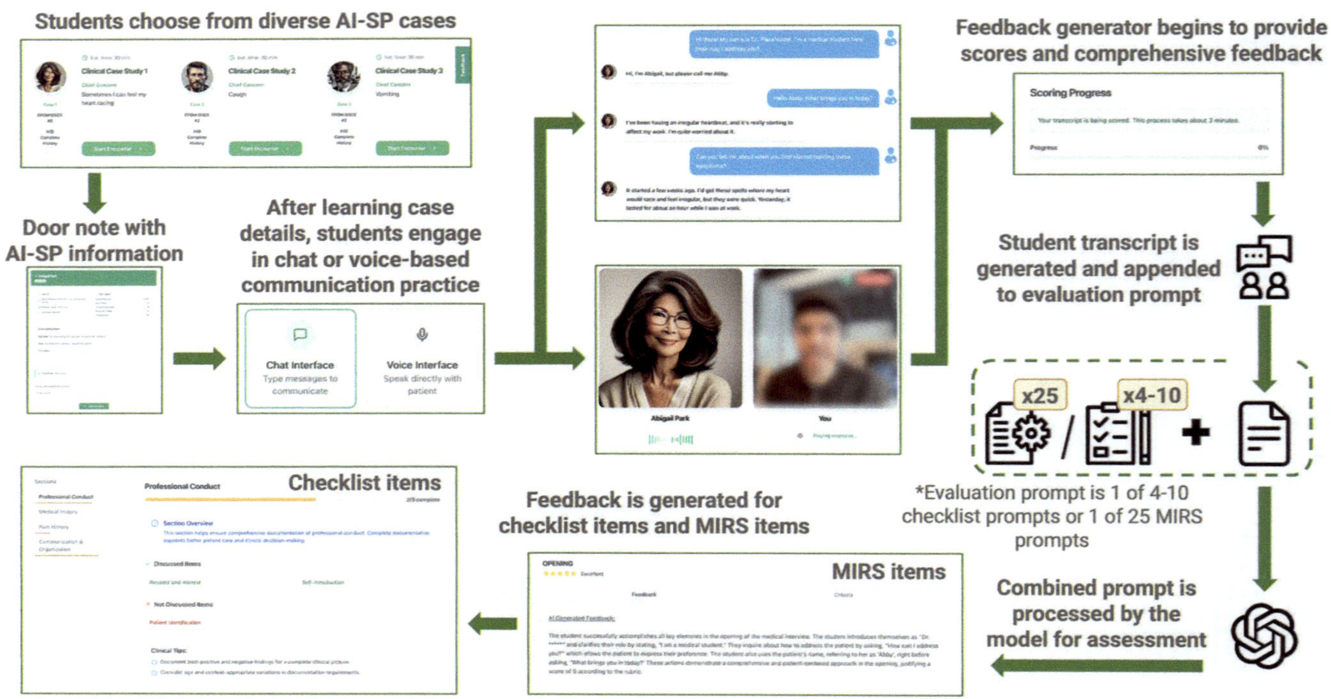

Fig. 4.2 Workflow of the MedSimAI platform. The system enables learners to select clinical cases, interact with AI-simulated patients via chat or voice, and receive AI-generated feedback based on checklists and rating scales. Reproduced from Hicke et al. [18], published in ArXiv Preprint ArXiv:2503.05793 (2025), under the Creative Commons Attribution 4.0 International License (CC BY), (https://creativecommons.org/licenses/by/4.0/)

as eye-tracking technology, are still being studied as a potential method to estimate levels of attention or cognitive load [21]. These measures may allow the AI system to note if a learner appears disengaged and suggest a shift in the learning modality, such as an interactive quiz to re-engage the at-risk learner.

Importantly, education using adaptive technology in medicine must be evidence-based and transparent. Educators confirm the effectiveness of these adaptive systems by measuring outcomes in performance compared to traditional teaching practices [13]. Adaptive learning can reduce the time it takes for learners to gain competency in certain skills without compromising quality. For example, the Perceptual and Adaptive Learning Module (PALM) for ECG learning significantly improved accuracy and fluency among learners in less than two hours of training, allowing them to perform at or above the level of peers who were one year ahead in training but had not used PALM [22]. However, faculty supervision was still important. Educators should review the AI-driven learning pathways to ensure that learners did not skip important content and that they achieved competency benchmarks, rather than relying solely on the algorithm's assessment.

In conclusion, adaptive and personalized learning with AI offers a tailored, efficient, and engaging learning experience that follows each learner's pathway. It is a move away from a one-size-fits-all model toward a competency-based advancement plan, where the student moves forward upon mastery rather than time spent. As these systems improve and adapt, the medical education experience may evolve to view education as a guided self-paced experience, with AI as the guide and safety net, creating a clinician who is well-informed and has experienced a model of personalized education that they can apply for their own patients in the future (similar to personalized medicine). However, as with all systems, the human element will remain—mentorship, professional judgment, and social learning dynamics are irreplaceable and will enhance the learning experience when cognition, social learning, and interactions are integrated with adaptive technology.

4.2.3 Simulation-Based Training and Virtual Patients

Clinical skills and decision-making are best learned by doing, but real-life practice opportunities are often limited by patient availability, supervision, and risk. AI-enhanced, simulation-based training provides immersive, repeatable clinical practice experiences through Virtual Reality (VR), Augmented Reality (AR), and computer-based simulation scenarios. Current medical simulators go far beyond static mannequins and provide a dynamic virtual patient environment for learners to practice procedures, history taking, and critical thinking skills in a safe learning space. AI propels these simulations by managing the predictive progression of the scenario (scenario branching), animating the responses of the virtual patient, and tracking the user's behavior to provide feedback [1].

For instance, in a VR surgical simulator, a trainee donned a headset and used haptic controllers to perform a simulated laparoscopic surgery; an AI engine in the simulator could react to the trainee's actions. For example, when the trainee made an erroneous maneuver, the simulator's AI engine analyzed the action in real time and provided immediate corrective feedback to guide performance improvement [23]. Bogar et al. [24] created a low-cost VR laparoscopic trainer for a standard peg-transfer task combined with an AI-based assessment system. They conducted a randomized trial with 60 students, comparing the VR laparoscopic skills simulator to a traditional box trainer. Their results indicated that the performance gains in surgical skill between VR-trained versus box-trained groups were similar, which would indicate equivalence in laparoscopic skills training using VR or the traditional method. Additionally, the AI assessment matched expert human evaluations 95% of the time and gave practice recommendations much faster. The main benefit of training using these kinds of simulators is the opportunity to practice repeatedly, with no risk to real patients, while allowing trainees to build muscle memory, gain proficiency, and improve clinical decision-making, skills that usually take many real cases to develop.

In addition to protocol-based simulators, AI also drives virtual patient encounters for history taking and clinical reasoning. Natural Language Processing (NLP) allows these virtual standardized patients to engage in realistic conversations. For example, a medical student may interview a computerized patient (on screen or via VR) with a presenting complaint and practice taking history in a conversational manner. Reiswich et al. [25] developed a conversational agent powered by NLP specifically for virtual patients to train medical students in history taking. Their chatbot agents do not follow a fixed scripted pathway; instead, ML is used to interpret free-text questions from students and respond appropriately. In a small test using a limited dataset (109 questions), all scores (recall, precision, F1) reached a level above 80%. This is an encouraging step toward creating more flexible and tailored virtual patient interviews using AI. In nursing education, Zhao et al. [26] reported a training program using a virtual patient designed to improve nursing interns' history-taking skills. They conducted a non-randomized controlled study with 90 nursing interns (44 using the virtual patient training, 46 controls) to evaluate its impact. Results showed that students who practiced with virtual patients achieved significantly greater improvements in history-taking skills compared to the control group. The nursing history assessment scores improved by an average of 29 points with the virtual patient compared to 9 points with standard training ($p < 0.001$). The authors concluded that virtual patients provide autonomous, repeatable practice that prepares students for clinical encounters. Each of these studies indicates that virtual patients can engage learners in realistic conversations while guiding relevant history taking. These applications allow medical and nursing trainees to practice clinical reasoning and communication skills with dynamic feedback, supplementing or replacing traditional in-person patient simulations in learning environments.

In medical training, team scenarios using VR also exist—multiple learners can join a shared virtual environment to train teamwork during an emergency [27, 28]. AI can simulate the environment and the patient, as well as control virtual team responses in the simulated setting. This provides opportunities for learners to train in interprofessional collaboration and communication in acute or emergent situations.

Additionally, metrics like leadership, clarity of communication, and adherence to protocols can be tracked for debriefing purposes.

In general, simulation-based training enhanced by AI provides a safe, reproducible, and varied clinical experience. It addresses the limitations of real-world training (such as limited patient availability and ethical challenges with high-risk interventions) and accelerates skills development. It allows failure without consequence—this means learners can learn from mistakes that, in reality, could cost lives, thereby building confidence and competence. Medical schools have begun to explore AI-enhanced simulations in different educational contexts, such as virtual anatomy labs, AR-guided surgical training, and immersive scenarios for emergency care. Evidence suggests that students who have participated in high-fidelity simulations are associated with improved technical performance in real clinical settings [29]. The challenge is to ensure these simulations are effectively integrated into curricula and that instructor training occurs to interpret AI performance data. As simulation technology improves, we may even see fully virtual clinical rotations in some areas, although patient exposure will remain a tenet of medical education.

4.2.4 AI in Assessment and Evaluation

Assessment is a significant aspect of medical education, including written tests, essays, and assessments of clinical skills. AI is being used to facilitate assessment in a more objective, efficient, and formative manner. One example is automated grading. ML models allow for automated scoring of written responses, including written clinical vignettes, essays, or short answers [30–32]. This may involve algorithms that use methodologies such as Latent Semantic Analysis (LSA) to evaluate the content of a medical student's response to a topic, such as differential diagnosis, based on comparison to a model answer or a corpus of medical literature [33, 34]. These systems determine whether key points are covered and provide a score or feedback to the student. Some studies have shown that AI systems that score essays do so with similar reliability to human graders while providing results instantly [34]. This mechanism means students can receive immediate feedback (from AI scoring systems) on practice essay examination questions, like the United States Medical Licensing Examination (USMLE), and can identify areas for improvement.

AI is also supporting the assessment of practical examinations. A particular instance is the Objective Structured Clinical Examination (OSCE), where students might rotate through different stations to perform tasks which may involve taking a history or interpreting a radiological image. Typically, a student's performance is assessed by examiners at each station or through the use of a checklist, usually carrying a higher degree of subjectivity and labor-management costs. With advancements in AI and Computer Vision (CV), assessing an OSCE station may be simplified through the use of video or audio recordings of the student in a space where they are performing certain tasks. For example, an AI program that incorporates speech recognition could transcribe the student's interview of the patient and check the patient interview against a complete list of questions to see if the student asked all the appropriate and important questions. This application of AI could serve as "silent examiners" to ensure the student did not neglect to ask any key item [35]. Similarly, in principle, for a station where the student is asked to interpret an imaging study or to identify anatomical structures, similar image recognition algorithms could be used to compare the student's interpretations or anatomical selections to the "correct" answer while aiding the rating process. A pilot project showed that computer vision could accurately track hand hygiene dispenser use in a hospital using depth sensors and Convolutional Neural Networks (CNNs), with accuracy similar to human observers [36]. Although this system was designed for a clinical environment, the general approach can be applied to develop an assessment system for an OSCE station that could be used to assess a student's technique of hand hygiene against a predetermined standard, for example, World Health Organization (WHO) hand hygiene guidelines. Assessing hand hygiene techniques is time-consuming and tedious for individual human examiners, and may be efficiently supported using AI.

Video analysis to assess surgical skills is becoming a commonplace practice in surgical training. Trainees need to be assessed for proficiency skills, which has historically been done by having a supervising surgeon fill out a checklist. With the help of AI, this assessment can be accomplished in a more granular and unbiased fashion by examining surgical video footage. AI can analyze the movement of instruments, hand tremors, economy of motion, and errors to assign a skill score in an objective manner. As an example, one study took video footage of surgeons performing a procedure and successfully classified skill level (expert vs. novice) with high accuracy [37]. This analysis can also highlight specific areas for improvement—for example, "the surgeon spends too long on a certain step" or "the surgical camera is misoriented too often"—and these findings can be reported back to trainees for focused practice. Additionally, as the AI system observes additional surgeries and surgical outcomes, it may even be able to predict which trainees will perform well in actual surgeries based on their simulation or practice performance, thereby informing individualized training focus.

Automated quiz construction and adaptive testing are another area of focus. AI can not only score assessments but create them, as well. Generative models are capable of generating plausible multiple-choice questions, or clinical vignettes, from textbook material or lecture transcripts [38, 39]. While this process requires human vetting, it can help diversify question banks and provide educators with a steady stream of new practice questions. Some systems push further; for example, if a student continues to get a concept wrong, automation can generate a new question on the spot to assess the concept slightly differently. An example of this is Gan et al. [40] who developed a personalized adaptive tutoring system that dynamically generates tailored remedial questions based on cognitive diagnostic assessment. Adaptive testing has evolved to use AI to determine subsequent question items based on the previous responses, honing in on the true level of proficiency [41, 42], which can greatly reduce the number of questions needed to accurately assess and generate a unique challenge for each student.

Lastly, it is important that fairness and bias mitigation in AI-driven assessment are addressed. AI models learn from data, and if we use past grading data or an already existing data set that includes bias (e.g., if there are different expectations for language fluency, or any subtle gender/racial bias in a clinical scenario), our AI will replicate that bias. For example, an automated scoring system may unintentionally reward the content of longer essays (length equals knowledge) or penalize a non-native English-speaking style even if the medical content is appropriate. To address this, developers should adjust algorithm priorities to focus on content rather than style and use diverse training data. In addition, human intervention should still be an important component of AI-augmented assessment— instructor reviews can be done following AI-generated assessments. Thus, we can achieve the benefits of AI consistency and efficiency, while coupling it with human judgement when necessary.

In conclusion, assessment tools powered by AI are making assessments more timely, customized, and potentially more objective. Automated scoring frees up faculty time and enables frequent formative assessments without extra grading burden, allowing students to receive more feedback for learning. However, educators still play a central role in interpreting the output of AI, offering mentorship as a result, and ensuring that the nuance of human performance (for example, the role of empathy or professionalism in an interaction with a patient, which AI may not capture) is incorporated into the overall assessment. With responsible use, AI has the potential to maintain high standards in assessment while achieving the ultimate goal of ensuring that students graduate competent and ready for independent practice.

4.2.5 AI in Curriculum Development and General Institutional Decision-Making

Developing a medical curriculum can be a difficult and challenging job with many variables: educational objectives, accreditation standards, faculty capacity to deliver, and student needs. With the introduction of AI and data analytics, administrators and curriculum committees may be able to use compelling, educationally based mechanisms to help inform curricular decisions. One application is the use of learning analytics dashboards that aggregate different related data across courses and clerkships [43]. These dashboards, that can be supported by AI, can notify and highlight overall performance trends and indices, including but certainly not limited to which topics are more difficult for many students or which teaching methods correlate with better outcomes. For example, if students were consistently performing poorly on questions relating to the pharmacology of antibiotics, the analytics may suggest a change in curricular or educational design, be it additional lecture hours or an additional unit/module. With the support of AI, curricular designers may be better positioned to examine actual performance data and use such evidence to inform curricular decisions, complementing traditional experience-based and qualitative approaches.

Additionally, AI can support scenario planning and forecasting workforce requirements. It can assist academic leaders in visualizing how changing healthcare trends will affect training requirements. For example, ML models can replicate workforce scenarios by forecasting the future distribution of specialists and generalists or by predicting demand in emerging fields such as telehealth and AI-assisted care. Alvarez et al. [44] created an ML system that accurately predicts medical students' future career specialties (e.g., primary care versus surgery). This example demonstrates how AI could help workforce planning for physicians. Such programs allow educators to identify potential specialty shortages and strategically develop training pipelines. National workforce assessments also use scenario-based modeling. For example, in the most current AAMC workforce report, the forecast for practicing U.S. physicians in 2030 projects a deficit of between 42,600 and 121,300 physicians, based on different scenarios [45]. These models help medical schools proactively expand training programs in areas with shortages (e.g., geriatrics or primary care).

AI could help align curricula with competency standards by automating the mapping of educational content to external reference points, such as accreditation standards or licensing examination blueprints. Zaki et al. [46], for example, developed a system that uses AI techniques, including NLP, to automate the mapping of Course Learning Outcomes (CLOs) to Program Learning Outcomes (PLOs), achieving over 83% precision in relation to expert mapping (manual mapping by an expert). This use of AI lowers human workload and subjectivity while consistently ensuring the alignment of curricula with standards for accreditation. In other cases, a structured computer-based model (not using AI) has been used by some institutions. Dexter et al. [47], for example, described a system that mapped a medical school curriculum to the USMLE Step 1 content outline using MeSH terms assigned manually by faculty, allowing faculty to visualize the coverage of content in their curriculum. Although these systems offer transparency and assist with curriculum review, they often require significant manual effort. Combination of AI automation with structured manual systems can help educators identify gaps, remove overlaps, and keep curricula aligned with modern healthcare needs more efficiently and accurately. This combined approach to evaluating curricula can facilitate ongoing improvement while balancing innovation with educational, regulatory, and institutional requirements.

AI could also support the development and curation of curriculum content in medical education. With the ever-increasing doubling of medical information, it is becoming increasingly difficult to know what to include (and exclude) in the curriculum. In 2020, medical knowledge was estimated to double every 73 days [48], and no one can keep up with that rate of knowledge acquisition. Educators are under more pressure than ever to incorporate new developments—new drugs, new research, new AI tools in clinical practice—and to limit content overload for their learners. In this environment, AI presents an opportunity to review substantial knowledge bases and curriculum data to help support content curation. As an example, topical NLP algorithms could potentially provide analytics of textbooks, clinical practice guidelines, or course syllabi to find important topics, duplicative information, or missing information. An AI-based solution could potentially review existing practices and determine that one of the many core topics, e.g., "ML in health care," was missed from a program. In this case, the curriculum committee would have data-driven insights to help determine where curricular content is lacking and create new material on important topics that are clinically relevant.

Another area is logistics optimization, such as a timetable creation or allocating faculty workloads. Logistics can be immense and often still need to be accomplished manually, taking multiple variables into consideration (room availability, clinical duty schedules, avoiding student conflicts, etc.). An academic timetable can be modeled as a very large constraint problem in which the AI optimization algorithm can search the problem space and provide solutions that meet the maximum requirements of consideration. Diallo and Tudose [49], for example, designed a scheduling system that generates conflict-free schedules using evolutionary algorithms and multi-objective optimization. The scheduling system utilizes aspects such as room capacity, instructor availability, and student preferences in producing schedules intended to maximize efficiency and minimize conflict. The end product of the scheduling system is a generated schedule intended to meet requirements while minimizing gaps and overlaps—a task that would take humans manual weeks to configure. Then, last-minute adjustments to a schedule, and their administrative burden and error likelihood, could also be quickly and easily made in an automated schedule.

Decision support frameworks powered by AI are also changing institutional policies around admissions and student support. Medical programs have started investigating AI models in admissions by screening applications and eventually determining which applicants will enter the program. In an example, a study used ML to analyze five years of admissions data (over 22,000 applications) to see if an algorithm could replicate and enhance the screening decisions [50]. Trained on admission decisions from prior years, the AI model had an Area Under a Curve (AUC) of 0.93 in predicting interviewees, matching human committees' decisions about 88% of the time. Notably, when this AI model was used alongside human screeners in a trial, the human + AI process achieved 96% decision accuracy. This suggests the potential for AI to make admissions screening more consistent while potentially eliminating inter-observer variability or unconscious bias among reviewers. Furthermore, the algorithm's explainability analysis demonstrated that it was using application features relevant to the school's defined rubric; knowing this gave the admissions committee trust in the merit-based evaluations of the AI. Still, schools using such tools keep humans in the evaluation process. AI can act as a pre-screening process that shortlists applicants or detects outliers, though in the end, admissions committees will review potential candidates based on holistic evaluative processes involving human readers.

In addition to admissions, AI is assisting in identifying students who may be at academic risk early in the program and providing support targeted to academic success. Predictive models can combine a range of data, such as variables before admission, course grades, examination results, and even engagement variables, to predict certain outcomes, such as performance on a USMLE board exam or likelihood of failing a course. Mastour et al. [51] created an Explainable AI (XAI) model to predict the performance of medical students on high-stakes comprehensive examinations at multiple institutions. Their model had high accuracy in predicting who would pass or fail, up to one year in advance. Because an advisor has this information, they may offer targeted support to individuals far in advance of licensing examinations, such as extra tutoring or support in adjusting study strategies.

Notwithstanding the possibilities, obstacles exist in utilizing AI for curriculum and institutional decision-making. Data quality is significant issue—student performance data may exist in discrete systems (exam systems, clinical rotation evaluations, etc.) that need to be transparently integrated. Privacy and ethical use of student performance data are extremely important—analytics should be used to support students and inform program improvement, not to punish or label students unfairly. Moreover, educators and administrators may need training to interpret analytics outputs. A dashboard could indicate that test scores have improved post-curriculum change, but does that actually mean the intervention worked? Human judgment will still be required to substantiate conclusions obtained through AI. Another challenge involves bias and equity. AI may highlight inequities (e.g., particular groups of students who are consistently underperforming in a segment of the curriculum), but it is the institution that will need to address whether and how it will respond in a fair and conscientious manner. For example, if data suggests that students with non-traditional backgrounds struggle more with standardized tests, the recommended solution could be increased mentorship or support, rather than simply redesigning the test. AI can point out the gaps, but it is the humans in the system who will need to be responsible for how they manage them in a student-centered way.

In conclusion, AI for curriculum design and educational governance is a means to drive institutional evolution. Instead of leaning solely on intuition or the slowly moving train of committee discussions, decisions can be based on real data and predictive modeling. The result is a curriculum that is more responsive to learners and to the current and future realities of medicine. AI, by streamlining logistics and resources, helps maintain an educationally sustainable environment for both faculty and learners. Ultimately, the goal is a learning ecosystem where continuous feedback (from learners, healthcare outcomes, and societal needs) loops back into curriculum improvements—a process well-suited to AI's strengths in data analysis. However, like clinical AI, the final decision rests with the human educator and leader who must balance these insights with individual professional judgment and professional values to design the best possible education for future healthcare workers.

4.3 AI in Healthcare Management

In addition to the benefits associated with direct patient care and training, AI is also a major game changer in the management of healthcare services. Healthcare management refers to administrative, operational, and policy-making activities that allow health systems to administer healthcare services efficiently—this includes everything from staffing a hospital and managing operating room schedules to managing supply chains and shaping health policy. These areas are rich in data and complexity and provide opportunities for AI to provide optimization and enhancement support for decision-making. This section reviews AI technologies that benefit hospital administration (as an example, scheduling, billing, and maintenance), facilitate predictive analytics for resource allocation, and enhance governance and healthcare policy decision-making at the system level. The management aspect of AI is of interest not only because of the promise of improved efficiency and cost savings but also as a means to improve safety, quality of care, and accessibility.

As we investigate specific areas, we will see similar ideas, such as the use of ML to forecast future needs (e.g., bed occupancy, supply usage), the use of NLP for automating documentation and conversations, and the use of artificial agents (e.g., chatbots or robots) to carry out administrative functions. Major health systems have begun to implement AI solutions, from Mayo Clinic's AI scheduling to Cleveland Clinic's AI command center, and they are demonstrating measurable improvements in operational performance [52, 53]. At the same time, this innovation raises important considerations about workforce training, managing change, data governance, and ethics. The following subsections describe examples of AI usage and evidence of efficacy in each operational aspect of healthcare management.

4.3.1 AI in Hospital Administration

Managing a hospital or clinic entails numerous administrative responsibilities, many of which consume a lot of time and have the potential for inefficiencies. AI is being utilized to automate and streamline administrative workflows with the aim of allowing staff to spend more time on patient-centered work. One particular use involves staff rostering and scheduling. Staff scheduling (for nurses, doctors, and technicians) is complicated by the need to accommodate staff preferences and requests, along with considerations of the skill mix of various providers, contractual obligations, and changing patient demand. AI algorithms are able to quickly create staff schedules that attempt to optimize coverage while minimizing overtime or gaps [53–55]. These systems use historical data to learn patterns (for example, the analytics involved in predicting that there will be an increase in visits to the emergency department on weekends and Monday evenings) and adjust staffing plans accordingly to provide extra coverage ahead of time. Predictive analytics may also allow managers to add shifts or move staff around based on periods of increased demand for services and generally lead to smoother operations. AI can also provide continually improved alternatives by learning and accounting for variables such as which shifts are most likely to have call-offs or by arranging staff into pods or support pools based on shared interchangeable skills, creating more resilient schedules for what is often a variable environment. Some hospitals have reported that the rostering process (for nurses in particular) with an AI tool reduced the hours of the nurse manager's and team managers' time spent identifying and producing schedules for a given day, as well as improving staff satisfaction by better matching the actual demand and workload requirements [53].

Another area of opportunity is operating room (OR) block scheduling. The OR is one of the most resource-depleting areas and wasted OR time or delays are often at a premium cost. AI-driven systems can take into consideration surgeon case length, turnover time, and available surgeon time to optimize utilization of OR time. AI systems can more accurately predict case length, whether through the use of historical data or even details like the individual surgeon or level of patient complexity. For example, if a surgeon is using block time for knee surgeries and those typically take longer than what may be specified in their block, the AI will automatically adjust future block scheduling to prevent delays in subsequent cases. Also, AI modules that are embedded in current OR case management software within existing OR systems have demonstrated increased OR utilization and allow the scheduling of additional OR cases, which contribute to improved hospital revenue and more efficient patient access [56, 57].

The use of AI is now also being applied to revenue cycle management, including billing and coding. Hospitals process thousands of claims, and with the thousands of medical billing codes, manual processes can introduce errors; approximately 10% of claims are denied by insurers each year due to coding errors or lack of documentation [58]. AI-enabled tools using NLP can now read clinical documentation and assign billing codes or verify that physician notes corroborate billed services [59]. These AI "coders" can learn from expert coders and update their knowledge base with new coding rules—contemporary AI systems allow expert coders to provide feedback, substantiating new perspectives or guidelines for the AI to code against [60]. For example, Kim et al. [59] developed an NLP-based model that could auto-generate surgical billing codes with near-human-level of accuracy in the assignment of Current Procedural Terminology (CPT) codes from operative notes. Kim et al. [58] introduced a Deep Learning (DL) framework ("Deep Claim") that mines historical claims to forecast the likelihood of insurer responses, which was able to identify 22% more claim denials at 95% precision compared with previous rule-based methods. Each of these AI-based efforts can transform the billing model from reactive to more proactive. By utilizing ML programs, systems flag likely denials for human review before submitting to the payer. Staff are then able to proactively fix issues noted in claims and curb delays or lost reimbursement. Evidence supports that hospitals utilizing AI have reported faster revenue capture and a reduction in staff burden, who have historically spent hours on chart reviews and manual coding. By streamlining coding and improving denial management, AI can automate the revenue cycle and improve financial performance in healthcare administration.

Another administrative advantage is intelligent document processing. Hospitals create many paper records—intake forms, consent forms, lab reports, and discharge summaries—and previously required manual data entry and manual filing of paper records. However, AI can now address these traditional tasks. For example, an AI program can process scanned referral letters by extracting patient-specific details and relevant clinical information from unstructured data, such as a doctor's written notes, and append that information into applicable hospital electronic systems [2]. This reduces errors in person-related documentation or entry and allows information to flow rapidly. Pandey et al. [61] designed an AI-based intelligent document management system, integrating CV and NLP methods to automate data extraction from hospital invoices, Aadhar cards, and PAN cards. One of the main objectives was to support accuracy and efficiency in functionalizing a variety of unstructured documents. Their NLP-CV hybrid approach demonstrated up to 97% accuracy in the processing of hospital invoices, and they emphasized its efficiency in the functionality of document processing and the incorporation of documents in general for healthcare updates and administrative purposes. Hospitals are employing document management systems to assist with processing insurance pre-authorizations and to provide a summary of the important points from multi-page specialist reports in a document that can be read at a glance to cross-check the multi-page reports.

AI virtual assistants and chatbot technologies are increasingly being implemented in hospitals to facilitate the management of routine patient interactions and inquiries. Administrative staff typically spend a considerable amount of time replying to frequently asked questions such as "What times can I visit?" or "How do I prepare for my MRI exam?" as well as calling to remind patients about appointments. AI-powered chatbots embedded in hospital websites or accessed over the phone can swiftly respond to frequently asked questions, guide patients through the process of scheduling appointments, and provide clinic information while easing the burden on administrative staff and expanding access to services. Studies show that these chatbots are becoming much more functional through the use of NLP and DL technologies. Khadija et al. [62] suggested a general architecture for AI-powered health chatbot systems that combines NLP-based dialogue systems with expert components to improve not only human-like conversations but also the generation of accurate responses. This architecture is displayed in Fig. 4.3, with the four parts being the Client Platform, APIs, NLP Engine, and Core Engine. In this context, the user will obtain access to the system via the Client Platform, which should be approachable while providing the absolute best user experience. When the user makes a request, it will be forwarded to the NLP Engine through the provided APIs. The NLP Engine is based on Natural Language Understanding (NLU) to process the request and convert it into a structured format that can be processed by the Core Engine. Once the data is structured, the Core Engine uses DL algorithms to determine the most appropriate response and sends that response back to the NLP Engine. Because the response that comes back from the Core Engine is not human-readable, the NLP Engine uses Natural Language Generation (NLG) to put the information in a form that makes sense to the user. The message is then sent back to the user via the Client Platform (using appropriate APIs). In addition to responding to questions, these AI chatbots can also send personalized reminders via text or voice call. AI can assess patient preferences and behaviors to determine the best timing and form of communication to enhance engagement and decrease missed appointments. By automating these routine forms of communication, an AI-powered virtual assistant allows hospital administrative staff to devote time to less routine and more complex transactions that require human presence and empathy.

Another significant use of AI in hospital administration is the predictive maintenance of medical devices. When hospitals have technical devices such as MRI

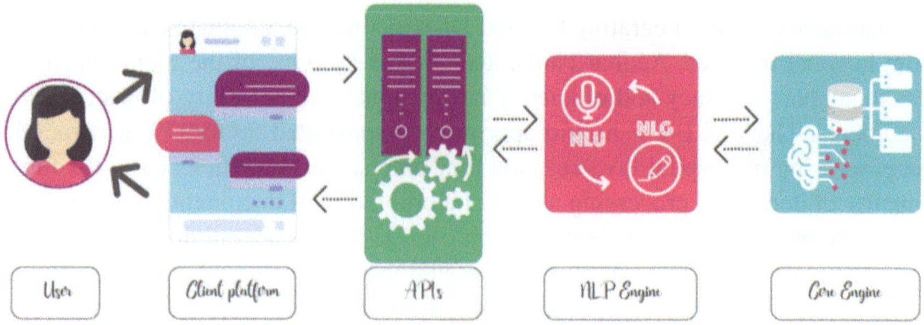

Fig. 4.3 General architecture of an AI-powered health chatbot. Reproduced from Khadija et al. [62], published in Procedia Comput Sci 191 (2021) 355–360, under the Creative Commons Attribution 4.0 International License (CC BY), (https://creativecommons.org/licenses/by/4.0/)

machines, ventilators, and infusion pumps, equipment downtime can happen unexpectedly and disrupt clinical workflows or put patient safety at risk. Clinical engineers use predictive algorithms by processing sensor data, maintenance logs, and information about usage to forecast when a device might fail or need routine maintenance. Zamzam et al. [63] designed an ML-based model for device failure prediction, specifically for medical device management. The model used data from 13,350 devices across 19 categories of equipment, while utilizing features to predict first failure events, failure-to-year ratios, and groups of failure functions. The purpose of their model was also to support maintenance decisions to enable remanufacturing and refurbishment with reliability and to extend service life. AI is also leveraged for smart facilities management for improved performance [2]. Hospitals have extensive and complicated systems where optimal conditions of temperature, humidity, and air quality need to be maintained for patient care, staff comfort, and the operation of sensitive equipment. Increasingly, AI systems are being utilized to control heating, ventilation, and air conditioning (HVAC) systems to optimize energy consumption while still maintaining the needed environmental parameters [64]. These AI-enabled facility management systems assist in lowering operational costs and overall environmental impact by dynamically adjusting energy consumption using real-time data, all within a safe environment for patients and healthcare workers.

In conclusion, AI in hospital operations focuses on the efficiency, accuracy, and forward-thinking of operational workflows. AI-driven changes reduce manual jobs, ensure consistency, and reduce errors. One example is the Cleveland Clinic's AI-powered Virtual Command Center, which provides a real-time dashboard for bed management, staffing, and OR scheduling across the system [53]. The Virtual Command Center, now operational, has transformed decision-making from manual and siloed to a coordinated and data-driven process. The pilot program improved patient flow, supported better alignment of nurse staffing with operational demand, and enhanced the usage of ORs. These improvements are no longer theoretical; they are being realized in practice. These are no longer just theoretical endeavors in a hospital administrative mindset—these are systems used to run hospitals smarter.

Human administrators and staff will, of course, still play a significant role in supervising these systems, handling exceptions to the data, and reporting on patient interactions that the machines cannot manage. However, the addition of AI to healthcare functions brings productivity gains, reducing drudgery and burden, and creating better opportunities to focus on strategy and patients. The main challenge going forward is change management—specifically, how staff are educated to use AI tools and how they build trust in their findings.

4.3.2 AI for Resource Allocation and Predictive Analytics

Healthcare systems live in a constant balance between limited resources (i.e., beds, staff, equipment, and medications) and variable demand. Predictive analytics developed with AI have the potential to be useful in predicting needs and improving the allocation of those resources. One particularly useful application is in forecasting bed capacity and managing patient flow. Hospitals experience peaks and valleys in patient census (for example, a greater volume of admissions on Mondays and seasonal surges such as during the flu season) and can now predict potential trends based on models developed from data [2, 65, 66]. A well-known success story occurred during COVID-19, when data-driven predictive tools helped hospitals with implementation planning by forecasting bed demand two or three days in advance. For example, Deschepper et al. [67] created a ward occupancy forecasting tool for use in a Belgian hospital, which—though based on conventional statistical models rather than AI—was able to produce reliable short-term forecasts of hospital bed demand while facilitating proactive capacity actions during COVID-19 surges. Such predictive models also have the potential to identify impending capacity problems even during normal, non-COVID circumstances. Corren et al. [68] mentioned that failure to predict bed availability is among the leading causes of planned surgical cancellations. They developed an ML model which was able to forecast next-day census with a median error of 7%, allowing surgical managers to plan and reschedule elective admissions or guide care teams in specific ward actions in advance. In summary, by embedding these models to anticipate patient demand, hospitals can avoid last-minute resource adjustments to create bed capacity.

Similarly related is the Emergency Department (ED), where predictive analytics improves patient flow and the utilization of resources. Brossard et al. [66] created a model to predict the hourly arrival of patients to the ED. Their model demonstrated a mean absolute error of only approximately 2.6 patients in tests conducted at two hospitals. They further suggested that integrating such a system into their ED operations could facilitate optimal staffing adjustments beforehand. Gafni-Pappas et al. [69] showed that ML models—for example, RFs and Gradient Boosted Machines (GBM)—slightly outperformed time-series methods in predicting daily visits to the ED. In their study, RFs produced the most accurate estimates of daily ED visits, performing better than common time series forecasting methods; "day of the week" was the strongest predictor of patient load, and weather variables were also a factor in predicting seasonal volume patterns. With access to AI-based forecasts, ED administrators can pre-adjust staffing levels to anticipate spikes in demand and lulls, resulting in better patient throughput and possibly reduced waiting times for care.

AI-based predictive analytics can be applied to supply chain and inventory management as well. Hospitals manage thousands of items that can be consumed (gloves, syringes, drugs, PPE, etc.), so it's essential to have a proper inventory system. In a traditional inventory system, there may be a simple threshold for ordering needed goods based on stock (e.g., if the stock of an item is less than X, order more of the item). AI methods produce far more sophisticated analyses that focus on forecasting useful consumption patterns and optimizing appropriate stock amounts [70]. ML models are certainly able to assess historical consumption, seasonal patterns in a hospital, patient volumes, and potentially real-time data (e.g., disease outbreaks) to produce a more accurate forecast of utilization. In fact, large health systems (Mayo Clinic, Cleveland Clinic, etc.) have already started using models to predict utilization to avoid seasonal shortages due to supply stop conditions [70]. Advanced approaches like Reinforcement Learning (RL) can learn optimal ordering policies by balancing stockout risk against waste [71]. Kaur and Prakash [72], for instance, developed an intelligent and adaptive inventory replenishment strategy for the pharmaceutical supply chain based on their model of deep RL with a continuous action space. Their model, based on a Markov Decision Process (MDP), optimizes order quantities dynamically while accounting for stochastic demand and lead times to minimize stockouts and medical waste. Fig. 4.4 depicts this technical approach to decision-making as it relates to inventory replenishment as an MDP problem, which allows an AI agent to adapt order sizes based on real-time systemic states. The system was shown to be robust across seasonal, non-seasonal, and epidemic conditions while being capable of supporting the resilient and sustainable availability of medicine. AI systems can also consider expiration dates and lead times. For example, Farrington et al. [73] trained an ML model with years of data from a hospital blood bank and demonstrated a potential reduction of expired platelet waste of ~14% without harming the available supply. Practically, hospitals implementing AI-based inventory platforms demonstrated a 30% reduction in stockouts, along with a supply chain cost reduction of as much as 20% [70]. Altogether, intelligent systems will continually learn and evolve within the constraints of finding the "sweet spot" for patient care—to have enough inventory delivered while minimizing expiration or excess inventory.

As a result of these AI tools, a shift from reactive, crisis-driven management to proactive and efficiently run operations has begun. Instead of responding to crises (no beds, running out of a drug, etc.), managers are given early warnings and even suggestions for prevention. This has led to benefits in real improvement metrics, such as reduced waiting times for patients, fewer cancellations of procedures due to missing supplies, and increased emergency preparedness. Another benefit is cost savings; more efficient use of resources creates lower overtime costs, and fewer emergency supply orders are needed, while expensive assets such as MRIs are more effectively utilized.

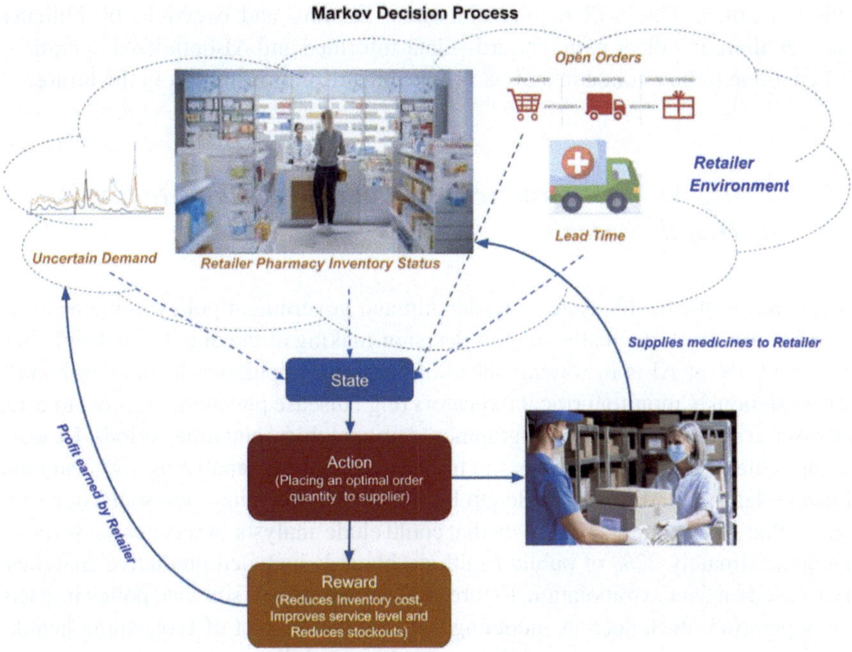

Fig. 4.4 Inventory optimization problem modeled as MDP, forming the foundation of the deep RL strategy used for adaptive pharmaceutical inventory management. Reproduced from Kaur and Prakash [72], published in Societal Impacts 5 (2025) 100109, © 2025, with permission from Elsevier

Nonetheless, the use of predictive analytics faces some challenges. Data silos can impede a holistic perspective; if the AI source does not receive data from all potential feed-in sources (for example, outpatient clinics and their potential impact on hospital admissions), the predictions will suffer. There are also challenges related to the trust and usability of the model; managers have to trust the model to place it into play and work it into their workflows. This can be addressed by initiating the AI as an advisory tool, building the confidence of users in the model based on its accuracy initially, and then gradually implementing the models into the decision-making process. Also, forecasting itself in health care is a challenge; there will always be unexpected events (e.g., a mass casualty incident or a disease outbreak). AI models can model typical variability but may not handle truly novel situations. AI models should be viewed as tools for enhancing human planning, not as an alternative to a contingency plan.

In summary, using AI-enabled predictive analytics in resource allocation is akin to providing the health system with near-future radar and autopilot. It enhances the system's resilience and effectiveness by anticipating needs and optimally responding. As algorithms improve and more real-time data are integrated into the system, the forecasts become sharper. One can start to think of a future where regional health systems coordinate based on a connected AI system, balancing loads so seamlessly that patients always receive timely care with minimal waiting, while preserving time and effort. This will require consistent refining and oversight by humans; however, there is a clear path forward—data-informed and AI-optimized operations will continue to be a fundamental part of healthcare administration in the future.

4.3.3 Using AI in Governance and Policy Decision-Making of Health Systems

AI is entering the health systems leadership and government policy domains as an informed tool to strategically support decision-making at the population level. One prominent use of AI is in staying ahead of prevalent population health dashboards that continuously monitor critical indicators (e.g., disease prevalence, access to care, and disease outcomes) across geographics, demographics, and time periods. Leaders are thus able to identify inequities and trends in advance by analyzing a vast amount of health data—e.g., Electronic Health Records (EHRs), claims, and social determinants—that show patterns of activity that could elude analysts. A recent review found that approximately 22% of public health dashboards included predictive analytics, often based on data extrapolation, to forecast future trends or simulate policy impacts at a population level, such as modeling the potential impact of broadening healthcare coverage in a community [74]. In turn, this capability utilizes data to facilitate evidence-based decisions with a clear lens on equity. For instance, Shi et al. [75] developed the Meaningful Integration of Data Analytics and Services (MIDAS) platform, which integrates multi-source health data into actionable insights to support policymakers. Pilot studies demonstrated the platform's ability to highlight regional health gaps and offer targeted interventions. The system architecture (Fig. 4.5) shows how the platform presents local, open, and social data streams with analytic and visualization tools for health decision-makers. Such analytic dashboards put health care leaders in a position to actively divert resources and implement harm reduction interventions for at-risk communities, leading to more equitable health outcomes.

AI methods can potentially support policy simulation and the assessment of budget impact forecasts. Typically, health systems and governments want to know "What if?" in relation to proposed changes to current policy. For instance, they may consider, "What if reimbursement changes enable patients to access that expensive new drug?" or "What if we invest in a diabetes prevention program today?" AI models may integrate epidemiological trends and clinical data, and account for economic conditions, to model these scenarios. Dritsakis et al. [76] reviewed data analytics tools designed specifically for policy making in noncommunicable disease, and they noted that many decision-support tools employed some form of predictive modeling to estimate long-term outcomes. Relying on predictive modeling, these tools can potentially function as practical policy simulation tools which allow decision-makers to modify inputs, examine best-case and worst-case outcomes of a policy decision, and assess use cases for decisions made in the real world. For example, simulations may deliver the

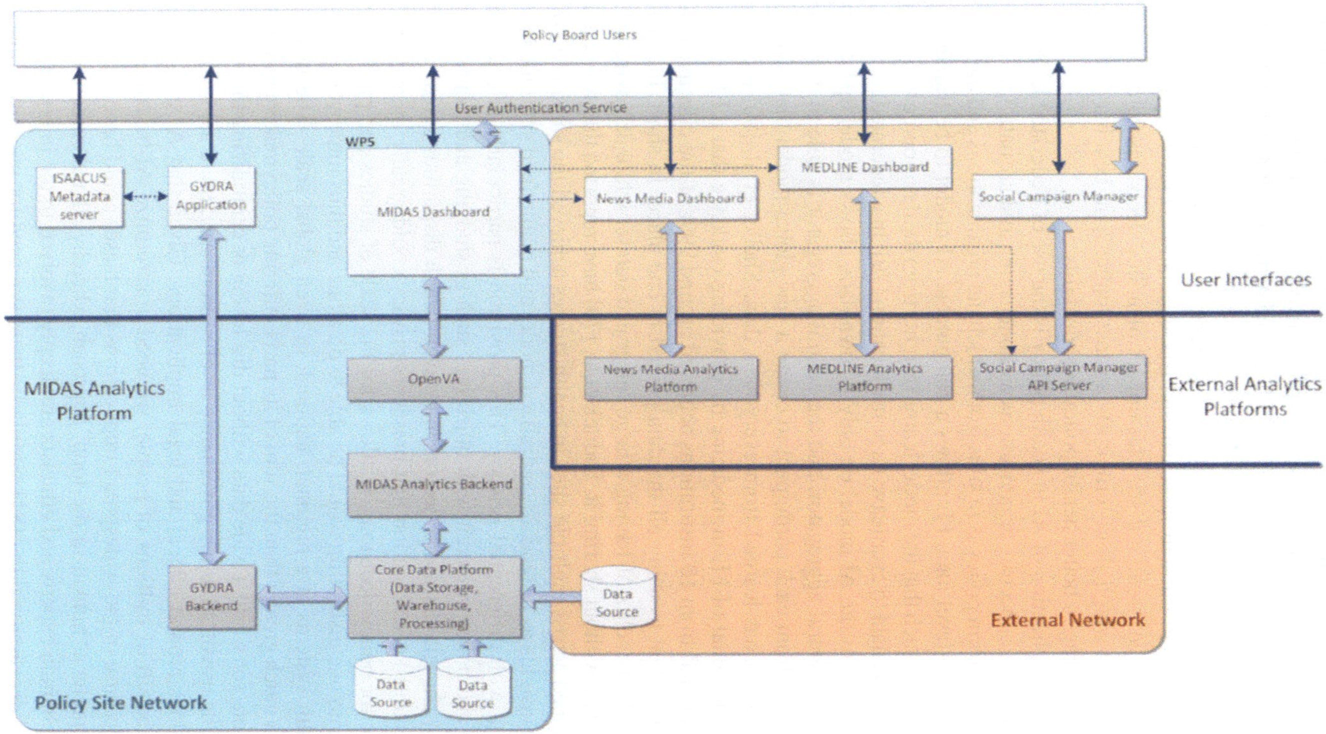

Fig. 4.5 System architecture of the MIDAS platform for health policy decision-making. The MIDAS platform integrates heterogeneous health-related data—such as local clinical data, open data, and social media inputs—within a modular architecture. Reproduced from Shi et al. [75], published in Front Public Health 10 (2022) 838438, under the Creative Commons Attribution 4.0 International License (CC BY), (https://creativecommons.org/licenses/by/4.0/)

message that if policymakers invest in a diabetes prevention program, acute complications will decrease, thereby achieving significant health care savings in the coming decade, which may support the funding of preventive policy. Emerging evidence supports this direction; Canfell et al. [77, 78] described platforms that currently offer descriptive, comparative, and geospatial analytics for precision public health, and mentioned that future systems are expected to integrate predictive features designed to inform policymakers through forecasts and risk estimation. This will help yield a long-term quantified fiscal and societal impact of policy decisions so decision-makers can properly weigh short-term costs against longer-term benefits of public health policy, resulting in better health policy sustainability.

A prospective application of AI in health policy is the use of Federated Learning (FL) as a method for connecting organizations without having to share data. Often, the data necessary to inform policy is in silos from which the organizations and agencies cannot share patient-level data. FL allows a computable AI model to be trained on distributed datasets, such that the model learns insights from the data source without a requirement for raw data to ever leave its home location [79]. In a federated network, each participant trains the AI model on only its own data, allows model updates to be sent back to a central aggregator, and the central aggregator is able to combine all model updates from each participant to create a new global model that is more powerful because it has learned from everyone's data. Sheller et al. [80] recently illustrated the potential of FL in medicine by providing evidence that a FL model utilizing data pooled from 10 institutions achieved around 99% of the effectiveness of a model equivalent to using all the data pooled in one place. In short, FL may offer many of the benefits of having a large integrated dataset while achieving the goal of using data without sharing it. Sadilek et al. [79] have reported that federated models developed across multiple sites in health studies achieved the same level of accuracy and insights as a standard centralized model and maintained strict locality of patient data with differential privacy. This provision is particularly relevant to public health and policy research with objectives such as studying and responding to pandemics, chronic disease trajectories, or even health disparities across many regions. AI-enabled collaboration that preserves privacy could greatly increase the evidence base for policy decisions. It allows for the scale of studies and predictive analytics that no one institution would be able to do alone and thus improves governance of health systems at a regional, national, or even global scale. The whole, through FL, is much greater than the sum of its parts, offering policymakers insights based on nation- (or world-) wide data without disclosing or centralizing that data.

Although the use of AI at the governance level is promising, there are a number of considerations around ethical and legal implications. Given that AI can make decisions on behalf of millions of people, we need to scrutinize AI-based recommendations because of the widespread implications that biases could have. For this reason, many prefer a "human-in-the-loop" approach, whereby AI makes recommendations while human experts and ethicists are deeply involved in the interpretation, judgment, and decision-making [81]. Similarly, there is a need for interdisciplinary policy groups that consist of data scientists, clinicians, and patients to direct AI-based approaches.

In addition, accessibility and public trust are also factors, especially if AI is engaged in invariably prioritizing who gets access to services or resources. People may be concerned about fairness. Therefore, it is necessary to be as transparent as possible in explaining how those AI tools work and what contributes to the decision-making process. For example, if an AI tool is employed to determine which geographic areas will receive additional vaccine doses during a shortage, there should be explicit communication that the order is based on criteria (i.e., outbreak risk), not discrimination.

To conclude, AI is a deeply impactful decision-support partner in the governance and policy context, interpreting broad and deep datasets to support policy that creates more efficient, equitable, and effective health systems. We are in the early stages of realizing the benefits, such as targeting interventions more effectively, managing risk proactively, and streamlining regulatory compliance. Moving forward, we will need to continue to refine XAI and ethical AI structures so that data governance improves human well-being and fairness. AI will never replace the need for wise health leadership, but it will facilitate greater transparency and foresight for health leaders.

4.3.4 AI in Regulatory Compliance and Fraud Detection

AI is establishing a transformative change in the oversight of regulatory compliance in the health sector. Historically, compliance teams could perform manual audits of only a small sample of records. The majority of issues would go unnoticed. AI now allows for automated, continuous review of all documentation as a way to close this gap in auditing and review. Even more powerful are advanced NLP algorithms that can review thousands of existing clinical documents, forms, and notes in real time to determine whether they have all of the required components of documentation, staff compliance, and follow documentation policies. No human can perform this process at anything close to that scale. These so-called "compliance assistants" are a continuous workhorse of review. For example, commercial platforms, such as CFlow, claim to provide AI-driven documentation review systems that identify inconsistencies, missing entries, and compliance issues in patient records, helping clinicians prevent errors and maintain reliable, high-quality data [82]. Datagrid, likewise, claims that its AI agents are capable of continuously auditing documentation practices to proactively identify potential compliance risks regarding the Health Insurance Portability and Accountability Act (HIPAA) and the General Data Protection Regulation (GDPR) [83].

In addition to auditing, AI is also aiding in drafting compliant documents. Wang et al. [84] reported on InformGen—an AI copilot designed to efficiently draft clinical informed consent documents consistent with regulations. InformGen ingests protocol documents and generates consent language that adheres to 18 core rules set forth by the FDA, documenting compliance just below 100% with those regulations (compared to more than 30% higher accuracy than a baseline model, GPT-4o). It generates in-line source citations for each document section, consistently yielding >90% veracity and traceability when combined with human oversight. This allows administrators to rely on AI for both reviewing existing consent documents and helping with new drafting and compliance administration while satisfying legal and ethical standards. The authors also urged caution regarding this practice. Oh et al. [85], for example, evaluated the effectiveness of using an LLM (ChatGPT-4o) to reformat surgical consent forms to ease patients' experience with them while preserving their content. They demonstrated that AI-edited (or -assisted) documents resulted in significantly easier readability but at the same time led to a reduction in the breadth and depth of surgical risk disclosures. While this suggests the potential for AI to create more patient-oriented consent forms, one must be careful not to sacrifice content that is consistent with regulation.

AI is also changing the field of privacy compliance through automated monitoring of EHR access logs. Providers in the health sector must comply with strict privacy laws; however, it is challenging to report or detect breaches or misuse of patient records using traditional monitoring methods in large hospital systems while complying with these laws. Meanwhile, AI has arrived on the scene to provide a means to enhance compliance. Algorithms can learn normal modes of EHR access and then discern and flag abnormal usage patterns indicating possible unauthorized access or snooping of patient records. For example, Hurst et al. [86] developed a supervised ML approach to detect insider threats in EHR logs in a hospital setting in the UK. They trained classifiers with labeled access data using a number of different methods and achieved a match accuracy rate of 98.96% with one method (SVM) detecting anomalous accesses to patient records. They recommended their method for proactive privacy monitoring. Using their method, if a hospital employee accessed an unusually high number of records, an alert could be instantly sent to the security officer, which could potentially uncover privacy breaches as they occur. Hurst et al.'s work [86] was similar in aim to a systematic review published in 2022, which found similar promise for ML protocols in privacy monitoring activities [87]. The systematic review concluded that monitoring records using ML provided a "more robust security mechanism for the sustainable management of EHR systems" through proactive detection of suspicious access. The systematic review also found that research on monitoring patient records for privacy and confidentiality using ML is in its infancy. In summary, AI serves as a constant, automated privacy officer to track unauthorized access and other suspicious events that human auditors (although thorough) may miss when properly auditing records. Hospitals can use AI-enabled anomaly detection tools to detect subtle patterns of misuse; for instance, a staff member accessing records of patients not under their care multiple times. By using a facility's specific usage patterns to develop its definition of what is "abnormal," the AI will gradually reduce false alarms, discovering authentic breaches more rapidly (thereby generating more useful alerts). This type of continuous monitoring and breach detection will support compliance with privacy regulations and help healthcare organizations more effectively protect patient confidentiality than current practices.

Easily the most clear-cut success has been in the area of fraud and abuse detection. Fraud in health care, from phantom billing to upcoding and kickbacks, costs the system tremendous amounts of money each year. In the U.S. alone, health care fraud is estimated to account for about 3%–10% of total health care expenditures [88]. AI offers powerful tools for fighting this fraud by reviewing billing data in ways that are not feasible to perform manually and at scale. Current fraud detection algorithms take in vast datasets of claims to learn the complex patterns or irregularities that are indicative of fraud.

New literature suggests a range of perspectives on this application. For example, Amponsah et al. [89] conceived a hybrid system by combining DTs with blockchain smart contracts to detect and prevent health care fraud in claims processing. This model achieved a classification accuracy of 97.96%, demonstrating that incorporating fraud detection rules within the blockchain system is feasible and can aid in secure claims processing and transparency. Prova [90] conducted a thorough comparison of different ML methods (e.g., RF, XGBoost, SVM, Isolation Forest, a DL model, and a stacking ensemble) on over 558,000 records. The stacking ensemble model emerged as particularly efficacious with 92.79% accuracy and 96.95% ROC-AUC (Area Under the Receiver Operating Characteristic Curve) score. Additionally, the study reported the development of a real-time fraud detection pipeline and model-retraining framework to ensure effectiveness against new tactics used to commit fraud, as well as a commitment to maintain model updates for changes in fraud situations. Agarwal [91] introduced an ML framework specifically for detecting fraud in medical claims insurance. Their results indicated significant improvement over traditional fraud detection methods. Nabrawi and Alanazi [92] created and validated a predictive fraud detection model capable of operating on health insurance claim data from Saudi Arabia. Comparing RF, logistic regression (LogReg), and ANNs, the RF had the highest accuracy at 98.21% and identified important predictors of fraud such as policy type, education, and age, suggesting it may benefit national health insurance setups.

Building upon these research efforts, public applications of AI-enhanced fraud detection have begun to demonstrate their effectiveness. For instance, the Centers for Medicare & Medicaid Services (CMS) employed unsupervised, rule-based data mining techniques to identify irregularities in healthcare claims. In addition, CMS datasets have been utilized to assess fraud risk using supervised ML approaches, such as DT models [92]. These systems operate continuously to assess vast sets of health care claims in real time and flag claims suspected of fraud for further investigation before payment occurs. This is a significant change in strategy because it transforms a system that relied on manual audit processes into a more efficient, preemptive, automated fraud detection system. AI is now playing an important and more powerful role in protecting governance in the health care system by enhancing human oversight with the speed and ability to recognize subtle patterns.

4.4 Conclusion

Although AI in health care is frequently associated with high-tech diagnostics or robotic surgery, the influence of AI in health care settings is more pervasive than this narrow association. In this chapter, we have focused on AI's role in two areas that are often not discussed but are extremely important foundations of our work: medical education and health care management. From students in classrooms to executives around the boardroom table, AI is providing people with the opportunity to make decisions more effectively, helping leaders and educators streamline processes, and giving learners classroom experiences that help them understand each person's unique role in the health care environment.

AI has additional requirements in education and management that help ensure its success in both areas of implementation. The first is data quality and availability. Whether examining student progress in education or forecasting patient flow in a clinic, AI depends on reliable, standardized, and real-time data that is accessible. Institutions of health care and education must work together to implement EHR systems that protect privacy while establishing a secure way to share data. Next is the need to develop a workforce that is AI-aware. Every student in health care education and every leader should work to understand what AI can do and what it cannot be expected to do. One reason for training for AI using simulations in health care curricula is to develop students' appropriate background knowledge for future practice.

Both fields, however, share similar challenges. First and foremost are bias and ethics. AI algorithms can, often unintentionally, reinforce societal inequalities—in grading, for example, if the data used to train AI systems is biased, or in resource allocation, if historical inequities are built into the system. This is precisely why it is extremely important to continuously audit AI systems, ensure data comes from diverse sources and includes multiple perspectives, and consult with experts in ethics, law, and the community. It is equally important to continue to provide human oversight and empathy. AI should not replace teachers' mentoring or doctors' ethical reasoning. Benefits are enhanced when AI and humans collaborate—with AI processing large quantities of data and performing repetitious tasks, while humans use ethical reasoning, complex decision-making, and emotional care.

Looking forward, we will see an even more connected and adaptive AI in education and management. For instance, FL allows hospitals and universities to jointly train AI models without disclosing sensitive data, enabling the global improvement of tools. We may have real-time adaptive systems soon that integrate learning and work into one experience. For instance, imagine a medical resident seeing a patient, and while she treats the patient, an AI assistant—part of the electronic medical record system—provides suggestions and explanations based on reasoning and evidence in real time. Or consider hospital systems that automatically revise workflows, like a self-driving hospital, targeting improved efficiency and safety. These advances offer great potential, but they also raise questions about governance. We must establish clear boundaries around what AI can alter autonomously, which changes should require a human's sanction or approval, and who is accountable when any AI decision impacts someone's well-being.

Overall, AI has the capability to substantially advance health care education and management in significant ways, allowing for more personalized learning, efficient care, and equitable systems. However, to fully realize its potential, we must continue to center human values and oversight. It is not what AI is capable of doing, but how we will deliberately and responsibly use it.

References

1. E.H.H. Rincón, D. Jimenez, L.A.C. Aguilar, J.M.P. Flórez, Á.E.R. Tapia, C.L.J. Peñuela, Mapping the use of artificial intelligence in medical education: a scoping review. BMC Med. Educ. **25**, 526 (2025)
2. S. Maleki Varnosfaderani, M. Forouzanfar, The role of AI in hospitals and clinics: transforming healthcare in the 21st century. Bioengineering **11**, 337 (2024)
3. W. Chen, Z. Shen, Y. Pan, K. Tan, C. Wang, Applying machine learning algorithm to optimize personalized education recommendation system. J. Theory Pract. Eng. Sci. **4**, 101–108 (2024)
4. N. Ghorashi, A. Ismail, P. Ghosh, A. Sidawy, R. Javan, AI-powered chatbots in medical education: potential applications and implications. Cureus **15**, e43271 (2023)
5. E. Waisberg, J. Ong, M. Masalkhi, A.G. Lee, Large language model (LLM)-driven chatbots for neuro-ophthalmic medical education. Eye **38**, 639–641 (2024)
6. G. Arun, V. Perumal, F.P.J.B. Urias, Y.E. Ler, B.W.T. Tan, R. Vallabhajosyula, E. Tan, O. Ng, K.B. Ng, S.R. Mogali, ChatGPT versus a customized AI chatbot (Anatbuddy) for anatomy education: a comparative pilot study. Anat. Sci. Educ. **17**, 1396–1405 (2024)
7. K. Sunmboye, H. Strafford, S. Noorestani, M. Wilison-Pirie, Exploring the influence of artificial intelligence integration on personalized learning: a cross-sectional study of undergraduate medical students in the United Kingdom. BMC Med. Educ. **25**, 570 (2025)
8. M.M. Mir, G.M. Mir, N.T. Raina, S.M. Mir, S.M. Mir, E. Miskeen, M.H. Alharthi, M.M.S. Alamri, Application of artificial intelligence in medical education: current scenario and future perspectives. J. Adv. Med. Educ. Prof. **11**, 133 (2023)
9. A.L.J. Martinez, K. Sood, R. Mahto, *Early Detection of At-Risk Students Using Machine Learning*, arXiv:2412.09483 (2024).
10. Y. Tsekhmister, T. Konovalova, B. Tsekhmister, Utilizing predictive analytics to identify at-risk students in digitalized medical education: a motivational perspective. Academia 3–24, (2024)
11. A. Almalawi, B. Soh, A. Li, H. Samra, Predictive models for educational purposes: a systematic review. Big Data Cogn. Comput. **8**, 187 (2024)
12. T. Bland, Enhancing medical student engagement through cinematic clinical narratives: multimodal generative AI–based mixed methods study. JMIR Med. Educ. **11**, e63865 (2025)
13. L. Simon-Campbell, J. Phelan, Effectiveness of an adaptive quizzing system as an institutional-wide strategy to improve student learning and retention. Nurse. Educ. **41**, 246–251 (2016)
14. E. Simon-Campbell, J. Phelan, Effectiveness of an adaptive quizzing system as a self-regulated study tool to improve nursing students' learning. Int. J. Nurs. Clin. Pract. **5**, 290 (2018)
15. R.A.M. Thompson, Y.B. Shah, F. Aguirre, C. Stewart, C.D. Lallas, M.S. Shah, Artificial intelligence use in medical education: best practices and future directions. Curr. Urol. Rep. **26**, 1–8 (2025)
16. N.B. Golchini, E. Passalacqua, L. Vaughn, R.-E. Abdulnour, T. Zack, S. Finlayson, Socratic AI: an adaptive tutor for clinical case based learning. MedRxiv 2025–2026, (2025)

17. Y. Xu, Y. Shao, J. Dong, S. Shi, C. Jiang, Q. Li, Advancing problem-based learning with clinical reasoning for improved differential diagnosis in medical education, in *Proceedings of the 2025 CHI Conference on Human Factors in Computing Systems* (2025), pp. 1–32
18. Y. Hicke, J. Geathers, N. Rajashekar, C. Chan, A.G. Jack, J. Sewell, M. Preston, S. Cornes, D. Shung, R. Kizilcec, *MedSimAI: Simulation and Formative Feedback Generation to Enhance Deliberate Practice in Medical Education*, arXiv:2503.05793 (2025)
19. The Role of AI in Personalized Learning | Claned, (n.d.). https://claned.com/the-role-of-ai-in-personalized-learning/ (accessed July 11, 2025)
20. Personalized Learning Platforms in 2025: AI In Education—eLearning Industry, (n.d.). https://elearningindustry.com/ai-in-education-personalized-learning-platforms? (accessed July 11, 2025)
21. H.M. Šola, F.H. Qureshi, S. Khawaja, AI eye-tracking technology: a new era in managing cognitive loads for online learners. Educ Sci (Basel) **14**, 933 (2024)
22. S. Krasne, C.D. Stevens, P.J. Kellman, J.T. Niemann, Mastering electrocardiogram interpretation skills through a perceptual and adaptive learning module. AEM Educ. Train **5**, e10454 (2021)
23. X. Ma, S. Wijewickrema, Y. Zhou, S. Zhou, S. O'Leary, J. Bailey, Providing effective real-time feedback in simulation-based surgical training, in *Medical Image Computing and Computer-Assisted Intervention– MICCAI 2017: 20th International Conference, Quebec City, QC, Canada, September 11-13, 2017, Proceedings, Part II 20* (Springer, 2017), pp. 566–574
24. P.Z. Bogar, M. Virag, M. Bene, P. Hardi, A. Matuz, A.T. Schlegl, L. Toth, F. Molnar, B. Nagy, S. Rendeki, Validation of a novel, low-fidelity virtual reality simulator and an artificial intelligence assessment approach for peg transfer laparoscopic training. Sci. Rep. **14**, 16702 (2024)
25. A. Reiswich, M. Haag, Evaluation of chatbot prototypes for taking the virtual patient's history. DHealth 2019–From EHealth to DHealth 73–80 (2019)
26. J. Zhao, H. He, J. Du, Y. Liu, Z. Li, L. You, K. Li, The effects of using virtual patients on the history-taking ability of nursing interns: a non-randomized controlled study. Nurse Educ. Pract. **59**, 103289 (2022)
27. M. Lehmann, J. Mikulasch, H. Poimann, J. Backhaus, S. König, T. Mühling, Training and assessing teamwork in interprofessional virtual reality-based simulation using the Team-STEPPS framework: protocol for randomized pre-post intervention study. JMIR Res. Protoc. **14**, e68705 (2025)
28. A.N. Neher, R. Wespi, B.D. Rapphold, T.C. Sauter, J.E. Kämmer, T. Birrenbach, Interprofessional team training with virtual reality: acceptance, learning outcome, and feasibility evaluation study. JMIR Serious Games **12**, e57117 (2024)
29. M.W. Schmidt, K.F. Köppinger, C. Fan, K.-F. Kowalewski, L.P. Schmidt, J. Vey, T. Proctor, P. Probst, V. V Bintintan, B.-P. Müller-Stich, Virtual reality simulation in robot-assisted surgery: meta-analysis of skill transfer and predictability of skill. BJS Open **5**, zraa066 (2021)
30. A.T. Cianciolo, N. LaVoie, J. Parker, Machine scoring of medical students' written clinical reasoning: initial validity evidence. Acad. Med. **96**, 1026–1035 (2021)
31. M.J. Gierl, S. Latifi, H. Lai, A. Boulais, A. De Champlain, Automated essay scoring and the future of educational assessment in medical education. Med. Educ. **48**, 950–962 (2014)
32. J. Kibble, J. Plochocki, Comparing machine learning models and human raters when ranking medical student performance evaluations. J. Grad. Med. Educ. **15**, 488–493 (2023)
33. T. Miller, Essay assessment with latent semantic analysis. J. Educ. Comput. Res. **29**, 495–512 (2003)
34. N. LaVoie, J. Parker, P.J. Legree, S. Ardison, R.N. Kilcullen, Using latent semantic analysis to score short answer constructed responses: automated scoring of the consequences test. Educ. Psychol. Meas. **80**, 399–414 (2020)
35. A.H. Shakur, M.J. Holcomb, D. Hein, S. Kang, T.O. Dalton, K.K. Campbell, D.J. Scott, A.R. Jamieson, Large *Language Models for Medical OSCE Assessment: A Novel Approach to Transcript Analysis*, arXiv:2410.12858 (2024)
36. A. Singh, A. Haque, A. Alahi, S. Yeung, M. Guo, J.R. Glassman, W. Beninati, T. Platchek, L. Fei-Fei, A. Milstein, Automatic detection of hand hygiene using computer vision technology. J. Am. Med. Inform. Assoc. **27**, 1316–1320 (2020)

37. S. Matsumoto, H. Kawahira, K. Fukata, Y. Doi, N. Kobayashi, Y. Hosoya, N. Sata, Laparoscopic distal gastrectomy skill evaluation from video: a new artificial intelligence-based instrument identification system. Sci. Rep. **14**, 12432 (2024)
38. S. Al Shuraiqi, A. Aal Abdulsalam, K. Masters, H. Zidoum, A. AlZaabi, Automatic generation of medical case-based multiple-choice questions (MCQs): a review of methodologies, applications, evaluation, and future directions. Big Data Cogn. Comput. **8**, 139 (2024)
39. M. Stadler, A. Horrer, M.R. Fischer, Crafting medical MCQs with generative AI: a how-to guide on leveraging ChatGPT. GMS J. Med. Educ. 41, Doc20 (2024)
40. W. Gan, Y. Sun, S. Ye, Y. Fan, Y. Sun, AI-tutor: generating tailored remedial questions and answers based on cognitive diagnostic assessment, in: *2019 6Th International Conference on Behavioral, Economic and Socio-Cultural Computing (BESC)* (IEEE, 2019), pp. 1–6
41. A. Ghosh, A. Lan, Bobcat: *Bilevel Optimization-Based Computerized Adaptive Testing*, arXiv: 2108.07386 (2021)
42. D.F. Mujtaba, N.R. Mahapatra, Artificial intelligence in computerized adaptive testing, in *2020 International Conference on Computational Science and Computational Intelligence (CSCI)* (IEEE, 2020), pp. 649–654
43. S. Kitto, H.L.M. Chiang, O. Ng, J. Cleland, More, better feedback please: are learning analytics dashboards (LAD) the solution to a wicked problem? Adv. Health Sci. Educ. **30**, 69–85 (2025)
44. D.V. Alvarez, M. Abbiati, A. Bornet, G. Savoldelli, N. Bajwa, D. Teodoro, Assessment of machine learning algorithms to predict medical specialty choice. MedRxiv 2023–2025, (2025)
45. X. Zhang, D. Lin, H. Pforsich, V.W. Lin, Physician workforce in the United States of America: forecasting nationwide shortages. Hum. Resour. Health **18**, 8 (2020)
46. N. Zaki, S. Turaev, K. Shuaib, A. Krishnan, E. Mohamed, Automating the mapping of course learning outcomes to program learning outcomes using natural language processing for accurate educational program evaluation. Educ. Inf. Technol. (Dordr) **28**, 16723–16742 (2023)
47. J. Dexter, G. Koshland, A. Waer, D. Anderson, Mapping a curriculum database to the USMLE Step 1 content outline. Med. Teach. **34**, e666–e675 (2012)
48. P. Densen, Challenges and opportunities facing medical education. Trans. Am. Clin. Climatol. Assoc. **122**, 48 (2011)
49. F.P. Diallo, C. Tudose, Optimizing the scheduling of teaching activities in a faculty. Appl. Sci. **14**, 9554 (2024)
50. G. Keir, W. Hu, C.G. Filippi, L. Ellenbogen, R. Woldenberg, Using artificial intelligence in medical school admissions screening to decrease inter-and intra-observer variability. JAMIA Open **6** (2023)
51. H. Mastour, T. Dehghani, E. Moradi, S. Eslami, Explainable artificial intelligence for predicting medical students' performance in comprehensive assessments. Sci. Rep. **15**, 23752 (2025)
52. Transforming Cardiac Surgery Scheduling at Mayo Clinic with Opmed.ai, (n.d.). https://www.opmed.ai/blog-posts/transforming-cardiac-surgery-scheduling-at-mayo-clinic-with-opmed-ai (accessed July 10, 2025)
53. How AI Assists With Staffing, Scheduling and Once-Tedious Tasks, (n.d.). https://consultqd.clevelandclinic.org/how-ai-assists-with-staffing-scheduling-and-once-tedious-tasks (accessed July 10, 2025)
54. Optimizing Labor Scheduling With Machine Learning, (n.d.). https://timeforge.com/industry-news/the-role-of-machine-learning-in-optimizing-labor-scheduling/ (accessed July 11, 2025)
55. Predictive Scheduling Adjustments: Leveraging Historical Data for Efficient Workforce Management in Healthcare Settings | Simbo AI - Blogs, (n.d.). https://www.simbo.ai/blog/predictive-scheduling-adjustments-leveraging-historical-data-for-efficient-workforce-management-in-healthcare-settings-3265330/ (accessed July 11, 2025)
56. Enhancing Operating Room Efficiency with AI: Insights into Improved Case Volumes and Investment Returns in Healthcare Facilities | Simbo AI - Blogs, (n.d.). https://www.simbo.ai/blog/enhancing-operating-room-efficiency-with-ai-insights-into-improved-case-volumes-and-investment-returns-in-healthcare-facilities-4018138/ (accessed July 11, 2025)
57. How Banner Health uses AI and automation to supercharge ORs, (n.d.). https://www.fiercehealthcare.com/ai-and-machine-learning/banner-health-doubles-down-ai-powered-automation-tech-modernize-its-or (accessed July 11, 2025)

58. B.-H. Kim, S. Sridharan, A. Atwal, V. Ganapathi, *Deep Claim: Payer Response Prediction From Claims Data with Deep Learning*, arXiv:2007.06229 (2020)
59. J.S. Kim, A. Vivas, V. Arvind, J. Lombardi, J. Reidler, S.L. Zuckerman, N.J. Lee, M. Vulapalli, E.A. Geng, B.H. Cho, Can natural language processing and artificial intelligence automate the generation of billing codes from operative note dictations? Global Spine J. **13**, 1946–1955 (2023)
60. K.P. Venkatesh, M.M. Raza, J.C. Kvedar, Automating the overburdened clinical coding system: challenges and next steps. NPJ Digit Med. **6**, 16 (2023)
61. M. Pandey, M. Arora, S. Arora, C. Goyal, V.K. Gera, H. Yadav, AI-based integrated approach for the development of intelligent document management system (IDMS). Procedia Comput. Sci. **230**, 725–736 (2023)
62. A. Khadija, F.F. Zahra, A. Naceur, AI-powered health chatbots: toward a general architecture. Procedia. Comput. Sci. **191**, 355–360 (2021)
63. A.H. Zamzam, K. Hasikin, A.K.A. Wahab, Integrated failure analysis using machine learning predictive system for smart management of medical equipment maintenance. Eng. Appl. Artif. Intell. **125**, 106715 (2023)
64. P.W. Tien, *Department of Architecture and Built Environment Faculty of Engineering Deep Learning-Powered Vision-Based Energy Management System for Next-Gen Built Environment* (2023)
65. R. El-Bouri, T. Taylor, A. Youssef, T. Zhu, D.A. Clifton, Machine learning in patient flow: a review. Prog. Biomed. Eng. **3**, 022002 (2021)
66. C. Brossard, C. Goetz, P. Catoire, L. Cipolat, C. Guyeux, C. Gil Jardine, M. Akplogan, L. Abensur Vuillaume, Predicting emergency department admissions using a machine-learning algorithm: a proof of concept with retrospective study. BMC Emerg. Med. **25**, 3 (2025)
67. M. Deschepper, K. Eeckloo, S. Malfait, D. Benoit, S. Callens, S. Vansteelandt, Prediction of hospital bed capacity during the COVID− 19 pandemic. BMC Health Serv. Res. **21**, 468 (2021)
68. Y.B. Corren, J. Merrill, R. Wilkinson, C. Cannon, J. Bickel, B.Y. Reis, Predicting surgical department occupancy and patient length of stay in a paediatric hospital setting using machine learning: a pilot study. BMJ Health Care Inform. **29**, e100498 (2022)
69. G. Gafni-Pappas, M. Khan, Predicting daily emergency department visits using machine learning could increase accuracy. Am. J. Emerg. Med. **65**, 5–11 (2023)
70. Smarter Healthcare: How AI Is Streamlining Healthcare Supply Chains, (n.d.). https://www.clearfunction.com/insights/how-ai-is-streamlining-healthcare-supply-chains (accessed July 14, 2025)
71. Deep Reinforcement Learning: A Game Changer for Healthcare Inventory Replenishment Strategies | Simbo AI - Blogs, (n.d.). https://www.simbo.ai/blog/deep-reinforcement-learning-a-game-changer-for-healthcare-inventory-replenishment-strategies-2748620/ (accessed July 14, 2025)
72. A. Kaur, G. Prakash, Intelligent inventory management: AI-driven solution for the pharmaceutical supply chain. Soc. Impacts **5**, 100109 (2025)
73. J. Farrington, S. Alimam, M. Utley, K. Li, W.K. Wong, *Many Happy Returns: Machine Learning to Support plAtelet Issuing and Waste Reduction in Hospital Blood Banks*, arXiv:2411.14939 (2024)
74. G. Stahlman, I. Yanovitzky, M. Kim, Design, application, and actionability of US public health data dashboards: scoping review. J. Med. Internet Res. **27**, e65283 (2025)
75. X. Shi, G. Nikolic, S. Fischaber, M. Black, D. Rankin, G. Epelde, A. Beristain, R. Alvarez, M. Arrue, J. Pita Costa, System architecture of a European platform for health policy decision making: MIDAS. Front. Public Health **10**, 838438 (2022)
76. G. Dritsakis, I. Gallos, M.-E. Psomiadi, A. Amditis, D. Dionysiou, Data analytics to support policy making for noncommunicable diseases: scoping review. Online J. Public Health Inform. **16**, e59906 (2024)
77. O.J. Canfell, K. Davidson, L. Woods, C. Sullivan, N.M. Cocoros, M. Klompas, B. Zambarano, E. Eakin, R. Littlewood, A. Burton-Jones, Precision public health for non-communicable diseases: an emerging strategic roadmap and multinational use cases. Front. Public Health **10**, 854525 (2022)

78. O.J. Canfell, Z. Kodiyattu, E. Eakin, A. Burton-Jones, I. Wong, C. Macaulay, C. Sullivan, Real-world data for precision public health of noncommunicable diseases: a scoping review. BMC Public Health **22**, 2166 (2022)
79. A. Sadilek, L. Liu, D. Nguyen, M. Kamruzzaman, S. Serghiou, B. Rader, A. Ingerman, S. Mellem, P. Kairouz, E.O. Nsoesie, Privacy-first health research with federated learning. NPJ Digit. Med. **4**, 132 (2021)
80. M.J. Sheller, B. Edwards, G.A. Reina, J. Martin, S. Pati, A. Kotrotsou, M. Milchenko, W. Xu, D. Marcus, R.R. Colen, Federated learning in medicine: facilitating multi-institutional collaborations without sharing patient data. Sci. Rep. **10**, 12598 (2020)
81. M.A. Camilleri, Artificial intelligence governance: ethical considerations and implications for social responsibility. Expert. Syst. **41**, e13406 (2024)
82. Automated Medical Documentation Review—Cflow, (n.d.). https://www.cflowapps.com/automated-medical-documentation-review/ (accessed July 16, 2025)
83. How AI Agents Automate Clinical Documentation Review for Clinical Managers | Datagrid, (n.d.). https://www.datagrid.com/blog/ai-agents-automate-clinical-documentation-review-clinical-managers (accessed July 16, 2025)
84. Z. Wang, J. Gao, B. Danek, B. Theodorou, R. Shaik, S. Thati, S. Won, J. Sun, *InformGen: An AI Copilot for Accurate and Compliant Clinical Research Consent Document Generation*, arXiv:2504.00934 (2025)
85. N. Oh, J. Kim, S. Park, S. An, E. Lee, H. Do, J. Baik, S.M. Gwon, J. Rhu, G.-S. Choi, Large language model-assisted surgical consent forms in Non-English language: content analysis and readability evaluation. J. Med. Internet Res. **27**, e73222 (2025)
86. W. Hurst, B. Tekinerdogan, T. Alskaif, A. Boddy, N. Shone, Securing electronic health records against insider-threats: a supervised machine learning approach. Smart Health **26**, 100354 (2022)
87. A.H. Seh, J.F. Al-Amri, A.F. Subahi, A. Agrawal, N. Pathak, R. Kumar, R.A. Khan, An analysis of integrating machine learning in healthcare for ensuring confidentiality of the electronic records. Comput. Model. Eng. Sci. **130**, 1387–1422 (2022)
88. D.W. Simborg, Healthcare fraud: whose problem is it anyway? J. Am. Med. Inform. Assoc. **15**, 278–280 (2008)
89. A.A. Amponsah, A.F. Adekoya, B.A. Weyori, A novel fraud detection and prevention method for healthcare claim processing using machine learning and blockchain technology. Decis. Anal. J. **4**, 100122 (2022)
90. N.N.I. Prova, Healthcare fraud detection using machine learning, in: *2024 Second International Conference on Intelligent Cyber Physical Systems and Internet of Things (ICoICI)* (IEEE, 2024), pp. 1119–1123
91. S. Agarwal, An intelligent machine learning approach for fraud detection in medical claim insurance: a comprehensive study. Sch. J. Eng. Technol. **11**, 191–200 (2023)
92. E. Nabrawi, A. Alanazi, Fraud detection in healthcare insurance claims using machine learning. Risks **11**, 160 (2023)

Chapter 5
AI in Dental Diagnostics

This chapter discusses the impact of Artificial Intelligence (AI) on improving diagnostics in dentistry. The chapter describes the ways in which AI-based tools are improving the analysis of dental images, the detection of oral diseases, and ultimately clinical decision-making. The chapter begins with an overview of how AI processes images of different modalities—radiographs, Cone-Beam Computed Tomography (CBCT), and intraoral images— and then assists clinician decision-making throughout the diagnostic process.

The chapter reviews AI's enhancement of imaging through denoising, segmentation, landmark detection, and 3D reconstruction, resulting in more accurate and consistent data from dental structures. The chapter extends this theme of performance improvement in detecting oral diseases through a review of AI in the detection of dental caries, periodontal disease, periapical lesions, oral cancers, and orthodontic conditions. The chapter continues with a review of AI within clinical decision-making support systems.

Practical implications are explored through a review of a few AI platforms (there are many commercial options), and the chapter finishes with limitations such as data bias and regulation, future possibilities (including Federated Learning (FL), teledentistry applications, and ethical issues). By summarizing the current evidence and use cases, the chapter highlights the significant impact of AI on diagnostic accuracy, workflow consistency, and equitable access to care in dentistry, reinforcing AI's role as a critical element in the development of science and practice in dentistry.

5.1 Introduction

An early and accurate diagnosis is the basis of dental practice, defining treatment outcomes and patient quality of life. Multiple dental diseases, from dental caries to benign and malignant oral cancers, have much better outcomes with early diagnosis

L. Tayebi et al., *Artificial Intelligence in Medicine and Dentistry*,
https://doi.org/10.1007/978-3-032-15977-9_5

compared to symptomatic or late-stage diagnosis. For example, the five-year survival rate for oral cancer is 83% when diagnosed early, but only 32% when diagnosed late [1]. However, traditional diagnostic techniques are limited in the discipline of dentistry. Visual-tactile exams and radiographic interpretations are inherently subjective and influenced by inter- and intra-clinician variability. One study reported that early caries could not be consistently identified on radiographs, with dentists showing major disparities in their interpretations [2]. Factors that can affect the interpretation of dental imaging include the experience level of the clinician, the quality of imaging, the light source, and levels of fatigue. Furthermore, even with periodontal assessments, very small modifications to probing technique can influence disease severity classification. These variations underline the importance of employing other tools to support clinicians in their assessments and decisions.

AI may provide a viable means of addressing this issue and potentially enhancing the diagnostic performance of the clinician. AI algorithms, in particular those using Machine Learning (ML) or Deep Learning (DL), learn to detect patterns and features in dental data better than humans, with superhuman levels of consistency. AI algorithms learn from radiographs, images, and patient records as part of big datasets and can identify subtle early signs of disease that the clinician may miss [1]. When diagnosing disease, AI does not become fatigued or biased in the same way that humans may, which could help standardize diagnostic results within and across practitioners. For example, AI algorithms for caries detection have shown equivalent performance to experienced radiologists when detecting lesions on bitewing radiographs [3–5]. Sometimes these AI algorithms even detect developmental proximal caries that a busy practice might find difficult to detect [6].

In addition to increasing accuracy, AI can help with efficiency and workflow in dental diagnosis. AI systems can automate routine tasks related to imaging—for example, they can help capture the best X-ray images or even pre-analyze images before the dentist sees them [7]. In pre-screening radiographs, AI can triage normal imagery from suspicious imagery to save the clinician time. One AI study had a sensitivity of ~99% in filtering out "normal" panoramic films [6] and acted as an extremely reliable gatekeeper for the dentist's attention on a small number of images that would likely indicate pathology. Not only does this type of automation reduce human error, but it also standardizes imaging and its analyses across practitioners. If practitioners use consistent techniques (e.g., AI giving recommended positioning or recommended exposure settings), the diagnostic images coming from an AI-assisted practice show less variability, which translates into increased reliability of interpretations.

Importantly, AI systems do this quickly—for example, a trained Neural Network (NN) can read an entire radiograph in seconds, flagging areas of interest to the dentist for confirmation. This approach allows for augmented intelligence, meaning AI's relentless pattern recognition occurs in conjunction with the clinician's intelligence. Thus, the dentist remains at the center of the decision-making process, and AI's role is that of a clever assistant, ensuring nothing is missed or overlooked and, to the extent possible, every diagnosis is made based on evidence. As such, AI should make dental diagnostics more sensitive (picking up problems at an earlier stage), more specific (fewer false alarms), and, in particular, more personalized by using larger datasets—ultimately allowing the dentist to improve outcomes for their patients through earlier, more accurate recognition of pathology. In conclusion, AI is providing dental diagnostics with untiring eyes and consistently offers an analytical perspective that should elevate the level of care offered by the profession.

This chapter concentrates on how AI can be used as a diagnostic aid in dentistry. Section 5.2 introduces the underpinnings of AI processes in dental diagnostics, followed by sections on specific sectors where AI is having an impact: dental imaging (Sect. 5.3) and dental diagnostic information related to oral diseases (Sect. 5.4: caries, periodontal disease, endodontic lesions, oral cancers, etc.). We then turn our attention to the role of AI-focused clinical decision support systems (Sect. 5.5), which harness and integrate diagnostic data to support and guide clinical decision-making. Section 5.6 reviews a number of AI-based dental diagnostic software applications available in the marketplace today, comparing their functionality and regulations. We then look at adoption barriers and future possibilities in Sect. 5.7. Conclusion remarks are presented in Sect. 5.8. In summary, this chapter illustrates how AI is assisting the scientific development of dental diagnosis and advancing dental practice—with the goal of earlier detection and more consistent, more accurate diagnoses in oral health care.

5.2 Foundations of AI in Dental Diagnostics

AI and ML techniques for dental diagnostic tools follow the same principles of data-driven pattern recognition. Essentially, the AI system learns from examples—specifically, large sets of data related to dentistry—in order to discover features related to health or disease. Chapter 1 addressed algorithms (NN architecture, training paradigms, etc.) in detail, so this chapter focuses on the applications of these techniques. Often in practice, to develop an AI diagnostic tool, the first step is to create a labeled dataset (for example, radiographs that are labeled as having caries or no caries), train an AI model to provide a mapping of inputs (the images) to outputs (the diagnosis), and finally evaluate performance on new examples. Most contemporary dental AI models use DL, usually Convolutional NNs (CNNs), to complete diagnostic tasks focused on images such as lesion detection [2]. These AI models progressively learn hierarchical features—for example, edges, textures, and shapes—which they can use to find pathologies like cavities or periapical radiolucencies on X-rays. NNs have also been used for learning structured data (e.g., replies to survey questions from dental patients, or, as with X-rays, analysis of images and text), but dental imaging diagnosis research has been dominated by CNN-based DL.

In fact, AI in terms of dental diagnostics is derived from many different data modalities, including:

- **2D radiographic images:** The most common input that dental AI models use is intraoral radiographs (bitewings, periapical films, etc.) and extraoral radiographs (e.g., panoramic orthopantomograms). These images reveal hard tissues such as tooth restorations, decay, and bone levels. Large annotated radiographic datasets (in some cases tens of thousands of images) have been used to train AI systems to detect carious lesions and other findings. Lee et al. [6] created an archive of ~ 23,000 panoramic radiographs to train a multi-condition anomaly model. The extensive use of radiographs in dental practice makes them an amenable domain for AI.

- **3D imaging:** CBCT scans provide a volumetric three-dimensional view of dental and craniofacial structures. AI models can analyze CBCT data to perform tasks such as segmenting teeth and alveolar bone, detecting pathological lesions in three dimensions, or assessing anatomical landmarks. 3D information is more complicated because it is higher dimensional, and AI models developed for 3D data are more computationally intensive. Although the dimensionality of 3D data certainly makes its application more complicated, DL models can yield astounding results—for example, fully automatic tooth and bone segmentation on CBCT volumetric data with Dice similarity coefficients > 0.90 [8]. Applications of AI in dental practice will be discussed in more detail in Sect. 5.3.
- **For clinical photographs and optical scans:** Diagnostics are increasingly being conducted using intraoral camera images and extraoral photos of the face (e.g., identifying gingival inflammation or evaluating features of malocclusion). AI is capable of identifying soft tissue lesions and orthodontic markers based on the images' color, texture, and shape features. Examples include capturing high-resolution oral photographs and training algorithms to identify gum disease [9, 10], as well as evaluating malocclusion from standardized smile photographs [11].
- **For textual and tabular data:** Electronic health records (EHRs) contain extensive patient information, including medical histories, demographic data, past diagnoses, and treatment outcomes. ML models can incorporate this data, often in combination with imaging data, for risk predictions (e.g., caries risk) or prognostic modeling. For example, a personalized medicine model might use an ML system that leverages a patient's age, diet, fluoride exposure, socio-medical history, and previous caries experiences to predict the incidence of caries in the future [12, 13]. These risk models provide clinicians with decision support by identifying patients assessed as high risk and suggesting preventive actions. Textual data may also include pathology reports or clinical notes that AI, via NLP, can use to correlate radiographic interpretations with a diagnosis.

Most AI diagnostic systems deal with data regardless of modality. Overall, let us map the process as indicative of a typical approach as defined by field workflow (Fig. 5.1): (1) data acquisition, (2) data processing, (3) AI analysis (diagnosis), and (4) clinical decision support output. The workflow illustrates the processing pipeline as appropriate to the task of radiographic caries. Step 1 is obtaining the relevant data (either taking an intraoral bitewing radiograph or obtaining a set of slices in CBCT). In the data acquisition process, there is a stage of pre-processing or raw data processing to improve quality and prepare the data for analysis [14]. Pre-processing is an important stage in image processing typical of AI-based classifiers and may include noise reduction (diminishing X-ray graininess), contrast

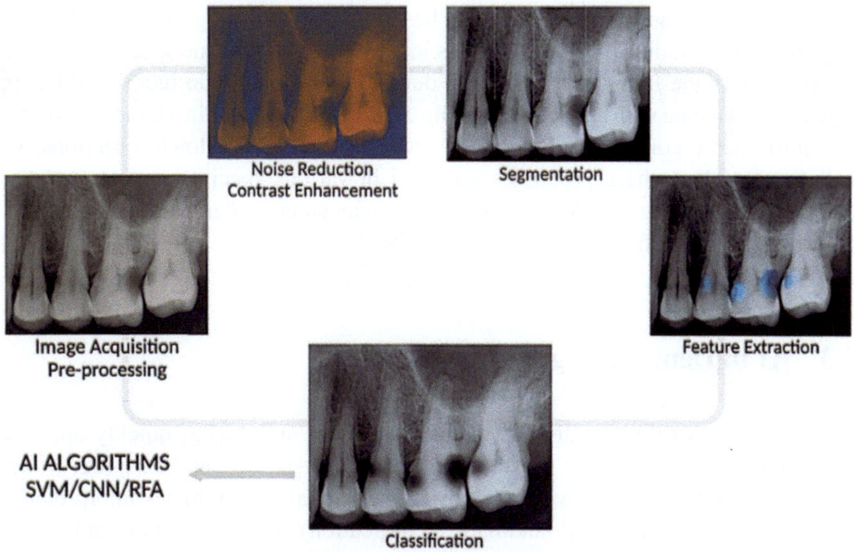

Fig. 5.1 General workflow of an AI-driven dental diagnostic system, illustrated for radiographic caries detection. Reproduced from Anil et al. [14], published in Cureus 15 (2023), under the Creative Commons Attribution 4.0 International License (CC BY), (https://creativecommons.org/licenses/by/4.0/)

enhancement (making lesions clearer), and other adjustments. These pre-processing steps also improve the signal-to-noise ratio for the AI algorithm. Fusing or aligning images from separate data acquisition sources can often be used to combine data for the AI algorithm—for example, using a transillumination image in conjunction with a radiograph may provide useful information. However, multi-modal fusion is still an emerging application in dentistry.

After pre-processing, the core AI analysis takes place. In imaging, this usually consists of segmentation (identifying pixel regions that correspond to anatomical or pathological structures) and classification (determining the presence, absence, or severity of a condition). For example, an AI might segment the outline of a tooth and then classify a region within that tooth as "caries" or "sound." The AI model then produces a diagnostic output—this could be a simple binary result (is there a cavity or not?), a multi-class categorization (Stage II vs. Stage III periodontitis), a continuous risk score, or a fully annotated image denoting all findings.

The last step is to implement this output into clinical decision support. Instead of replacing the dentist's judgment, the goal of current AI systems is to support it. In practice, that means the AI output is communicated to the clinician in a usable manner, such as an alert in the software if an incipient lesion is detected or a visual representation on the radiograph indicating the locations of concern. The dentist can then use this information with a "second opinion" approach to help make their diagnosis. The workflow is typically iterative—the dentist may collect more information (an additional image, clinical test, etc.) based on the AI's suggestions, and the AI may be able to modify its analysis if it is integrated in a real-time space.

At its core, the foundations of AI in dental diagnostics lie in merging different types of dental data with advanced learning algorithms arranged in a logical sequence that mirrors the conventional diagnostic workflow. In the following sections, we will examine how these principles are used in various specific contexts, starting with dental imaging applications (image enhancement, segmentation, etc.) and progressing to specific disease detection tasks.

5.3 AI in Dental Imaging

Imaging plays a role in nearly all dental diagnoses, and AI has quickly emerged as a force multiplier for the enhancement and analysis of dental imaging. In this section, we will discuss how AI improves image quality, automates interpretation (including segmentation and landmark identification), and deliver new and unique ways of acquiring data such as 3D reconstructions. These applications span modalities—including intraoral radiographs and intraoral cameras, panoramic radiographs, CBCT, and extraoral facial photographs.

5.3.1 Image Enhancement and Preprocessing

Enhancing images is one of the earliest applications of AI in imaging. Details may become obscured by noise, low contrast, and artifacts on dental radiographs. AI-based image enhancement approaches, often utilizing DL filters, can help render radiographs clearer by attenuating noise while preserving edges or, conversely, by altering and improving contrast in a contextually aware manner. Traditional approaches such as Gaussian smoothing and histogram equalization are common [14], but learning-based approaches can outperform them by learning the specific noise characteristics of dental X-rays. Furthermore, an NN trained on paired low-dose and normal-dose CT images can learn to mitigate noise in low-dose images while simultaneously improving image quality [15], which allows users, such as clinicians, to utilize diagnostic information while exposing patients to significantly less radiation. Improved image quality increases diagnostic accuracy—for example, AI has a better chance of detecting a periapical lesion if the radiograph is clearer with better contrast. Moreover, preprocessing is often the first step in any AI pipeline (as shown in Fig. 5.1) to ensure that segmentation or detection algorithms receive better input to work from.

5.3.2 *Automated Segmentation of Anatomical Structures*

Segmenting images—i.e., outlining regions of interest such as teeth, restorations, or bone—is a laborious process that AI can perform with great reliability and precision. In image series such as panoramic and periapical radiographs, AI segmentation can separate each tooth from the series and mark each surface where the bone levels are. CBCT images allow segmentation to be performed volumetrically, or over three dimensions, outlining all tooth surfaces and bone locations simultaneously. Recent studies have shown remarkable results in segmenting large CBCT datasets. For example, a fully automatic DL system developed by Cui et al. [8] segmented all teeth and the alveolar bone on more than 4,900 CBCT scans, yielding an average Dice score of 91.5% for teeth and 93.0% for bone—essentially on par with experienced radiologists. Figure 5.2 shows an example of this segmentation performed directly by AI on CBCT images compared with two human experts. This accuracy is clinically valuable because, in this study, AI was reliably able to outline the boundaries of teeth and alveolar bone nearly as well as a human and complete the segmentation process in a few seconds rather than the hours required by humans. The advantage is twofold: processing images quickly is time-efficient and eliminating human variability in measurements (e.g., different bone heights or different lesion sizes) provides consistency across practitioners.

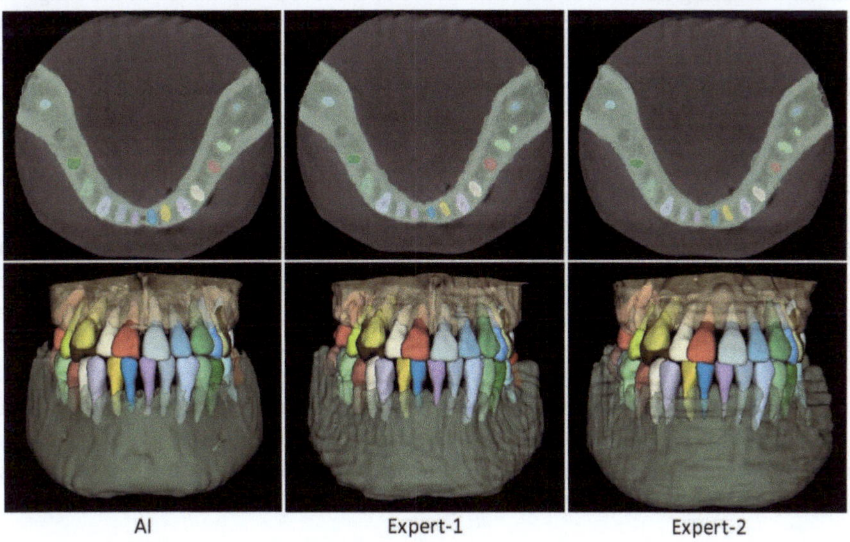

Fig. 5.2 Example of AI-performed segmentation on 3D dental imaging data (CBCT), compared with two human experts. The AI output closely matches expert segmentations. Across 4,938 scans, the AI achieved comparable accuracy (e.g., 0.5% improvement in terms of average Dice similarity coefficient), while significant improvement in efficiency (i.e., 500 times faster). Reproduced from Cui et al. [8], published in Nature Communications 13 (2022) 2096, under the Creative Commons Attribution 4.0 International License (CC BY), (https://creativecommons.org/licenses/by/4.0/)

AI-based segmentation is also important for detecting pathologies. Algorithms can segment lesions of chronic apical periodontitis on periapical radiographs or cysts and tumors on CBCT slices [16]. Abdolali et al. [17] developed a system that automatically segments maxillofacial cysts found on CBCT images. This segmentation work was the first part of their subsequent classification of cyst type. Similarly, segmentation of dental caries on bitewings—or essentially outlining the decay on the image—has also been attempted with DL models (e.g., U-Net versions) that highlight decayed pixels for the dentist's attention [18, 19]. AI segmentation translates pixels into areas of meaning (tooth, lesion, bone, etc.). It converts raw images into structured data, enabling measurement (e.g., dimensions of a lesion, percentage of bone loss) and supporting potential diagnosis.

5.3.3 Landmark Detection and Measurements

Apart from general segmentation, AI also takes the next step by identifying specific anatomical landmarks within images. In orthodontics and orthognathic surgery procedures, cephalometric analysis is performed by identifying many specific points on lateral cephalograms (e.g., Nasion, A-point, B-point, Gonion, etc.). Numerous AI models have been developed to automate the detection of cephalometric landmarks, and an increasing number of these models can achieve mean errors in the range of 1–2 mm, coming very close to human-level performance [20–22]. One example is by Codari et al. [23], who applied a computer-aided system on cephalograms derived from CBCT images to place landmarks. In the context of dental implant planning and assessment with CBCT, AI can also identify the mandibular canal path—an important structure to avoid—using unsupervised or supervised learning. Kim et al. [24], for instance, utilized clustering methods to categorize different paths taken by the mandibular canal in 3D, which can help clinicians evaluate how close nerves may be to their planned surgical sites. Landmark detection can facilitate automation of measurement; for example, AI can locate the cementoenamel junctions and the bone crest on a radiograph, then identify the bone level and automatically measure periodontal bone loss. In one study, a deep network was utilized to identify reference points in periapical images, which allowed measurement of bone level percentages and degrees of periodontal staging that were in substantial agreement with expert evaluation [25]. This automation of measurement may streamline periodic oral exams in the near future, with AI handling the dull measuring tasks while the dentist focuses on interpretation and treatment planning.

5.3.4 3D Reconstruction and Multi-Modal Imaging

Another application is using AI to gather and integrate imaging data into newer and more informative formats. For example, Huang et al. [26] derived lateral cephalometric images from CBCT scans using DL, effectively creating a virtual projection that replicates a cephalometric image without the individual needing a separate radiograph. This is helpful in cases where a CBCT exists, but a cephalometric image is required for orthodontic assessment. Conversely, researchers have attempted to derive 3D information from 2D images. Generative models are capable of producing a 3D dental arch model from two bitewing radiographs or even simple 2D photographs by learning what typical anatomical structures look like. Although not yet precise enough for clinical use, these reconstructions could potentially assist with diagnostics (e.g., visualizing the depth of possible occlusal caries in three dimensions from a bitewing).

Multi-modal AI refers to algorithms that use different types of data inputs—for example, a radiograph and an intraoral photograph—and combine them for a richer analysis. An example of integrated multi-modal diagnostics would be combining radiographs and patient history. An AI may only indicate moderate bone loss on a radiograph as "periodontitis likely" if the patient's EHR documents additional risk factors such as prior tobacco use or medical conditions like diabetes. The possibilities in dentistry remain in their infancy, but much like in general medicine, integrated models demonstrate the ability to draw upon multiple sources to make conclusions. In many cases, multi-modal AI has greater performance than single-source models, as utilizing imaging, lab results, and other variables leads to superior outcomes and recommendations, validating the importance of integrated multi-modal approaches.

5.3.5 Real-Time and Chairside Tools

An immediate benefit of AI for imaging is speed—numerous algorithms can analyze a captured image within seconds of acquisition. This is key to creating real-time diagnostic aids that can be incorporated into daily practice. For example, after taking a bitewing radiograph, a computational overlay might appear moments later, highlighting a lesion in the proximal regions of a tooth that is suspicious for radiolucency. Product development is finally bearing this out, as seen with offerings from Pearl's Second Opinion and Overjet (see Sect. 5.6). These products integrate with dental imaging software and analyze newly acquired images in real time [14]. Programs have also been prototyped for real-time caries detection from intraoral (small handheld) camera images [27]. As the dentist scanned with the camera, it was reported that the AI could identify white-spot lesions or regions of plaque on screen or in live video feeds.

A variation of this concept is research into AI-guided dental implant placement. These systems use both live 3D tomographic imaging (CBCT) and optical 3D trackers to alert the clinician if the drill angle is incompatible with a vital structure. It begins to feel like an AI-enhanced version of surgical navigation [28]. Although these are still experimental implementations, they suggest a future where AI acts as a digital assistant to the clinician during procedures, rather than simply serving as a pre- or post-operative tool. For chairside AI tools to be accepted widely, they need to be highly user-friendly, fast, and seamlessly integrated into workflows. If successfully implemented, AI can enhance efficiency (by absorbing image review tasks) and improve consistency (helping ensure no findings are overlooked), all while keeping the patient in the chair.

In conclusion, we find that AI has already effectively penetrated the dental imaging sequence—from before the image is taken until the diagnosis is made. It can clean up images to enhance clarity and detail, detect and segment regions of interest, measure and identify landmarks, and, simultaneously with image analysis, reconstruct and fuse images to provide enhanced understanding. The next section will transition from the general imaging tasks discussed so far to the diagnostic application of AI aimed at specific diseases or conditions. However, as we will see, many of those applications fundamentally rely on the imaging AI capabilities described in this section. For example, when an AI program detects dental caries on a radiograph, it is, in effect, executing a specialized image segmentation/classification task (caries vs. healthy) for a tooth region, building on the capabilities established here.

5.4 Oral Disease Diagnosis by AI

AI systems have shown very good performance at detecting multiple oral diseases and conditions, arguably at the specialist level. In this section, we address how AI is used in the diagnosis of common dental and orofacial diseases. We first provide a general overview of how AI models detect pathological features using a more general format across a spectrum of imaging modalities. We then examine how these models can be used to identify various conditions, including dental caries, periodontal disease, periapical and endodontic lesions, oral cancer and other potentially malignant lesions, other soft tissue pathologies, and malocclusion or orthodontic diagnoses. In many instances, AI algorithms can interpret radiographic or photographic data to identify pathologies with speed and consistency, and act as a supplementary diagnostic tool. We also review available data comparing AI performance to human expert capacity to demonstrate the current capabilities and limitations of AI systems.

5.4.1 General AI-Based Disease Detection from Dental Images

X-rays are an essential part of dental diagnosis, and radiographic imaging is the place where AI has made its largest impact. Dentistry creates a variety of imaging types—intraoral X-ray images (periapical and bitewing radiographs), extraoral panoramic, cephalometric for orthodontics, and 3D images such as CBCT. Each imaging modality has great visual information encoded, and AI algorithms have been created to interpret all of these modalities [29]. Most of the literature so far has focused on 2D X-ray images, as this is the imaging method most widely used by clinicians [30–32]. AI models (extensively CNNs) have been trained to analyze intraoral radiographs, so caries (tooth decay) can be detected in enamel or dentin [33, 34], periapical darkening indicating endodontic infections [35], or even root fractures [36]. For example, on bitewing X-rays, AI will highlight little interproximal cavities that could be similar to overlapping shadows, which might be indistinguishable to the human eye [19]. Similarly, on periapical films, AI can illustrate areas of periapical darkening suggesting the early stages of an abscess or cyst [37]. The image-analysis systems are a second set of eyes, scanning every millimeter of the radiograph with unwavering focus.

Panoramic radiographs have benefitted remarkably from AI because they document the whole mouth in a single film. A panoramic dental image shows all the teeth, the jaws, the sinuses, and the joints, from a large field of view of diagnostic information [6]. It is difficult even for an expert to examine panoramic images for all possible pathologies (impactions, cysts, tumors, bone loss, etc.). Here, AI-driven detection systems are useful because they can process the complete image in seconds, and ML models can automatically diagnose numerous conditions at once. For example, Lee et al. [6] trained a DL model on approximately 23,000 labeled panoramic images to detect the presence of 17 types of dental anomalies—ranging from impacted and/or supernumerary teeth to residual root and secondary caries. These labeled images are examples of the type of data used (Fig. 5.3). As depicted in Fig. 5.4a, their detection model had four elements. First, the DICOM panoramic images were converted to PNG format, then the anomalies were detected using trained Faster R-CNN models [38]. The models located possible areas of interest by drawing bounding boxes around suspected anomalies (Fig. 5.4b). As indicated in Fig. 5.4c, boxes that fell outside anatomically relevant areas, such as carious lesions outside of a dental region, were removed to promote accuracy. The last step involved converting boxes into polygons, as demonstrated in Fig. 5.4d. This resulted in more precise localization of anomalies while also allowing clinicians to determine not only the type and location of anomalies detected but also their shape and extent. For example, early-stage proximal caries and periapical radiolucency could be detected—conditions that require careful examination to identify even by clinicians—thus demonstrating the early diagnostic potential of AI. Figure 5.4e demonstrates their detection model. This AI model was capable of scanning panoramic images and leaving the normal ones behind with around 99% sensitivity. Therefore, nearly all cases with anomalies were detected [6]. This broad anomaly screening is incredibly useful—a typical algorithm could first make a sweep on any standard imaging and succeed in alerting the dentist to elements that require further attention.

AI is also advancing into other dental imaging techniques. For example, intraoral photographs can be assessed by AI for issues such as measuring dental plaque or lesion detection on soft tissues [29]. Emerging imaging methods, like near-infrared transillumination and imaging based on fluorescence—which can image early enamel

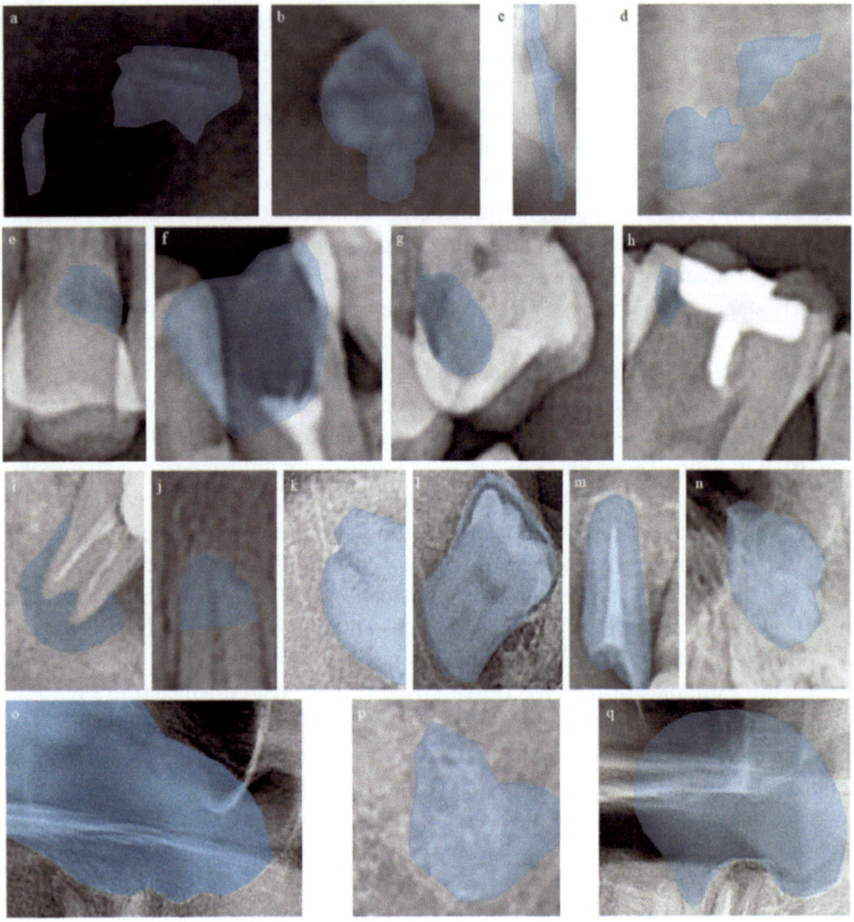

Fig. 5.3 Examples of labeled 17 dental anomalies: **a** calcified carotid atherosclerotic plaque, **b** lymph node calcification, **c** ossification of stylohyoid ligament, **d** tonsillar calcification, **e** cervical caries or abrasion, **f** dental caries or coronal defect, **g** proximal caries, **h** secondary caries, **i** periapical radiolucency, **j** external root resorption, **k** tooth overlapped with mandibular canal, **l** impacted tooth, **m** residual root, **n** supernumerary tooth, **o** mucosal thickening on maxillary sinus, **p** radiopacity in jaw, and **q** retention pseudocyst on maxillary sinus. Reproduced from Lee et al. [6], published in Scientific Reports 12 (2022) 5172, under the Creative Commons Attribution 4.0 International License (CC BY), (https://creativecommons.org/licenses/by/4.0/)

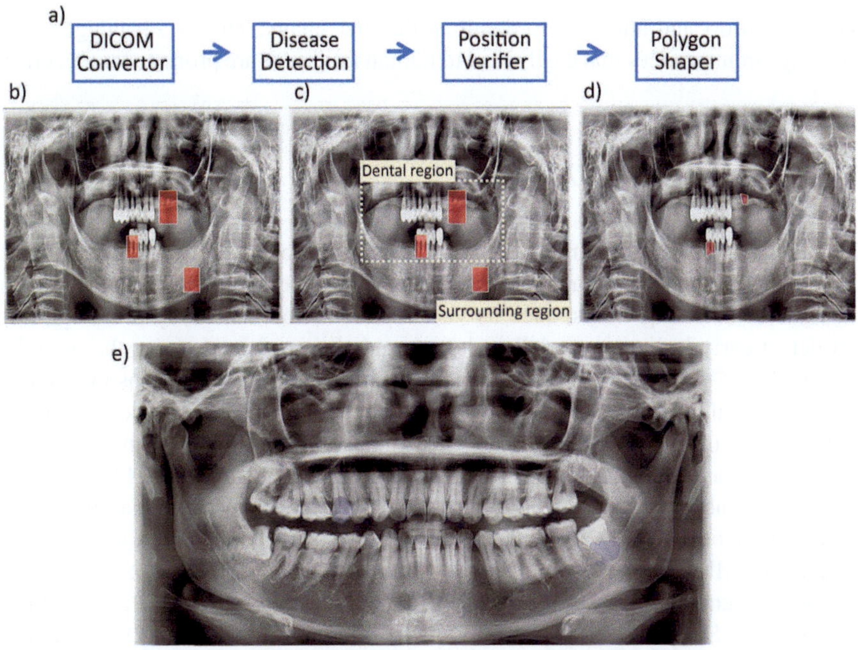

Fig. 5.4 AI-driven anomaly detection on panoramic X-ray images, developed by Lee et al. [6]: **a** overview of the four-stage detection model, **b** output from the disease detection stage, highlighting suspected regions with bounding boxes, **c** position verification step, where anatomically implausible detections—such as carious lesions outside the dental region—are filtered out, **d** polygon refinement stage, providing more precise delineation of anomaly boundaries, and **e** final output example of the model. Reproduced from Lee et al. [6], published in Scientific Reports 12 (2022) 5172, under the Creative Commons Attribution 4.0 International License (CC BY), (https://creativecommons.org/licenses/by/4.0/). Font style and text size were adjusted for improved readability; the figure content is unchanged

demineralization or bacterial activity—will produce images that AI can analyze to detect early carious lesions in a non-invasive manner. Three-dimensional dental images from CBCT scans present greater complexity (due to massive data per scan), but earlier models of AI have been used to automatically segment anatomical features or structures (e.g., the canals used in endodontics or the nerve canals in the jaw) and even detect lesions in 3D. The versatility of AI across these imaging modalities is seen in a recent review, which evaluated a wide range of NN models that commonly used to detect teeth, restorations, caries, endodontic treatments, and more, on alternative datasets of dental images [29]. AI algorithms' ability to adapt to various imaging conditions—from basic 2D X-rays to complex 3D scans—is indicative of their potential as general-purpose dental image interpreters. Importantly, AI's performance in image assessment does not diminish with repetitive work or increased image complexity. For example, an algorithm would assess the tenth image of the day with the same effort and attention to detail as the first image. This is advantageous in imaging circumstances that easily lead to human fatigue or are prone to human error.

5.4.2 Dental Caries Diagnosis

Dental caries is one of the most common diseases globally, and early detection of caries is one of the key areas for potential AI assistance in diagnostics. Traditional methods of detecting caries, such as visual examination and X-ray imaging, may not detect early lesions, especially when there is interproximal caries that may be obscured on X-ray images. AI techniques, especially CNNs, have demonstrated enormous potential to detect carious lesions through the use of intraoral photographs as well as X-ray images. Early studies on caries detection used mainly conventional AI methods applied to dental X-ray imaging. For example, Jusman et al. [39] used K-Nearest Neighbors (K-NN) and Support Vector Machines (SVM) to classify dental caries. In a separate study, Jusman et al. [40] classified dental caries by Multi-Layer Perceptron (MLP) model. Several other studies [41–43] examined NN-based models for caries diagnosis tasks. These models were shallower than modern DL architecture. For example, Sornam et al. [42] proposed a method for dental caries classification. They used Gray-Level Co-occurrence Matrix (GLCM) analysis for feature extraction and applied a Linearly Adaptive Particle Swarm Optimization (LA-PSO) algorithm to optimize a NN's learning rate. Patil et al. [43] introduced a preprocessing workflow based on Morphological Principal Component Analysis (MPCA), followed by classification using NN. Geetha et al. [41] combined feature extraction from GLCM with the gray-level difference method and then compared SVM, K-NN, and NN classification performance, finding that NNs achieved the highest classification accuracy. Collectively, these studies demonstrate the variety of classical ML and shallow NN approaches applied to caries classification and provide the background for many more advanced DL-based approaches developed in recent years.

DL, particularly CNNs, have had a significant impact on improving caries detection. Models based on CNN, without manpower involvement, learn the important features from image data so that the detection of pathology/early lesions is more reliable and sensitive. Various deep CNN architectures have been developed for radiographic caries detection; researchers trained many CNNs on panoramic and bitewing radiographs to classify and localize carious lesions. For example, Bayrakdar et al. [4] proposed a model that used CNN algorithms with U-Net and VGG-16 architecture to automatically segment and detect caries. Their system was tested on 621 anonymized bitewing radiographs and was found to reliably and efficiently detect carious lesions based on the metrics of F-measure, precision, and sensitivity. Lee et al. [44] trained a deep CNN with 3,000 periapical radiographs to automatically detect dental caries with a performance level comparable to experienced dentists (sensitivity in the high 80s% and specificity in the high 80s%). Casalegno et al. [45] proposed a CNN method based on near-infrared transillumination imaging, yielding Area Under the Receiver Operating Characteristic Curve (AUC-ROC) of 83.6% and 85.6% for occlusal and proximal caries, respectively. Cantu et al. [3] used a U-Net-based CNN on 3,686 bitewing radiographs and reported an accuracy of 80% for carious lesion detection. Lakshimi and Chitra [46] used a deep CNN and graph-cut method on 1,700 panoramic dental images, achieving 98.6% detection accuracy. Kumari et al. [47] proposed a hybrid ResNeXt–RNN network that classified tooth images as carious vs. non-carious with an accuracy of 93.67%. Singh and Sehgal [48] proposed a deep CNN-LSTM model based on periapical images for the detection and diagnosis of carious lesions with a G.V. Black classification system, utilizing a Dragonfly optimization algorithm to improve classification performance. Leo and Reddy [49] developed a hybrid NN that combined Deep NNs (DNNs) with stacked sparse auto-encoders and Artificial NNs (ANNs) in a logistic regression (LogReg) context. The hybrid NN was able to effectively classify caries levels across classification performance measures. There was also a unique application of semi-supervised learning to a dental use case developed by Qayyum et al. [2]. They trained a caries detector from an initial group of dentist-annotated dental images on a small subset of images and additional data with no annotations, similar to practices in the real world. Their results indicated high performance with an Area Under a Curve (AUC) of ~0.94 when evaluating for carious teeth even with limited dentist-annotated datasets. More importantly, their work demonstrated that even with unlabeled X-rays, AI can learn from structure in the non-annotated data to help detect dental caries.

Multiple comparative studies have investigated the relative performance of various AI models for the purpose of detecting caries. For example, in Refs. [50, 51], ResNet-50, ResNet-18, DenseNet-121, and EfficientNet-B0 were compared for binary classification tasks. Similarly, other studies [31, 52, 53] compared architectures such as AlexNet, VGG-16, and MobileNetV2 to achieve the same binary classification. Beyond binary classification, a handful of studies explored multiclass lesion classification. Lian et al. [54] performed an initial segmentation step, followed by classification of lesions using DenseNet-121 to classify three levels of caries depth. Zhu et al. [55] and Dayı et al. [56] introduced novel DL methods that classified multiple stages of carious lesions, while Kim et al. [57] implemented a NN that located carious regions and determined the severity of carious lesions in coronal, proximal, and cervical areas, reporting the fastest detection results using the Faster R-CNN framework. Imak et al. [58] used multi-input CNNs that took both raw images and enhanced images as inputs, or ensemble models that combined outputs of multiple CNNs, achieving results of 99.13% accuracy, 98% sensitivity, 100% specificity, and 100% precision in classifying teeth as carious or non-carious based on periapical radiographs.

AI has the ability to assess caries detection modalities beyond radiographs. Specifically, researchers are testing how intraoral photographs can be utilized for caries screening. Deeply trained CNNs can evaluate high-quality oral photos for potential decay on the surfaces. For example, Fig. 5.5 is from the study by Kühnisch et al. [34], who completed a study in which a CNN categorized teeth in clinical photos as no caries, non-cavitated caries, or cavitated caries. They were able to detect caries with an accuracy of ~92.5% (sensitivity 89.6% and specificity 94.3%). While intraoral photos are not yet used routinely for diagnostic purposes, findings such as these demonstrate the potential of AI to allow intraoral photographs to be used as screening tools for caries in patients when radiographs cannot be obtained.

Overall, DL models now consistently show the same accuracy as experienced clinicians in identifying dental caries on common imaging modalities. As training datasets grow and models evolve, AI-enhanced caries diagnoses are ready to be fully integrated into everyday clinical practice to help clinicians in the early management and treatment of dental caries.

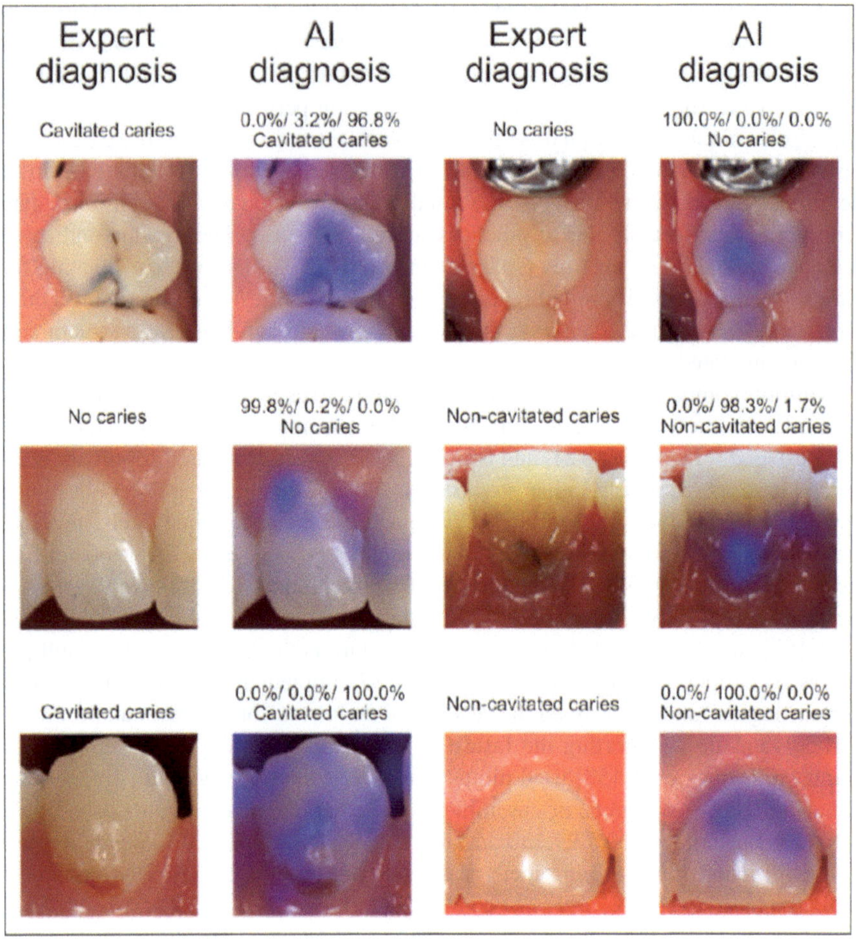

Fig. 5.5 Example intraoral images used for caries detection and corresponding saliency maps highlighting regions of diagnostic relevance (in blue), as identified by the AI model. These outputs illustrate both the interpretability and diagnostic precision of CNNs in clinical image analysis. Reproduced from Kühnisch et al. [34], published in Journal of Dental Research 101 (2022) 158–165, © 2022, with permission from Sage Publications

5.4.3 Periodontal Disease and Alveolar Bone Loss

Various AI-based detection methods have been proposed for use in periodontal diseases (gingivitis and periodontitis) [59–61]. Standard periodontal assessment involves (1) clinical measurements (probing depths or attachment loss) and (2) radiographic evaluation of alveolar bone levels. With AI, the evaluation process can be automated, made more efficient, and improved overall. Algorithms can be used on dental radiographs to detect certain signs of periodontitis, including loss of alveolar bone. By examining the contours and density of alveolar bone in many patients, AI can suggest focused areas for clinicians' review based on the identified areas of bone loss. While AI periodontal assessment cannot replace human clinicians, it may represent a more thorough and quantitative assessment of periodontal health by measuring bone levels for each tooth on a radiograph in a consistent manner [7, 62, 63]. Early research provides evidence that AI is capable of distinguishing between radiographs based on categorical periodontal severity (no, mild, moderate, and severe, based on bone loss) with good agreement with expert periodontists [64]. This can help ensure that periodontal disease is assessed, diagnosed, and treated at early points in the disease, which can help prevent tooth loss.

There are many studies in literature that have applied CNNs to assess periapical and panoramic radiographs for measuring crestal bone levels and have found comparable performance to expert reviewers [65, 66]. Krois et al. [67] trained a DL model with thousands of panoramic dental radiographs to classify the level of bone loss and found substantial agreement with periodontists in classifying the severity of the cases. Kabir et al. [25] described an integrated AI framework that first performed tooth segmentation and numbering on full-mouth intraoral radiographs, then measured bone levels in association with the new periodontal staging system. The AI's bone loss measurements translated into correct periodontitis stage classification with approximately 90% accuracy.

Beyond imaging, AI is addressing gingival condition detection using optical imaging. Gingivitis—inflammation of the gums—is observable by visual evidence of redness, swelling, and plaque. Researchers have developed DL models that detect gingival states of inflammation, as well as the presence of dental calculus and plaque, from traditional color photographs of the mouth. Figure 5.6 shows one example: a multi-task CNN that classifies an image for gingivitis and simultaneously maps localizations of problem areas [9]. The model was trained on a total of 3,932 photos of mouth collected from 625 patients and produced AUC scores of 87.11% for detecting gingivitis and 80.11% for calculus and plaque. Specifically, the model was capable of creating localization heatmaps that indicate where gingival inflammation or deposits exist, with visual explanations of its predictions. After outperforming general-purpose CNNs on these tasks, the model illustrated how DL can effectively be adapted for large-scale, non-invasive periodontal screening. It is noteworthy that patients may soon have smartphone apps allowing them to capture a photo of their gums and receive an AI-supported pre-diagnosis for gingivitis or to determine if a dental visit is needed. For example, Garg et al. [68] developed a lightweight CNN

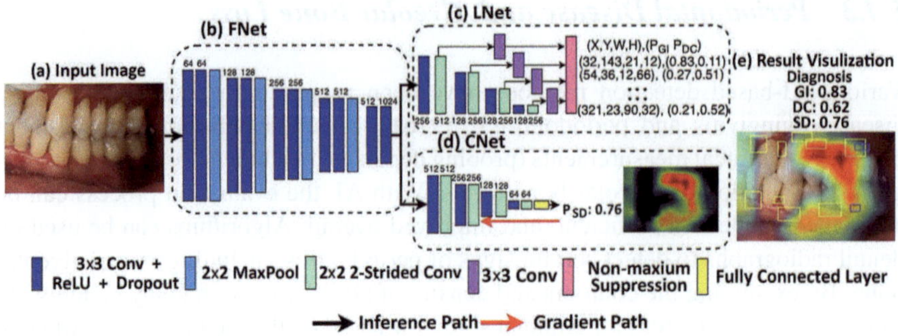

Fig. 5.6 Example of an AI model analyzing an oral photograph to detect gingival disease. The multi-task CNN outputs both the probabilities for diagnosis, as well as the locations of the detections with heat-maps and bounding boxes (GI = gingivitis, DC = dental calculus, SD = soft deposits). Reproduced from Li et al. [9], published in Scientific Reports 11 (2021) 16,831, under the Creative Commons Attribution 4.0 International License (CC BY), (https://creativecommons.org/licenses/by/4.0/). Font style and text size were adjusted for improved readability; the figure content is unchanged

(MobileNetV3) in a mobile app for detecting calculus and demonstrated accuracy exceeding 72%. While a larger ResNet34 model increased accuracy to ~82%, this suggests the inherent trade-off between model complexity and the ability to run it on mobile and portable devices.

AI can help not only in detecting disease presence but also in staging periodontal disease. For example, Chang et al. [69] created a DL model that not only detected periodontal bone loss on radiographs but also staged periodontitis severity, with performance comparable to periodontists. This means that AI can classify how extensive the disease is (slight, moderate, or severe periodontitis) as well as potentially track disease progression over time.

As a whole, AI systems now cover the range of periodontal diagnostic procedures—from detecting gingivitis in photographs, to quantifying bone loss and calculus detection on X-rays, to segmentation of diseased areas. These AI systems have demonstrated accuracy that is often clinically equivalent to that of a human and hold valuable potential for improving early periodontal problem identification. With increasing numbers of image datasets (photographic, radiographic, etc.) and increasing diversity in populations represented in datasets, we expect even more sophisticated periodontal AI systems will emerge. Such AI could be embedded within dental practice management software or new patient smartphone apps to facilitate consistent and regular monitoring of periodontal health outside of the dental office.

5.4.4 *Periapical and Endodontic Lesion Detection*

Identification of periapical radiolucencies (which typically indicate periapical infections or periapical cysts) is another area wherein ML models help diagnostics. These lesions can be subtle and may be easily missed on radiography, especially if they are small or obscured by anatomical structures. Models have been developed to survey X-rays and identify probable periapical lesions [70–72]. For example, a DL system may outline the periapical portions, delimiting the radiolucent area at the root apices, and even attempt to distinguish between different etiologies (e.g., granuloma vs. cyst vs. scar). A study by Yilmaz et al. [73] examined computer-aided diagnosis that successfully differentiated periapical cysts from keratocystic tumors on CBCT, with impressive reliability and accuracy in the 90% range. In another example, Lee et al. [6] developed an AI system that detected periapical lesions on panoramics as part of a multi-anomaly detector, where the model achieved 99% sensitivity in filtering out normal images (i.e., identifying or flagging any image that had anomalies, including periapical lesions). Clinically, this means that AI may serve as a triage approach in identifying and reporting the presence of periapical lesions, justifying and prompting recall of patients for further assessment and/or treatment of the periapical region.

In endodontics in particular, there is growing interest in using AI to assess the quality of root canal treatments via X-rays as well [74, 75]. At the diagnostic stage, the presence of a dark area at the root tip (a possible abscess or cyst) is significant, and AI could provide an objective measure of lesion size and density. Moreover, by using unsupervised ML methods to analyze patterns of the mandibular canal, an expanding lesion might be correlated with increased risk of nerve involvement if there is significant non-uniform growth [24]. Therefore, AI can ensure that no "hidden" lesion is missed on radiographs and can offer standardization to the often arbitrary and inconsistent process of radiographic periapical diagnosis.

5.4.5 *Oral Cancer and Oral Lesions*

In the field of oral medicine, AI is being used for the detection of Oral Potentially Malignant Disorders (OPMDs) and oral cancers from captured images. The ability to detect Oral Squamous Cell Carcinoma (OSCC) early—often by identifying the presence of suspicious lesions such as erythroplakia or leukoplakia—improves outcomes; however, general dental practitioners often struggle with recognizing subtle signs in the early stages. AI tools that use DL applied to photographic images have demonstrated capability in assisting with this issue. For example, a study conducted in 2020 developed a deep CNN that could analyze photographic images of oral mucosal lesions and achieved approximately 90% sensitivity in differentiating early OSCC lesions from their benign equivalents [76]. Chauveron et al. [77] reviewed recent studies utilizing automated AI approaches to detect OSCC and noted impressive performance, with consistently reported sensitivity above 85% and accuracy over 90% from datasets averaging about 1,000 images.

Most recently, Li et al. [1] developed an AI model to analyze images taken from a portable electronic oral endoscope specifically for cancer detection. In their work, they implemented a U-Net approach to segment the lesion area and subsequently employed a ResNet-34 classifier, achieving a precision of 96% on the test set for identifying cancerous lesions (recall was much lower, with an F1 score of ~ 0.58). Figure 5.7 shows an example of such a system, comparing an AI-predicted mask to the true lesion area on intraoral images. In some studies, AI assists in very early oral cancer detection—empowering low-resource situations by using smartphone cameras and cloud-based back-end analysis methods [78, 79].

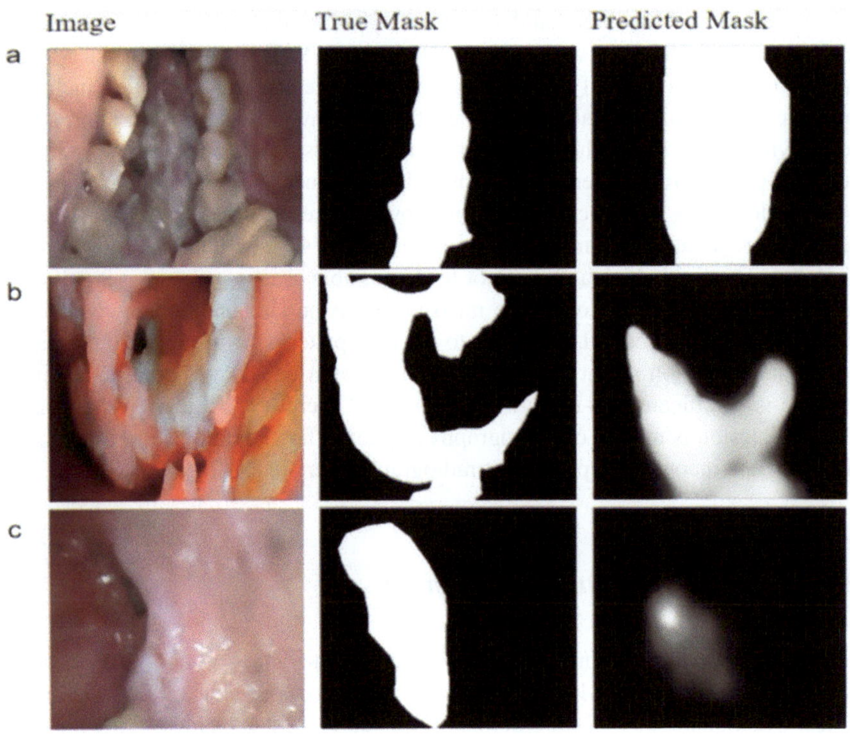

Fig. 5.7 AI-based detection of oral cancer from intraoral images, showing a comparison of ground truth vs. model prediction for lesion segmentation. Each row **a, b, c** represents a different oral lesion case. In each row, the left image is the original intraoral photograph of the lesion, the middle image is the true mask (expert-annotated area of the lesion, shown in white), and the right image is the AI model's predicted mask for the lesion (white areas are predicted as cancerous). **a** The predicted mask shows some differences compared to the true mask. **b** The prediction differs slightly, likely due to complex or unclear lesion boundaries. **c** An example of a more significant mismatch between the predicted and true masks, highlighting areas where the model's predictions need further refinement. Reproduced from Li et al. [1], published in BMC Oral Health 24 (2024) 1468, © 2024, with permission from Springer Nature

While AI cannot serve as a biopsy (the gold standard for definitive diagnosis), it can be an effective screening and triage tool. For example, an AI app for detecting oral lesions could be used by general dentists or even health workers to capture oral lesion images. If AI suggests a "high-risk" flag, the lesion could then be referred swiftly for specialist review and biopsy [79, 80]. In addition, AI can help reduce false reassurance. It has been established that generalists frequently underdiagnose or misdiagnose many oral lesions, but an AI system— after being trained on many cancers and precancer images—may highlight subtle but concerning features that a clinician might otherwise overlook, such as a small red patch on the lateral tongue.

5.4.6 Other Soft Tissue Lesions

In addition to cancer, the oral cavity is host to various soft tissue lesions (benign tumors, ulcerative lesions, fungal infections, etc.) that AI may be able to detect. There are a number of studies, for example, that use AI to classify conditions such as aphthous ulcers, lichen planus, and candidiasis from photographs [81–83]. In addition, several studies report that CNN-based models have reached rates of 90% + accuracy when classifying tongue lesions and conditions from photographic datasets [84, 85]. This suggests that AI could be very useful for oral medicine specialists.

Another interesting use case is assessing gingival health. AI models have been created with gingival images that can classify levels of inflammation (healthy vs. gingivitis vs. periodontitis) based on the color or texture of the gingiva [59, 86]. One of these models achieved greater than 90% accuracy in classifying gingivitis from intraoral photographs [86]. Rana et al. [87] took a different perspective and developed an automated segmentation process for gingival disease classification from oral images, essentially outlining areas of gingival response such as redness and swelling in photos. This has the potential to provide an objective measure of gingival inflammation over time.

Importantly, AI can also identify dental plaque on teeth using high-definition images or photos of teeth with disclosing agents [88, 89], and has the potential to score oral hygiene levels for both patient education purposes and clinical studies. Although these applications are less mature than radiographic assessments, they indicate a vision of a future where a full oral screening (hard and soft tissues) could be augmented by AI—a patient's gum health, plaque amounts, and mucosal lesions could be automatically assessed based on an image sequence of standard mouth photos or a standard intraoral scan.

5.4.7 Malocclusion and Orthodontic Diagnosis

Traditionally, understanding the presence and classification of malocclusion (Class I, II, III, etc.) has been a qualitative skill; however, AI is bringing quantitative methodology to this field. Using various datasets of orthodontic records (photographs, cephalograms, dental casts), AI models have been able to learn to identify features of malocclusion and classify the cases. Kim et al. [90] utilized a deep CNN model to classify skeletal relationships from lateral cephalograms, with the AI model achieving a high level of agreement (kappa ~ 0.91) with standard Ceph measurements for Class I/II/III classification. In terms of case classification, their AI achieved ~ 0.94 sensitivity and ~ 0.96 accuracy, exceeding prior automated Ceph analysis software. Kim et al. [91] engaged a multi-channel CNN on 3D CBCT data to classify skeletal malocclusion classes and achieved > 90% accuracy for each class.

In addition to skeletal class, AI has also been utilized on panoramic radiographs to identify impacted canines or enumerate supernumerary teeth [92–94]. In the 3D realm, there are systems analyzing either digital orthodontic models or CBCT data to classify arch forms and the degree of crowding. For instance, Ryu et al. [95] applied DL to categorize the degree of dental crowding with promising results, with a mean error comparable to that of orthodontists.

In the context of malocclusion, AI can quickly process an extensive array of diagnostic records and produce an initial classification and even suggest subsequent treatment. Orthodontic diagnosis is inherently multifactorial in terms of data (Ceph + pano + photos + models), and it seems AI is going to provide us with the ability to combine this information. In fact, commercial software is now being produced that will automatically deliver cephalometric analyses and treatment simulations. CephX (ORCA Dental AI) automatically marks optimal cephalometric landmarks and provides growth forecast superimpositions to assist clinicians in diagnosis and treatment sequencing. They have regulatory approval for these capabilities [96–98].

When we evaluate AI performance vs. human experts in these domains, the common conclusion is that AI is often at least as good as a typical expert and more reliable, but not necessarily better than the best expert in all cases. In the case of caries and bone loss detection, AI's higher sensitivity means it detects more true lesions (and in some cases, produces more false positives). Dentists may be more specific (fewer false positives), but they might miss borderline cases; therefore, benchmarking against AI can help alleviate that issue. AI's performance on more complex processes involving cephalometric landmarking or tooth segmentation is unequaled, because AI completely avoids the chances of human error and, of course, is faster. In areas of more "subjective" diagnosis and evaluation, such as oral lesion evaluation, the accuracy of AI will depend on the training data (if it has good-quality, biopsy-proven, labeled data, then AI will provide high accuracy; if it does not, then AI's performance will be less than acceptable).

Importantly, it is worthwhile to point out the benefits of integrating AI with clinical expertise, rather than using AI alone. Evidence tends to suggest that the accuracy of diagnosis is much better supported when clinicians have an AI tool to consult.

Put another way, the combination of human expertise and AI pattern recognition can work better than relying on either one alone. Experiential evidence based on radiology already exists and holds in dental diagnostics anecdotally—using AI as a support tool has led to more correct calls by dentists (especially in edge cases such as incipient lesions or subtle bony changes). So, it can be safely concluded that our goal is not putting AI up against dentists; the goal is to integrate AI into the diagnostic workflow to improve the level of care across the board.

We will examine how this integration can be achieved in the following section on clinical decision support systems, and we will also address implementation struggles, such as ensuring AI works well across representative patient populations and imaging condition domains to prevent biases. But as an evolution snapshot circa 2025, there is already evidence that AI is detecting nearly all common dental diseases as well as, or even better than, specialists in research conditions, and real-world use of AI capability and competence is constantly being added to clinical solutions.

5.5 AI in Clinical Decision Support

Clinical decision support systems for dentistry are computerized interactive software programs that aid practitioners in making decisions regarding diagnosis and treatment. AI has added new capabilities to dental decision support systems, particularly on the diagnostic side. In essence, an AI-based decision support system can take input from a variety of patient data, including images, history, and clinical findings, and provide the dentist with a prompt and/or alert that brings attention to its findings, including identifying a probable condition, predicting the likely risk for future disease, and/or providing clinicians with an explanation for any suggestions based on patient information. This section illustrates how AI-based decision support capabilities are incorporated for diagnostic issues.

5.5.1 Risk Prediction and Personalized Diagnostics

Decision support does not only include determining current status—AI is also being utilized to predict future oral health risks and deliver personalized diagnostics. Caries risk assessment is a key example. CAMBRA, one of the traditional approaches, identifies caries risk using professional judgment and patient responses to questionnaires to classify people as low, moderate, or high caries risk. On the other hand, ML can identify patterns of data that would otherwise go unnoticed by human judgment. By analyzing variables including social determinants of health, medical history, dietary information, fluoride exposure, etc., an ML system can construct individual risk profiles that may trigger an early intervention [12].

For example, Kang et al. [13] presented an ML system, "DCP," that utilized features like age, gender, and past caries experience to identify people at high risk for developing dental caries. Ramos-Gomez et al. [99] conducted a similar study to assess early childhood caries risk based on caregiver responses using a Random Forest (RF) algorithm, also providing predictive information regarding the presence of active caries, as well as assessing the presence of caries history for children aged 2–7. Sadegh-Zadeh et al. [100] expanded on this line of inquiry by comparing different models based on data from 780 parent–child pairs, and found that the RF and MLP models were optimal for identifying children at increased risk, reinforcing the benefits of modeling diversity in pediatric risk stratification. Similarly, Park et al. [101] explored national health survey data from over 4,000 children to model caries risk using several ML approaches.

These studies illustrate the capacity of AI to improve traditional caries risk assessment methods by strengthening predictive frameworks based on behavioral and demographic data along with clinical data. The potential of AI to move us away from traditional diagnostic modes, via data-driven and individualized diagnostic approaches, offers substantial opportunities for improving early intervention practices in dental care.

5.5.2 EHR Integration and Comprehensive Support

To maximize the effectiveness of AI decision support, it must be part of the clinician's work process and, ideally, built into practice management or EHR software. In this situation, the AI system has the appropriate access to the patient's file in the EHR (with appropriate privacy controls) and ideally requires the ability to read and write relevant information. For example, as the dentist reviews the chart of the patient, there is an "AI summary" pane that may say: "Last X-ray: no abnormalities; Caries risk: low; Periodontal risk: moderate (evidence of gingivitis noted at last exam); Oral cancer screening: 1 photograph flagged for review." Imagine that this dashboard summary provides immediate, at-a-glance decision support for the clinician before the dentist even begins the exam.

Some products are moving toward this ideal. For example, Overjet's dental AI reported that its platform integrates with practice management systems and can automatically extract and analyze all radiographs [102]. Another example could be AI that listens to conversations between the clinician and patient, then transcribes any notes (Denti. AI has an FDA-cleared device to transcribe dental conversations [103]). Transcription isn't diagnosis, but it does fulfill the task of contributing data that the AI algorithms can index (like recording a patient's complaints of sensitivity, which an AI may link to radiographic findings). AI that is integrated can also guarantee that decision support is offered in the right place and at the right time. For instance, when picking patients for recall, it could prompt staff by saying: "Patient X is due for a full-mouth series. It's been 5 years," or "Patient Y had a watch on tooth 18; maybe we should consider an X-ray to check it." Providing prompts like this could increase adherence to diagnostic protocols and follow-ups.

A key new frontier in decision support is explainability—making the AI's rationale transparent to the user. In healthcare, the importance of explainability cannot be overstated, both in terms of trust and legality; clinicians need to understand why the AI is telling them something before they can responsibly take action. Explainability can take many forms—saliency maps, heatmaps, or class activation maps—showing the areas of an image that contributed to the AI's decisions. For example, if the AI said, "possible fracture on root of tooth 12," an explainable approach would highlight the specific area of the root with a heatmap and fracture line that led to the conclusion. This transparency gives the dentist an opportunity to confirm the finding. Figure 5.8 is an example of Explainable AI (XAI) via class activation maps in an orthodontic scenario; in this example, it shows the areas that the AI model "looked" at in cephalometric images when classifying jaw relationships. In the successful classifications, the AI's attention (the red zones) was on the relevant areas (the jaws or occlusion), while in the failure case, it was either all over the image or focused on totally irrelevant areas (which showed the AI was confused) [90]. These visualizations help the clinician discern whether the basis of the AI appears plausible or misaligned due to image artifacts or confounding factors. In conclusion, explainability is a crucial element of AI decision support that preserves human oversight and trust.

5.5.3 A Case Scenario for an AI Decision Support in Action

A great way to demonstrate this is through a case example. Let's take the new patient exam, where the dentist has taken a panoramic radiograph and intraoral photos. The AI clinical decision support system immediately flags that there are green markers on several teeth for calculus, a red marker at an upper molar root tip indicating a possible periapical lesion, and an asymmetry in a mucosal patch on the tongue based on facial photographs. It also extracts information from medical history (identifying that the patient has Type II diabetes, a risk factor for periodontal conditions). It flags: "Generalized moderate calculus noted; could be prudent to have a complete periodontal assessment. Suggest a pulp vitality test (and diagnosis regarding tooth #15); also shows a radiolucency at the apex." Additionally: "Unusual lesion in photo; could be prudent to further evaluate." The dentist, with this awareness prompt, pursues further examination and identifies subgingival calculus, bleeding, with the intraoral AI-calculus detection assisting in quick identification of a preliminary periodontal diagnosis. The dentist does a pulp test on tooth #15, identifying it as non-vital, confirming a need for endodontic treatment that could not have waited. The dentist examines the lesion on the tongue and might take the step of referring the patient for a biopsy, perhaps capturing a dysplastic change in the early phase. In this case, the AI did not make any decisions, but it ensured that the dentist would not miss any of these findings and that the decisions the dentist made had evidence, where applicable, and were prioritized.

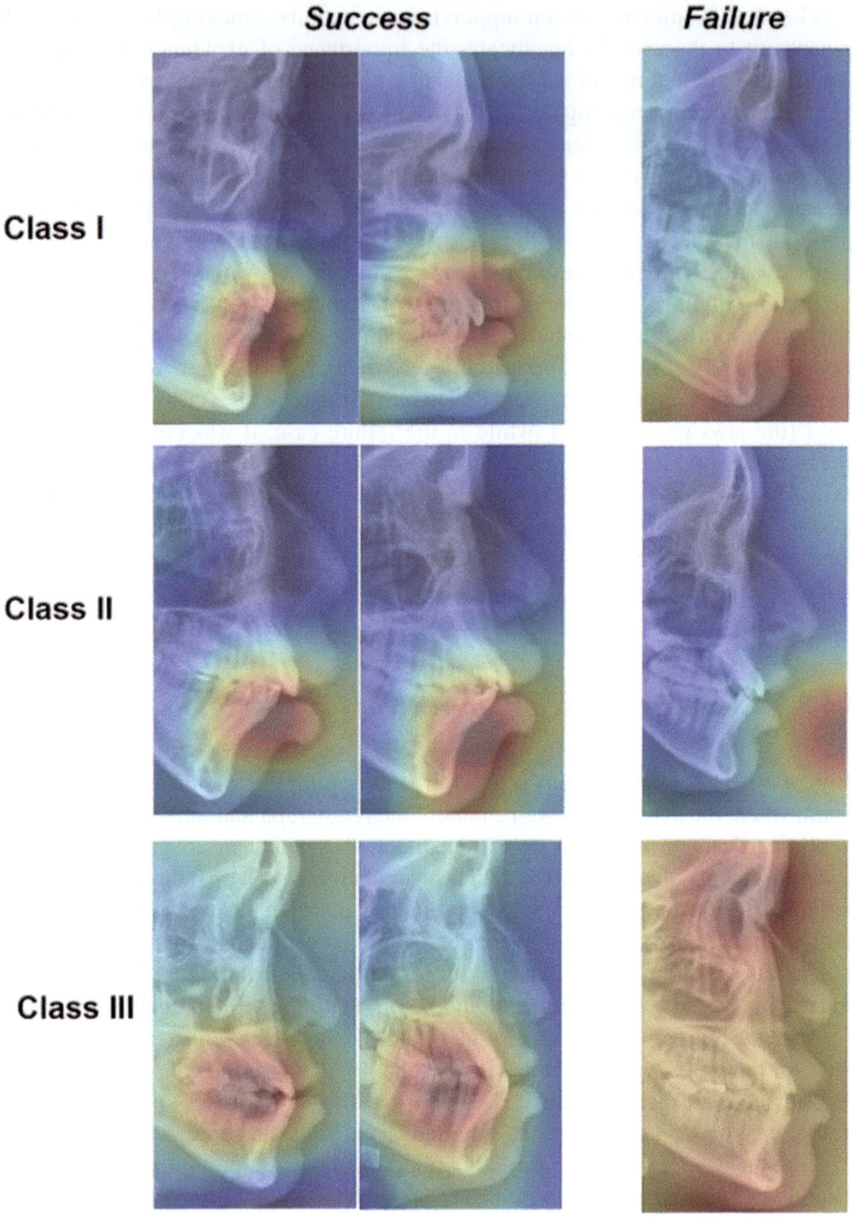

Fig. 5.8 Class activation maps illustrating XAI in a diagnostic context. The figure shows where the AI model is focusing its attention. Reproduced from Kim et al. [90], published in Scientific Reports 12 (2022) 11,659, under the Creative Commons Attribution 4.0 International License (CC BY), (https://creativecommons.org/licenses/by/4.0/)

Lastly, we should mention that human oversight is important. In any situation, the dentist is ultimately responsible for the final diagnosis and treatment plan, regardless of how advanced the AI may be. AI in decision-making is similar to an assistant—knowledgeable, but not perfect. The dentist should have the ability to appraise the decision-making of the AI, whether the information was generated by a human colleague or an AI system. For example, if an AI indicates "cavity here," and the dentist has no radiographic or clinical evidence of a cavity, they should trust their judgment and possibly obtain a second human opinion or imaging. It is the dentist, for instance, who appreciates that they know the patient's story and context—something an AI may not account for (AI does not have the ability to consider patient symptoms unless specifically identified, such as describing pain, etc.). As a result, effective engagement of AI decision support is dependent on establishing a balance—specifically, perceiving this system qualitatively as an assistant, and not as a way to yield an audited outcome without using judgment. The role that explainability plays in this stance (as we have discussed previously), and aspects of how the system is set up to function (such as having the AI suggest or highlight a particular diagnosis rather than automatically charting a diagnosis without the clinician reviewing it first), are crucial.

In summary, AI in clinical decision support for dental diagnostics holds promise for improving consistency, highlighting omissions, predicting risks, and overall augmenting the clinical decision process. Technology has the potential to analyze imaging in combination with EHR data to provide broader context. Technology will have the most impact when integrated seamlessly into clinical workflows and processes, and when the system is transparent in providing the rationale supporting its suggestions. The next Sect. (5.6) will provide some insights into actual commercial systems currently available to implement many of these capabilities, and later in Sect. 5.7 we will discuss challenges including accuracy, validity, bias, and acceptance by clinicians. But, whether we like it or not, we have seen that AI is becoming a co-pilot for dentists to elevate the standard of care for diagnostic care across all clinical settings.

5.6 Commercial AI-Based Diagnostic Software in Dentistry

Over the past years, several specific AI software tools have been designed and released for use in dental practices as part of the transition from research into clinical reality. These AI tools usually augment either radiographic viewing software or software used to keep track of the details of a dental practice, acting as an AI assistant during the patient exam to aid the evaluator. Three noteworthy examples include [14, 102–107].

- **Pearl® (Second Opinion):** an FDA-cleared, AI-based radiographic interpretation tool that is leading the transformation of dental diagnostics. Pearl's platform analyzes dental X-ray images provided by the dentist and identifies multiple common pathologies of interest with delineated annotations in a matter of seconds. The powered core of Pearl integrates an advanced DL model trained on millions of dental radiographs from hundreds of sources to provide reliable and consistent identification of features such as caries, periapical lesions, and periodontal bone loss. Pearl essentially generates a visual "second opinion" for the dentist and highlights areas on the image that may represent a cavity between teeth, a change in bone level, or similar findings. By bringing precision and consistency to radiographic analysis, Pearl helps standardize diagnostic quality and experience across practitioners and clinics. The key goal of Pearl is never to replace the dentist's clinical judgment, but to ensure that details are not overlooked—it is an aid designed to reduce the risk of human error or oversight. In practice, when a dentist takes bitewing images during a check-up, Pearl can almost immediately mark any questionable lesions for the dentist to review. This can be particularly useful for new clinicians or when reviewing difficult images. The end result is improved accuracy and confidence, with the dentist remaining in control of the final diagnosis.

- **Overjet:** another FDA-cleared AI product designed for dental radiograph analysis. Overjet software integrates with digital radiography systems to analyze images in real time, often even before the dentist has a chance to chart their findings. Utilizing DL algorithms trained on thousands of dental X-rays, Overjet can identify and quantify various conditions such as caries and periodontal bone loss. Overjet doesn't just mark a cavity—it may also provide an estimated depth of the lesion, or quantify a tooth's bone support in millimeters. This adds a quantifiable dimension to diagnostics. With more detail comes improved objectivity and consistency. Observers have noted that Overjet can help tremendously with inter-observer reliability, since it provides a standardized set of analyses that every dentist can rely on. In a busy multi-doctor office, Overjet ensures that whether Dr. A or Dr. B interprets a patient's X-ray, the process is consistent and comparable to the same criteria. It serves as an efficient and consistent diagnostic assistant, and many clinicians use Overjet's output to explain findings to patients (e.g., showing the areas highlighted by AI directly on the X-ray). Through its attention to detail and standardization, Overjet has established itself as one of the leaders in applying AI to dental diagnostics.
- **Denti.AI®:** Denti.AI offers a collection of AI-enabled applications for dentistry, including Denti.AI Detect—an FDA-cleared radiographic analysis platform—and additional tools such as a voice-based charting function. In October 2023, Denti.AI Detect received FDA 510(k) clearance as a full imaging solution to support clinicians in identifying common dental conditions (e.g., carious lesions, periapical lesions, and bone loss) on intraoral and panoramic radiographs. Notably, Denti.AI Detect is the first AI application to receive FDA clearance for disease detection on panoramic images. Clinical studies showed that its use contributed to a 26% increase in treatment opportunities identified by dentists in participating practices. Denti.AI Detect also integrates with the previously approved Denti.AI Auto-Chart (approved in 2022), which automatically charts restorations, crowns, root canals, implants, and missing teeth. Together, these tools enhance diagnostic

accuracy, speed charting, and optimize workflows when integrated with Practice Management Systems (PMS). Like Pearl and Overjet, Denti.AI provides outputs and analyses that inform clinical decisions; however, the responsibility to interpret findings in the patient's context and make the ultimate diagnostic decision remains with the dentist.

Early reports from practices using such tools indicate a positive effect on diagnostic catch-rates (finding problems that might otherwise have gone undiagnosed). Additionally, for patient communication, many patients find it engaging and convincing to see AI-flagged X-rays, which often increases their trust in the diagnosis and their follow-through with the dentist's recommended treatment. Collectively, these tools underscore that AI is assistive technology. All operate under the understanding that the human dentist ultimately takes final responsibility, while AI plays the role of guide and analytical support [14]. As AI tools become more commonplace, it is likely that software such as Pearl, Overjet, and Denti.AI will become as ubiquitous in dental offices as digital X-ray sensors—quietly operating in the background and contributing to the quality of care.

5.7 Challenges and Future Directions

In this section, we discuss the challenges related to the use of AI in dental diagnostics, including data bias, transparency, regulatory and legal issues, and workflow integration. We then outline future research directions for AI, such as improving explainability and justification of AI outputs, applying FL to expand the reach of AI without compromising privacy, using AI to support tele-dentistry, and designing and implementing ethical dental AI systems.

5.7.1 Challenges

Data bias and fairness: A fundamental struggle in AI is that biased data biases the model. In dentistry, a given example could be that if the AI was trained on radiographs from one demographic, or one clinic setting, it may perform less well on other demographics or dental imaging contexts. For example, if the AI was trained predominantly on pediatric patients, the differences in anatomy and presentation of lesions seen in the radiographs of pediatric patients differ from what is seen in adults. If the AI had not seen children's presentations, it would miss caries on primary teeth and may lack confidence with images of mixed dentition. There are differences in imaging modalities and quality as well. For example, the AI may have done well on radiographs produced from a digital sensor, yet not transfer well to those produced from a film radiograph, or if trained predominantly on high-resolution images, it will not produce equally credible results when faced with lower-resolution images.

We can avoid data bias issues by ensuring the training dataset is as representative as possible, including age, ethnicity, severity of disease, sources of images, and so on [14]. An example of a documented bias in medical AI was the poorer performance of tools in underrepresented minorities. In the field of dental AI, we could say we build a model that attempts to predict risk for periodontitis; without a developer being aware, if the training dataset had most of the smokers grouped in the periodontitis group, it could pick up on a proxy, such as "presence of nicotine staining" in the teeth in the photo, that may not generalize or may be biased against certain patients.

Bias is also relevant to the quality of the labels. If a "gold standard" incorporated human biases—for instance, if a group of people had consistently been undertreated in the past (or at least not treated the same as others)—AI can learn those human biases. For example, it is important for developers to regularly audit their models by looking at error distributions across sub-groups (groups that should be treated differently, like children versus adults). Good practice would also include keeping diversity in test sets and potentially employing techniques like re-weighting or data augmentation to mitigate skewed distributions that will emerge in the test set. Fairness implies that a model should work similarly for all patients. In our example—would you want an AI that is outstanding for the adult population but clearly under-detects caries in the child population, or vice versa? It will be important for regulators and those in research, and the dental community more widely, to be aware of potential bias in emerging AI systems. If, for example, a dentist notices a pattern that the AI consistently performs poorly with radiographs taken from a specific X-ray unit, any feedback should be shared with developers to improve the reliability and fairness of the system.

Model transparency and the "black box" problem: Many AI models, particularly DNNs, exist as black boxes. They work in a manner that is not easily understandable or interpretable; they make decisions based on "reasoning" we cannot easily discern. This lack of transparency is particularly troublesome in the healthcare setting, where we need to understand the reasoning of a decision made with DL every bit as much as the decision itself. The XAI techniques mentioned earlier, such as class activation maps, provide some visibility into areas the model is attending to [90].

However, true transparency is ultimately challenging, as a network may be reasoning based on pixels that associate with a disease without humans seeing a clear behavior or pattern. For example, an AI could potentially learn a very subtle gray-level pattern in radiographs that indicates early caries. The decomposition of a processing pathway could be flagged as an area of reasoning, but a dentist could still conclude, "I'm not sure why those pixels matter." Trust is the obstacle here, and it shouldn't be so difficult to design our AI-trained pathways to limit interpretation and build trust with users. We could constrain the decision pathways of AI to improve interpretability and trust. For example, rather than a single-step monolithic CNN, we could use a two-step process, first interpreting the image via segmentation, and then classifying the representation based on segmentation.

One way to sidestep plain vanilla black-box AI is to use rule-based AI or hybrid approaches with domain knowledge. The rules could state interpretable things such as "if bone loss exceeds 30% in more than two teeth, periodontitis is probable," which is interpretable. The drawback is that you might be missing out on the complete potential of unconstrained ML and this will create tension—the best models could also be the least interpretable or explainable. The dental space might find a happy medium—using AI for tasks where the black-box concept is acceptable (e.g., measuring something automatically or flagging an area for you to look at) while retaining the final diagnosis with a human who can rationalize it. In other words, let AI enhance vision, perception, and cognitive processing, but let the human apply reasoning to make the final judgment. That way, even though the AI is an opaque box, it's running implied AI as advanced triage or added value, not as an autonomous diagnostician. Regardless, greater transparency will be an important goal—and an even more important consideration for AI that gives recommendations such as "extract vs. endo," which have implications that should be backed by a rationale.

Regulatory and legal considerations: The introduction of AI into clinical practice raises questions regarding liability and regulatory approval. If an AI misses a diagnosis, and the dentist also misses the same diagnosis, who is responsible if harm is caused? Generally, liability will fall on the practitioner—current regulations envision AI as just another tool (e.g., an X-ray unit, probe, or other diagnostic/therapeutic tool). The dentist is responsible for using the tool appropriately, which will generally mean the dentist is liable for the diagnoses made ultimately [108]. Practitioners should stay involved (always verify AI findings) to be aware of any risks.

Regulators, such as the FDA, expect evidence for safety and efficacy of AI tools—we have seen that multiple dental AI (as well as other AI technologies) have moved through this process. One particular regulatory issue with AI is with "adaptive," or self-learning, AI. The FDA clears the "locked" version of AI algorithms (the version tested); if the algorithm "learns" from cataloged data such as cases and histories, this adaptive algorithm may form a new device classification requiring clearance. This poses a regulatory problem, as one of the advantages of AI is to improve through learning as more cases are analyzed—for instance, more accurately analyzing future radiographs. However, continuous change makes certification very difficult. A potential intermediate approach may be periodic updates (similar to software updates) that undergo validation.

Another regulatory piece is data privacy, and any training and subsequent use of an AI system typically requires large amounts of patient data, requiring adherence to Health Insurance Portability and Accountability Act (HIPAA) and similar regulations. Approaches like FL have been developed for AI training without aggregating patient data in one location, which is more privacy protective.

Workflow integration and human factors: From a human point of view, the introduction of AI into dental clinic workflows is certainly not simple. Some form of change management is necessary. Dental teams will need training in interpreting AI outputs, communicating them with patients, and balancing the extent to which they are relying on the technology. Alert fatigue might be one of the obstacles. Sometimes, when the AI flags too many findings deemed irrelevant, users may find themselves ignoring its suggestions, much like how many software alerts are disregarded out of habit. Calibration is essential, as an AI system's sensitivity and specificity may need to be adjusted so that they achieve the best results for clinical practice. Such settings may even be adapted to individual clinics. For example, some offices may instruct the AI to be less sensitive to caries detection to avoid false positives that would cause undue concern for patients, while others might want to maximize sensitivity.

Making sure that the AI can be used at the proper workflow stage is another concern in workflow integration. By the time the dentist begins an exam, for example, the AI analysis should be ready rather than still processing. Speed often becomes a demand for computing infrastructure (be it cloud or local). In fact, some offices have experienced slow networks that delayed AI results, frustrating the end user. Hence, integration must factor in some IT solutions: good internet, and maybe local AI servers.

One more factor would be human trust: Studies from other fields have shown that when AI systems make a small number of errors, users tend to either over-trust the system (considering all outputs correct) or under-trust it by discarding its results after just one or two demonstrated errors. Training and experience yield calibrated trust—dentists would initially double-check all AI suggestions, then through consistency, they could discern when to rely on them or be skeptical. Developing that very nuanced understanding is crucial and suggests that AI tools may need guidance on their known limitations.

5.7.2 *Future Directions*

Explainable and human-centric AI: AI systems in the near future will become transparent and interactive. One trend is to build explainable interfaces for AI software, giving a brief textual explanation for each prediction. This means that there would be a natural language explanation for the output, making the result easy to understand. Likewise, the AI may also show a few similar instances from the past. For example: "This looks like Lesion X; here are some images in a database that were confirmed to be the same." This offers the dentist some context. Such features build trust and comprehension.

FL and data collaboration: Collecting very large and diverse datasets while ensuring patient privacy remains the biggest hurdle to advancing dental AI. FL is the process by which an AI model can be trained on data from multiple institutions without that data ever leaving the institution. For instance, 100 dental clinics could collaborate in training a caries detection model by locally calculating updates to the model on their own images, then sending those updates, rather than the raw images, to a central server where they are aggregated into a better model. This approach has the potential to unlock access to huge quantities of data that are currently siloed in practice management software. It also addresses privacy because patient images do not leave local servers. Dental software companies can provide dental software plugins for FL, whereby clinics opt to contribute to a common AI model and receive the improved model periodically. This would provide assurance that AI is being trained with an ever-larger, up-to-date distribution of data, e.g., new conditions (if a new type of restoration or material comes into practice, the AI would become aware of how to handle it). The challenge is organizing such efforts, ensuring standardization of local labeling of data, and managing any legal/ethical approval required for use of patient data for model training.

AI and tele-dentistry: Tele-dentistry grew especially when in-person consultations were limited (for example, during the COVID-19 pandemic). AI can enhance tele-dentistry as it enables remote diagnosis. For example, a patient can upload smartphone photos of a lesion or have an intraoral scan via a home device; AI can filter those in advance and either give a preliminary diagnosis or highlight which tele-consults are a priority. In areas or countries that lack dental professionals, an AI triage system could support non-dental healthcare workers in deciding which patients to refer—just as AI is used in tele-dermatology to screen skin lesions for possible cancer. Already, there are startups that offer AI-based smartphone applications for evaluating the alignment of teeth (for orthodontic follow-up) [109, 110] or cavity checkups [111] with the help of specialized camera adapters. The future might involve patients routinely using an AI app at home that reports back to them saying, "All good, no apparent issues," or "Possible cavity starting on upper left—suggest you see a dentist." Dentists would need to be included in signing off on such consumer-facing devices, but if done right, this could add significantly to preventative treatment and early diagnosis.

Ethical Collaboration and Design: As dental AI becomes more ubiquitous, ethical concerns must drive its design. That entails secure treatment of patient data (robust anonymization, cybersecurity that guards against AI systems getting hacked), protection of patient autonomy and consent (patients should at least be informed when AI is used in their diagnosis and possibly allowed access to the AI-derived results if they want such a record). One more ethical issue is the narrowing of the digital divide—not every clinic, especially those in rural or low-income areas, may be in a position to pay for the latest AI. AI could serve to widen healthcare disparities if it is not accessible. Interdisciplinary partnerships among industry, professional societies, and academia can help by potentially developing some open-source AI software to make available for use by all at low cost (for basic diagnostic assistance) or subsidizing deployments in underserved communities. Professional dental societies can also set standards for the use of AI so that quality is ensured and abuse is prevented (e.g., alerting against too much dependency or use of experimental apps).

Multi-modal AI decision-making: Another exciting area of future research is multi-modal AI decision-making, combining radiographic interpretation with patient history, genetic data, saliva biomarkers, and more to provide a full diagnostic or risk assessment. For example, consider an AI that takes into account radiographs and EHR data and suggests: "Patient has several risk factors for aggressive periodontitis, and the radiographic pattern of bone loss looks aggressive; refer to specialist." Such integrated guidance would be highly beneficial and is not far off as AI techniques that can handle heterogeneous data improve.

Continual learning systems: The future will most likely involve continual learning systems using AI that get better the more a specific clinic uses them. For example, if the dentist repeatedly marks AI-suggested false positives as "not a cavity," the system could learn the nuance of that clinic's imaging or that dentist's thresholds and adapt.

That's hard because of regulatory constraints (technically an adapted device would be considered new), but perhaps local adaptation might be allowed if it's within some safety margins. More work must be done to figure out how to allow safe adaptation of AI without losing control.

In conclusion of this section, while current AI systems are already highly performant, careful testing must be done to maintain and improve their performance in actual conditions. The problems of bias, transparency, and integration are being tackled proactively by the community. All future advancements should make AI more collaborative, transparent, and equitable. Vision is an AI-facilitated dental practice in which technology assists at each step, ranging from screening and diagnosis through patient education and follow-up, without undermining the core position of the dentist's human judgment and expertise.

5.8 Conclusion

AI is ushering in a new age of dental diagnostics—one of greater consistency, productivity, and even enhanced accuracy in the identification of oral health issues. In this chapter, we have discussed how AI is being applied throughout the spectrum of dental diagnostics, from imaging analysis to clinical decision support, and we have examined today's reality and tomorrow's trajectory for these technologies.

In short, accurate and prompt diagnosis is essential in dentistry, and AI offers tools to overcome some of the limitations of traditional methods. Educated on large sets of radiographs, images, and clinical histories, AI systems are able to recognize disease patterns with incredible speed and objectivity. In Sect. 5.2, we set out the pillars of dental AI—ML algorithms that take in various forms of data (2D X-rays, 3D scans, text data) and integrate with a diagnostic workflow from image capture to final decision support. Understanding this pipeline is required to better understand how much AI can be made to fit into existing practices. For instance, the instant an X-ray is obtained, AI can pre-process it, scan it for any abnormality, and display the findings to aid the dentist in arriving at a decision.

Section 5.3 highlighted that AI has found particularly firm roots in dental imaging applications. We might see that AI algorithms can enhance images (e.g., filtering radiographs to clean them of noise), outline anatomical structures such as teeth and bone on 2D and 3D images with accuracy comparable to experts [8], and identify landmarks and measurements automatically that used to occupy much clinician time. Intraoral cameras, panoramic radiographs, and CBCT scans, even facial scans, are now being augmented by AI—whether through real-time caries detection using an intraoral camera or automatically performed cephalometric analysis for orthodontic treatment planning. The ability of AI to reconstruct 3D models and integrate information from different imaging modalities enables more complete diagnostics; for example, a combination of a CBCT and a facial scan can be used to analyze both hard and soft tissue harmony. Real-time chairside devices, though still in the work, demonstrate the promise of AI providing feedback in real-time during patient examination.

In Sect. 5.4, we discussed some of the oral diseases and how AI can help in identifying them. AI is now able to correctly identify dental caries on radiographs, often identifying lesions that go unnoticed by dentists [6], and does so consistently from patient to patient. In periodontal disease, AI can measure bone levels on X-rays and even classify periodontitis, standardizing an area that has otherwise been prone to subjective variation [25]. We also saw how AI is being used to diagnose periapical lesions, with some models being capable of distinguishing between classes of lesions on CBCTs [17]—a task that typically requires expert judgment. Importantly, AI is branching out into oral medicine and can assist in screening for oral cancer or other mucosal lesions by examining clinical images [1]. Orthodontic diagnosis benefits as well, as AI diagnoses malocclusion from X-rays or pictures and automates measurements, allowing orthodontists to focus more on treatment planning than on plotting points. Throughout these examples, we are comparing AI against human ability and have found that under controlled testing, AI will match or slightly beat average expert performance in specialized tasks (like detecting a cavity), although the marriage of AI and dentist remains the optimal scenario.

Section 5.5 discussed the integration of AI into a clinical decision support system. Rather than viewing AI as an isolated diagnostician, we view it as part of a human-AI combined team. AI can provide real-time alerts (e.g., "possible calculus on lower molars" while doing a prophy exam), risk assessments (i.e., utilizing big data to suggest who is likely to develop new caries or who is at risk of periodontal deterioration [12]), and even help synthesize patient data into a shared body of information. XAI and human oversight were emphasized as essential—the dentist is the decision-maker and AI's role is to inform and aid. By making AI's reasoning more transparent (e.g., heatmaps or an explanation in textual form), we ensure that clinicians can evaluate AI's suggestions and maintain their trust. Decision support AI already has proven to have the potential to reduce missed diagnoses, increase the speed at which we chart and document, and offer another layer of comfort for patients and providers. Patients like to have a "high-tech" second opinion involved in their treatment, while providers appreciate the added safety it brings.

We then examined commercial AI systems in Sect. 5.6 using the examples of Pearl, Overjet, and Denti.AI. These are not just laboratory prototypes—they have received FDA clearance and are being used in "real-world" practice. They encapsulate the move in dental diagnostics research towards practical application, that is, evidence that AI in the context of diagnosis has progressed beyond theory as an aid for clinicians. Each system offers clear utility and each behaves differently. They are also responsive to systems of regulation—as now a number of AI tools have received regulatory approval to the extent that they are safe and effective as a clinical aid. The uptake is increasing, and tools like the examples we discussed in the chapter gain further development by being integrated with ways of working within practice.

Section 5.7 was dedicated to the important cautionary perspective—on the key challenges involved in the implementation of AI systems, but also on future directions for responsible and effective integration. Challenges such as data bias require effort and management—AI needs to be fair and effective for all patient demographics. We have also discussed transparency concerns, and how different XAI approaches can help. The regulatory and legal landscape will keep evolving—and an important take-away is the idea that AI is a clinician-directed tool, not a replacement for clinicians. Integration aspects of AI remind us that tech adoption is as much about people as it is about software. Training and trust, as well as workflow design, all need consideration to maximize AI benefits.

In the future, AI will likely become even more integrated and pervasive in dentistry—pervasive in that it can quietly assist nearly every diagnostic process, and integrated in that it becomes seamless, natural, and intuitive to use. We can think of this as similar to the way drivers brake without thinking about how their anti-lock braking system works—drivers just trust that it works, and in fact, it works quickly and accurately. Similarly, AI in dentistry will have the potential to become a trusted assistant, working quietly behind the scenes. Increased integration and use of AI will likely occur in preventive dentistry, as well as in public health—analyzing community-level datasets to implement approaches to health disparities—and in education, where dental students may incorporate AI feedback into their instructional program to make an 'interpretation' of a radiograph by using AI, and through AI, increase the student's learning curve. Federated and collaborative AI development may help democratize these types of tools across the planet, not just in high-end dental clinics but in any situation where this type of digital dentistry infrastructure exists, whether a simple health facility or a high-performance setting.

In summary, AI technology in dental diagnostics has tremendous potential to improve oral health care. Patients will benefit from earlier detection, more harmonious diagnosis, and possibly lower costs via improved efficiencies of care. For dental practitioners, it has the potential to minimize routine functions as well as offer some reassurance that nothing has been overlooked, allowing practitioners to truly focus on their clinical decision-making in interpreting and communicating complex information and decision-making with the patient—things that AI cannot really do. On the other hand, when the time is ripe to start integrating AI into the delivery of dental diagnostics, a salient consideration will be to assess how we can do that and still maintain ethical practice, due diligence, and criticality with AI, and above all, how we center the dentist-patient relationship. AI is a strong aide, but not a magic bullet. Ultimately, the clinical judgment of a human dentist and their ability to foster empathic therapeutic relationships and rapport remain irreplaceable.

In conclusion, the future of dental diagnostics will likely feature a partnership between the human practitioner and AI, with each playing to the other's strengths; however, as has been indicated, the best diagnostic tool may not be AI in isolation, but the dentist using AI—combining human intuition and knowledge with AI's exactitude. If we responsibly embrace AI and other technologies as they evolve, the dental profession can improve the quality of patient care, pave the way for proactive, precise, and patient-centered dentistry, and obtain better health outcomes while doing so. Ultimately, the responsibility now falls on us—the dental profession (clinicians, developers, regulators, educators)—to continue the conversations and collaborations so that AI is advanced and implemented in ways that truly advance science, education, and clinical practice in dentistry. There will be no shortage of new and exciting advancements in the coming years, and the chapters of dental history yet unwritten will involve AI as a key player in the story of enhancing oral health for all.

References

1. L. Li, C. Pu, J. Tao, L. Zhu, S. Hu, B. Qiao, L. Xing, B. Wei, C. Shi, P. Chen, Development of an oral cancer detection system through deep learning. BMC Oral Health **24**, 1468 (2024)
2. A. Qayyum, A. Tahir, M.A. Butt, A. Luke, H.T. Abbas, J. Qadir, K. Arshad, K. Assaleh, M.A. Imran, Q.H. Abbasi, Dental caries detection using a semi-supervised learning approach. Sci. Rep. **13**, 749 (2023)
3. A.G. Cantu, S. Gehrung, J. Krois, A. Chaurasia, J.G. Rossi, R. Gaudin, K. Elhennawy, F. Schwendicke, Detecting caries lesions of different radiographic extension on bitewings using deep learning. J. Dent. **100**, 103425 (2020)
4. I.S. Bayrakdar, K. Orhan, S. Akarsu, Ö. Çelik, S. Atasoy, A. Pekince, Y. Yasa, E. Bilgir, H. Sağlam, A.F. Aslan, Deep-learning approach for caries detection and segmentation on dental bitewing radiographs, Oral Radiol (2022) 1–12.
5. W. Panyarak, K. Wantanajittikul, W. Suttapak, A. Charuakkra, S. Prapayasatok, Feasibility of deep learning for dental caries classification in bitewing radiographs based on the ICCMSTM radiographic scoring system, Oral Surg Oral Med Oral Pathol. Oral Radiol. **135**, 272–281 (2023)
6. S. Lee, D. Kim, H.-G. Jeong, Detecting 17 fine-grained dental anomalies from panoramic dental radiography using artificial intelligence. Sci. Rep. **12**, 5172 (2022)
7. A.M. Batra, A. Reche, A new era of dental care: harnessing artificial intelligence for better diagnosis and treatment, Cureus **15** (2023)
8. Z. Cui, Y. Fang, L. Mei, B. Zhang, B. Yu, J. Liu, C. Jiang, Y. Sun, L. Ma, J. Huang, A fully automatic AI system for tooth and alveolar bone segmentation from cone-beam CT images. Nat. Commun. **13**, 2096 (2022)
9. W. Li, Y. Liang, X. Zhang, C. Liu, L. He, L. Miao, W. Sun, A deep learning approach to automatic gingivitis screening based on classification and localization in RGB photos. Sci. Rep. **11**, 16831 (2021)
10. Y. Liu, Y. Cheng, Y. Song, D. Cai, N. Zhang, Oral screening of dental calculus, gingivitis and dental caries through segmentation on intraoral photographic images using deep learning. BMC Oral Health **24**, 1287 (2024)
11. H. Zhang, C. Liu, P. Yang, S. Yang, Q. Yu, R. Liu, The concept of AI-assisted self-monitoring for skeletal malocclusion. Health Informatics J. **30**, 14604582241274512 (2024)
12. B.T. Çiftçi, F. Aşantoğrol, Utilization of machine learning models in predicting caries risk groups and oral health-related risk factors in adults. BMC Oral Health **24**, 430 (2024)
13. I.-A. Kang, S. Ngnamsie Njimbouom, K.-O. Lee, J.-D. Kim, DCP: prediction of dental caries using machine learning in personalized medicine, Applied Sciences **12** (2022) 3043
14. S. Anil, P. Porwal, A. Porwal, Transforming dental caries diagnosis through artificial intelligence-based techniques, Cureus **15** (2023)
15. Y. Ma, B. Wei, P. Feng, P. He, X. Guo, G. Wang, Low-dose CT image denoising using a generative adversarial network with a hybrid loss function for noise learning. IEEE Access **8**, 67519–67529 (2020)
16. K. Hung, C. Montalvao, R. Tanaka, T. Kawai, M.M. Bornstein, The use and performance of artificial intelligence applications in dental and maxillofacial radiology: A systematic review. Dentomaxillofacial Radiology **49**, 20190107 (2020)
17. F. Abdolali, R.A. Zoroofi, Y. Otake, Y. Sato, Automatic segmentation of maxillofacial cysts in cone beam CT images. Comput. Biol. Med. **72**, 108–119 (2016)

18. S. Ying, B. Wang, H. Zhu, W. Liu, F. Huang, Caries segmentation on tooth X-ray images with a deep network. J. Dent. **119**, 104076 (2022)
19. S. Lee, S. Oh, J. Jo, S. Kang, Y. Shin, J. Park, Deep learning for early dental caries detection in bitewing radiographs. Sci. Rep. **11**, 16807 (2021)
20. M.-J. Kim, Y. Liu, S.H. Oh, H.-W. Ahn, S.-H. Kim, G. Nelson, Automatic cephalometric landmark identification system based on the multi-stage convolutional neural networks with CBCT combination images. Sensors **21**, 505 (2021)
21. R. Chen, Y. Ma, N. Chen, L. Liu, Z. Cui, Y. Lin, W. Wang, Structure-aware long short-term memory network for 3D cephalometric landmark detection. IEEE Trans. Med. Imaging **41**, 1791–1801 (2022)
22. A. Gupta, O.P. Kharbanda, V. Sardana, R. Balachandran, H.K. Sardana, Accuracy of 3D cephalometric measurements based on an automatic knowledge-based landmark detection algorithm. Int. J. Comput. Assist. Radiol. Surg. **11**, 1297–1309 (2016)
23. M. Codari, M. Caffini, G.M. Tartaglia, C. Sforza, G. Baselli, Computer-aided cephalometric landmark annotation for CBCT data. Int. J. Comput. Assist. Radiol. Surg. **12**, 113–121 (2017)
24. Y.H. Kim, K.J. Jeon, C. Lee, Y.J. Choi, H.-I. Jung, S.-S. Han, Analysis of the mandibular canal course using unsupervised machine learning algorithm. PLoS ONE **16**, e0260194 (2021)
25. T. Kabir, C.-T. Lee, L. Chen, X. Jiang, S. Shams, A comprehensive artificial intelligence framework for dental diagnosis and charting. BMC Oral Health **22**, 480 (2022)
26. Y. Huang, F. Fan, C. Syben, P. Roser, L. Mill, A. Maier, Cephalogram synthesis and landmark detection in dental cone-beam CT systems. Med. Image Anal. **70**, 102028 (2021)
27. B. Ding, Z. Zhang, Y. Liang, W. Wang, S. Hao, Z. Meng, L. Guan, Y. Hu, B. Guo, R. Zhao, Detection of dental caries in oral photographs taken by mobile phones based on the YOLOv3 algorithm. Ann Transl Med **9**, 1622 (2021)
28. K.P. Huynh, G. Mangui, From Tradition to Technology: Robotic Artificial Intelligence in Dental Implantology, Cureus **16** (2024)
29. S.S. Alharbi, H.F. Alhasson, Exploring the Applications of Artificial Intelligence in Dental Image Detection: A Systematic Review. Diagnostics **14**, 2442 (2024)
30. A.A. Al Kheraif, A.A. Wahba, H. Fouad, Detection of dental diseases from radiographic 2d dental image using hybrid graph-cut technique and convolutional neural network, Measurement **146** (2019) 333–342
31. M.M. Lakshmi, P. Chitra, Classification of Dental Cavities from X-ray images using Deep CNN algorithm, in: 2020 4th International Conference on Trends in Electronics and Informatics (ICOEI)(48184), IEEE, 2020: pp. 774–779
32. F. Liu, L. Gao, J. Wan, Z.-L. Lyu, Y.-Y. Huang, C. Liu, M. Han, Recognition of digital dental X-ray images using a convolutional neural network. J. Digit. Imaging **36**, 73–79 (2023)
33. E.Y. Park, H. Cho, S. Kang, S. Jeong, E.-K. Kim, Caries detection with tooth surface segmentation on intraoral photographic images using deep learning. BMC Oral Health **22**, 573 (2022)
34. J. Kühnisch, O. Meyer, M. Hesenius, R. Hickel, V. Gruhn, Caries detection on intraoral images using artificial intelligence. J. Dent. Res. **101**, 158–165 (2022)
35. S. Sadr, H. Mohammad-Rahimi, S.R. Motamedian, S. Zahedrozegar, P. Motie, S. Vinayahalingam, O. Dianat, A. Nosrat, Deep learning for detection of periapical radiolucent lesions: a systematic review and meta-analysis of diagnostic test accuracy. J. Endod. **49**, 248–261 (2023)
36. P. Yang, X. Guo, C. Mu, S. Qi, G. Li, Detection of vertical root fractures by cone-beam computed tomography based on deep learning. Dentomaxillofacial Radiology **52**, 20220345 (2023)
37. U. Pul, F. Schwendicke, Artificial intelligence for detecting periapical radiolucencies: a systematic review and meta-analysis, J. Dent. (2024) 105104.
38. S. Ren, K. He, R. Girshick, J. Sun, Faster r-cnn: Towards real-time object detection with region proposal networks, Adv Neural Inf Process Syst **28** (2015)
39. Y. Jusman, M.K. Anam, S. Puspita, E. Saleh, S.N.A.M. Kanafiah, R.I. Tamarena, Comparison of dental caries level images classification performance using knn and svm methods, in: *2021*

IEEE International Conference on Signal and Image Processing Applications (ICSIPA), IEEE, 2021: pp. 167–172
40. Y. Jusman, A. Widyaningrum, S. Puspita, Algorithm of Caries Level Image Classification Using Multilayer Perceptron Based Texture Features, in: *2022 IEEE International Conference on Cybernetics and Computational Intelligence (CyberneticsCom)*, IEEE, 2022: pp. 168–173
41. V. Geetha, K.S. Aprameya, D.M. Hinduja, Dental caries diagnosis in digital radiographs using back-propagation neural network. Health Inf. Sci. Syst. **8**, 1–14 (2020)
42. M. Sornam, M. Prabhakaran, A new linear adaptive swarm intelligence approach using back propagation neural network for dental caries classification, in: *2017 IEEE International Conference on Power, Control, Signals and Instrumentation Engineering (ICPCSI)*, IEEE, 2017: pp. 2698–2703.
43. S. Patil, V. Kulkarni, A. Bhise, Algorithmic analysis for dental caries detection using an adaptive neural network architecture, Heliyon **5** (2019)
44. J.-H. Lee, D.-H. Kim, S.-N. Jeong, S.-H. Choi, Detection and diagnosis of dental caries using a deep learning-based convolutional neural network algorithm. J. Dent. **77**, 106–111 (2018)
45. F. Casalegno, T. Newton, R. Daher, M. Abdelaziz, A. Lodi-Rizzini, F. Schürmann, I. Krejci, H. Markram, Caries detection with near-infrared transillumination using deep learning. J. Dent. Res. **98**, 1227–1233 (2019)
46. M.M. Lakshmi, P. Chitra, Tooth decay prediction and classification from X-ray images using deep CNN, in: *2020 International Conference on Communication and Signal Processing (ICCSP)*, IEEE, 2020: pp. 1349–1355
47. A.R. Kumari, S.N. Rao, P.R. Reddy, Design of hybrid dental caries segmentation and caries detection with meta-heuristic-based ResneXt-RNN. Biomed. Signal Process. Control **78**, 103961 (2022)
48. P. Singh, P. Sehgal, GV Black dental caries classification and preparation technique using optimal CNN-LSTM classifier. Multimed Tools Appl **80**, 5255–5272 (2021)
49. L.M. Leo, T.K. Reddy, Learning compact and discriminative hybrid neural network for dental caries classification. Microprocess. Microsyst. **82**, 103836 (2021)
50. A. Fariza, R. Asmara, M.O.F. Rojaby, E.R. Astuti, R.H. Putra, Evaluation of Convolutional Neural Network for Automatic Caries Detection in Digital Radiograph Panoramic on Small Dataset, in: *2022 International Conference on Data and Software Engineering (ICoDSE)*, IEEE, 2022: pp. 65–70.
51. F. Oztekin, O. Katar, F. Sadak, M. Yildirim, H. Cakar, M. Aydogan, Z. Ozpolat, T. Talo Yildirim, O. Yildirim, O. Faust, An explainable deep learning model to prediction dental caries using panoramic radiograph images, Diagnostics **13** (2023) 226
52. A. Choudhary, G. Raj, A.P. Agrawal, H. Sawhney, P. Nand, D. Bhargava, An effective approach for classification of dental caries using Convolutional Neural Networks, in: *2021 10th International Conference on System Modeling & Advancement in Research Trends (SMART)*, IEEE, (2021), pp. 204–209
53. S. Vinayahalingam, S. Kempers, L. Limon, D. Deibel, T. Maal, M. Hanisch, S. Bergé, T. Xi, Classification of caries in third molars on panoramic radiographs using deep learning. Sci. Rep. **11**, 12609 (2021)
54. L. Lian, T. Zhu, F. Zhu, H. Zhu, Deep learning for caries detection and classification. Diagnostics **11**, 1672 (2021)
55. H. Zhu, Z. Cao, L. Lian, G. Ye, H. Gao, J. Wu, CariesNet: a deep learning approach for segmentation of multi-stage caries lesion from oral panoramic X-ray image, Neural Comput. Appl. (2023), 1–9.
56. B. Dayı, H. Üzen, İ.B. Çiçek, Ş.B. Duman, A novel deep learning-based approach for segmentation of different type caries lesions on panoramic radiographs. Diagnostics. (2023); **13**: 202, https://doi.org/10.3390/DIAGNOSTICS13020202 (n.d.)
57. C. Kim, H. Jeong, W. Park, D. Kim, Tooth-related disease detection system based on panoramic images and optimization through automation: development study. JMIR Med. Inform. **10**, e38640 (2022)

58. A. Imak, A. Celebi, K. Siddique, M. Turkoglu, A. Sengur, I. Salam, Dental caries detection using score-based multi-input deep convolutional neural network. Ieee Access **10**, 18320–18329 (2022)
59. M. Revilla-León, M. Gómez-Polo, A.B. Barmak, W. Inam, J.Y.K. Kan, J.C. Kois, O. Akal, Artificial intelligence models for diagnosing gingivitis and periodontal disease: A systematic review. J. Prosthet. Dent. **130**, 816–824 (2023)
60. S. Patil, T. Joda, B. Soffe, K.H. Awan, H.N. Fageeh, M.R. Tovani-Palone, F.W. Licari, Efficacy of artificial intelligence in the detection of periodontal bone loss and classification of periodontal diseases: a systematic review. J. Am. Dent. Assoc. **154**, 795–804 (2023)
61. A. Polizzi, V. Quinzi, A. Lo Giudice, G. Marzo, R. Leonardi, G. Isola, Accuracy of artificial intelligence models in the prediction of periodontitis: a systematic review, JDR Clin Trans Res **9** (2024), 312–324.
62. P. Cholan, L. Ramachandran, S.G. Umesh, A. Tadepalli, S. Palanisamy, The impetus of artificial intelligence on periodontal diagnosis: a brief synopsis, Cureus **15** (2023)
63. A. Fatima, I. Shafi, H. Afzal, I.D.L.T. Díez, D.R.-S.M. Lourdes, J. Breñosa, J.C.M. Espinosa, I. Ashraf, Advancements in dentistry with artificial intelligence: current clinical applications and future perspectives, in: Healthcare, MDPI, 2022: p. 2188
64. J.-H. Lee, D. Kim, S.-N. Jeong, S.-H. Choi, Diagnosis and prediction of periodontally compromised teeth using a deep learning-based convolutional neural network algorithm. J Periodontal Implant Sci **48**, 114 (2018)
65. N. Ameli, M.P. Gibson, I. Kornerup, M. Lagravere, M. Gierl, H. Lai, Automating bone loss measurement on periapical radiographs for predicting the periodontitis stage and grade. Frontiers in Dental Medicine **5**, 1479380 (2024)
66. R.P. Danks, S. Bano, A. Orishko, H.J. Tan, F. Moreno Sancho, F. D'Aiuto, D. Stoyanov, Automating periodontal bone loss measurement via dental landmark localisation, Int. J. Comput. Assist. Radiol. Surg. **16** (2021) 1189–1199
67. J. Krois, T. Ekert, L. Meinhold, T. Golla, B. Kharbot, A. Wittemeier, C. Dörfer, F. Schwendicke, Deep learning for the radiographic detection of periodontal bone loss. Sci. Rep. **9**, 8495 (2019)
68. A. Garg, J. Lu, A. Maji, Towards earlier detection of oral diseases on smartphones using oral and dental rgb images, ArXiv Preprint ArXiv.2308 (2023).
69. H.-J. Chang, S.-J. Lee, T.-H. Yong, N.-Y. Shin, B.-G. Jang, J.-E. Kim, K.-H. Huh, S.-S. Lee, M.-S. Heo, S.-C. Choi, Deep learning hybrid method to automatically diagnose periodontal bone loss and stage periodontitis. Sci. Rep. **10**, 7531 (2020)
70. J. Liu, X. Liu, Y. Shao, Y. Gao, K. Pan, C. Jin, H. Ji, Y. Du, X. Yu, Periapical lesion detection in periapical radiographs using the latest convolutional neural network ConvNeXt and its integrated models. Sci. Rep. **14**, 25429 (2024)
71. M. Boztuna, M. Firincioglulari, N. Akkaya, K. Orhan, Segmentation of periapical lesions with automatic deep learning on panoramic radiographs: an artificial intelligence study. BMC Oral Health **24**, 1332 (2024)
72. R. Pauwels, D.M. Brasil, M.C. Yamasaki, R. Jacobs, H. Bosmans, D.Q. Freitas, F. Haiter-Neto, Artificial intelligence for detection of periapical lesions on intraoral radiographs: comparison between convolutional neural networks and human observers, oral surg oral med oral pathol. Oral Radiol. **131**, 610–616 (2021)
73. E. Yilmaz, T. Kayikcioglu, S. Kayipmaz, Computer-aided diagnosis of periapical cyst and keratocystic odontogenic tumor on cone beam computed tomography. Comput. Methods Programs Biomed. **146**, 91–100 (2017)
74. S.B. Khanagar, A. Alfadley, K. Alfouzan, M. Awawdeh, A. Alaqla, A. Jamleh, Developments and performance of artificial intelligence models designed for application in endodontics: A systematic review. Diagnostics **13**, 414 (2023)
75. M. Hung, M.W. Voss, M.N. Rosales, W. Li, W. Su, J. Xu, J. Bounsanga, B. Ruiz-Negrón, E. Lauren, F.W. Licari, Application of machine learning for diagnostic prediction of root caries. Gerodontology **36**, 395–404 (2019)

76. Q. Fu, Y. Chen, Z. Li, Q. Jing, C. Hu, H. Liu, J. Bao, Y. Hong, T. Shi, K. Li, A deep learning algorithm for detection of oral cavity squamous cell carcinoma from photographic images: A retrospective study, EClinicalMedicine **27** (2020)
77. J. de Chauveron, M. Unger, G. Lescaille, L. Wendling, C. Kurtz, J. Rochefort, Artificial intelligence for oral squamous cell carcinoma detection based on oral photographs: A comprehensive literature review. Cancer Med. **13**, e6822 (2024)
78. M. García-Pola, E. Pons-Fuster, C. Suárez-Fernández, J. Seoane-Romero, A. Romero-Méndez, P. López-Jornet, Role of artificial intelligence in the early diagnosis of oral cancer. A scoping review, Cancers (Basel) **13** (2021) 4600
79. V. Vinay, P. Jodalli, M.S. Chavan, C.S. Buddhikot, A.M. Luke, M.S.H. Ingafou, R. Reda, A.M. Pawar, L. Testarelli, Artificial intelligence in oral cancer: a comprehensive scoping review of diagnostic and prognostic applications. Diagnostics **15**, 280 (2025)
80. K. Warin, S. Suebnukarn, Deep learning in oral cancer-a systematic review. BMC Oral Health **24**, 212 (2024)
81. G. Keser, İŞ Bayrakdar, F.N. Pekiner, Ö. Çelik, K. Orhan, A deep learning algorithm for classification of oral lichen planus lesions from photographic images: A retrospective study. J. Stomatol Oral Maxillofac Surg. **124**, 101264 (2023)
82. M. Zhou, W. Jie, F. Tang, S. Zhang, Q. Mao, C. Liu, Y. Hao, Deep learning algorithms for classification and detection of recurrent aphthous ulcerations using oral clinical photographic images. J. Dent. Sci. **19**, 254–260 (2024)
83. A. Tiwari, N. Gupta, D. Singla, J.R. Swain, R. Gupta, D. Mehta, S. Kumar, N. Gupta Sr, Artificial intelligence's use in the diagnosis of mouth ulcers: A systematic review, Cureus **15** (2023)
84. M.H. Talu, S. Coşgun-Baybars, Ç. Danacı, S. Arslan-Tuncer, from image to diagnosis: convolutional neural networks in tongue lesions, journal of imaging informatics in medicine (2025), 1–11
85. B. Tiryaki, K. Torenek-Agirman, O. Miloglu, B. Korkmaz, İY. Ozbek, E.A. Oral, Artificial intelligence in tongue diagnosis: classification of tongue lesions and normal tongue images using deep convolutional neural network. BMC Med. Imaging **24**, 59 (2024)
86. R.C.W. Chau, G.-H. Li, I.M. Tew, K.M. Thu, C. McGrath, W.-L. Lo, W.-K. Ling, R.T.-C. Hsung, W.Y.H. Lam, Accuracy of artificial intelligence-based photographic detection of gingivitis. Int. Dent. J. **73**, 724–730 (2023)
87. A. Rana, G. Yauney, L.C. Wong, O. Gupta, A. Muftu, P. Shah, Automated segmentation of gingival diseases from oral images, in: *2017 IEEE Healthcare Innovations and Point of Care Technologies (HI-POCT)*, IEEE, (2017), pp. 144–147
88. W. You, A. Hao, S. Li, Y. Wang, B. Xia, Deep learning-based dental plaque detection on primary teeth: a comparison with clinical assessments. BMC Oral Health **20**, 141 (2020)
89. A. Ramírez-Pedraza, S. Salazar-Colores, C. Cardenas-Valle, J. Terven, J.-J. González-Barbosa, F.-J. Ornelas-Rodriguez, J.-B. Hurtado-Ramos, R. Ramirez-Pedraza, D.-M. Córdova-Esparza, J.-A. Romero-González, Deep learning in oral hygiene: automated dental plaque detection via YOLO frameworks and quantification using the O'Leary index. Diagnostics **15**, 231 (2025)
90. H.-J. Kim, K.D. Kim, D.-H. Kim, Deep convolutional neural network-based skeletal classification of cephalometric image compared with automated-tracing software. Sci. Rep. **12**, 11659 (2022)
91. I. Kim, D. Misra, L. Rodriguez, M. Gill, D.K. Liberton, K. Almpani, J.S. Lee, S. Antani, Malocclusion classification on 3D cone-beam CT craniofacial images using multi-channel deep learning models, in: *2020 42nd Annual International Conference of the IEEE Engineering in Medicine & Biology Society (EMBC)*, IEEE, (2020), pp. 1294–1298
92. B. Beser, T. Reis, M.N. Berber, E. Topaloglu, E. Gungor, M.C. Kılıc, S. Duman, Ö. Çelik, A. Kuran, I.S. Bayrakdar, YOLO-V5 based deep learning approach for tooth detection and segmentation on pediatric panoramic radiographs in mixed dentition. BMC Med. Imaging **24**, 172 (2024)

93. Y. Mine, Y. Iwamoto, S. Okazaki, K. Nakamura, S. Takeda, T. Peng, C. Mitsuhata, N. Kakimoto, K. Kozai, T. Murayama, Detecting the presence of supernumerary teeth during the early mixed dentition stage using deep learning algorithms: A pilot study. Int. J. Paediatr. Dent. **32**, 678–685 (2022)
94. S. Minhas, T.-H. Wu, D.-G. Kim, S. Chen, Y.-C. Wu, C.-C. Ko, Artificial intelligence for 3d reconstruction from 2d panoramic x-rays to assess maxillary impacted canines. Diagnostics **14**, 196 (2024)
95. J. Ryu, Y.-H. Kim, T.-W. Kim, S.-K. Jung, Evaluation of artificial intelligence model for crowding categorization and extraction diagnosis using intraoral photographs. Sci. Rep. **13**, 5177 (2023)
96. ORCA Dental AI's Cephx.com Secures FDA Clearance for AI Cephalometric Analysis Platform, (n.d.). https://cephx.com/orca-dental-ai-cephx-com-secures-fda-clearance-for-ai-cephalometric-analysis-platform/ (accessed May 26, 2025)
97. NEWS—Instant Cephalometric Analysis Powered by AI | CephX, (n.d.). https://cephx.com/our-news/ (accessed May 26, 2025)
98. AI Services: Automatic Cephalometric Analysis | cephX, (n.d.). https://cephx.com/cephalometric-analysis/ (accessed September 17, 2025)
99. F. Ramos-Gomez, M. Marcus, C.A. Maida, Y. Wang, J.J. Kinsler, D. Xiong, S.Y. Lee, R.D. Hays, J. Shen, J.J. Crall, Using a machine learning algorithm to predict the likelihood of presence of dental caries among children aged 2 to 7. Dent J (Basel) **9**, 141 (2021)
100. S.-A. Sadegh-Zadeh, A. Rahmani Qeranqayeh, E. Benkhalifa, D. Dyke, L. Taylor, M. Bagheri, Dental caries risk assessment in children 5 years old and under via machine learning, Dent J (Basel) 10 (2022) 164
101. Y.-H. Park, S.-H. Kim, Y.-Y. Choi, Prediction models of early childhood caries based on machine learning algorithms. Int. J. Environ. Res. Public Health **18**, 8613 (2021)
102. Seamless Dental AI Integration for Your Practice. Overjet Dental AI, (n.d.). https://www.overjet.com/blog/how-to-integrate-dental-ai-software-into-your-practice (accessed May 21, 2025)
103. A. Lal, A. Nooruddin, F. Umer, Concerns regarding deployment of AI-based applications in dentistry–a review. BDJ Open **11**, 27 (2025)
104. Second Opinion by Pearl Review. Dental AI Assisted Diagnostics!, (n.d.). https://instituteofdigitaldentistry.com/ai/second-opinion-by-pearl-ai-assisted-dental-radiography-review/?srsltid=AfmBOopvphdUzSiQJ3JqFjDCVNFdhorrbChkD0lso9dwalY54hcD7aVX (Accessed May 20, 2025)
105. Pearl—Elevating Dental Care with AI, (n.d.). https://www.hellopearl.com/ (Accessed May 15, 2025)
106. Overjet - The #1 Dental AI Platform for Providers & Payers, (n.d.). https://www.overjet.com/ (accessed May 15, 2025).
107. AI-Powered Dental Scribe, Perio Charting and X-Ray Diagnostics, (n.d.). https://www.denti.ai/ (Accessed May 15, 2025)
108. F. al Schwendicke, W. Samek, J. Krois, Artificial intelligence in dentistry: chances and challenges, J. Dent. Res. **99** (2020) 769–774
109. Home - DentalMonitoring, (n.d.). https://dentalmonitoring.com/ (accessed May 23, 2025).
110. Virtual Care AI, Invisalign Provider, (n.d.). https://www.invisalign.com/provider/align-digital-platform/virtual-care-ai (Accessed May 23, 2025)
111. N. Al-Jallad, O. Ly-Mapes, P. Hao, J. Ruan, A. Ramesh, J. Luo, T.T. Wu, T. Dye, N. Rashwan, J. Ren, Artificial intelligence-powered smartphone application, AICaries, improves at-home dental caries screening in children: Moderated and unmoderated usability test. PLOS Digital Health **1**, e0000046 (2022)

Chapter 6
AI in Dental Treatment

This chapter will provide a detailed overview of how Artificial Intelligence (AI) technologies are becoming a part of dental treatment planning and procedures. It identifies the impact AI-driven algorithms are having on personalizing treatment plans for unique patient characteristics and attributes from health data so that more predictive, optimized care journeys can be created. In restorative dentistry and prosthodontics, AI-enabled design and fabrication tools enhance fit, aesthetics, and the possibility with which restorations, including fillings, crowns, and dentures, are completed. Orthodontics benefits from AI through robust planning of the right sequence of tooth movements and more accurate prediction of treatment duration and outcomes. The chapter also looks at some of the applications of AI in endodontics, where Machine Learning (ML) aids in discovering complex root canal anatomies to assist in clinical decision-making and in emerging robotic systems that improve precision. In surgical disciplines such as implantology and oral surgery, AI facilitates pre-surgical planning, computer-guided implant placement, and even surgical procedures that utilize robotics to achieve enhanced accuracy and safety. Periodontal therapies are also increasingly becoming personalized, as AI analyzes the patient's risk factors to generate recommendations for interventions such as laser therapy and tissue regeneration. Furthermore, the chapter highlights AI's role in post-treatment monitoring and patient engagement through smart monitoring of healing, teledentistry follow-ups, and patient education resources focused on interactive learning. Together, these advances represent the emerging role of AI in changing the world of contemporary dentistry towards an optimal level of smarter, safer, and patient-centered care.

6.1 Introduction

Modern dental procedures frequently require complex processes and accurate tolerance levels, enabling even small errors to be detrimental to the outcomes. The procedures include varied tasks, from designing a crown that fits the unique bite of a patient

L. Tayebi et al., *Artificial Intelligence in Medicine and Dentistry*,
https://doi.org/10.1007/978-3-032-15977-9_6

to precision surgical extractions that depend on proximity to crucial structures. The complexities involved in dental treatment demand a high degree of precision and planning that has traditionally relied heavily on the skills and experience of clinicians. Effective use of AI is growing in importance in the field of dentistry and is continuously evolving into an innovative partner, offering additional options that improve treatment personalization, procedural accuracy, and long-term results in ways that human clinicians cannot necessarily replicate as easily. AI algorithms can examine vast data sets and increasingly subtle patterns at a rapid speed that are impractical for humans, thus allowing for more calculation-based decision-making in treatment planning and execution. Consequently, the integration of AI technologies can enable dental professionals to personalize treatment approaches and enhance the precision and predictability of clinical procedures [1].

The previous chapter in this book described the role of AI in diagnosis and how intelligent systems support the detection of dental disease from imaging and other information. This discussion is now extended to treatment applications of AI, including how AI is applied after a diagnosis is made to plan therapies, perform procedures, and improve care during recovery. We will highlight that AI can impact almost all aspects of dental specialties once treatment begins, from developing a personalized care plan for the patient to the restoration or surgical procedure and into the post-treatment follow-up and patient involvement. By limiting the discussion to treatment (while leaving the diagnostic content discussed earlier), we can take a deeper and more focused dive into the use of AI to inform clinical decision-making after the problem is diagnosed.

AI is able to provide support for dental treatment in a number of ways, including (1) using patient-specific data (e.g., health history, details about anatomy, genetic information) to provide a focused treatment plan personalized for that patient [2], (2) powering automation and accuracy in treatment delivery, e.g., guiding robotic devices or providing clinicians with immediate decision support regarding care, thereby minimizing human error and differences between clinicians [3], (3) providing predictive modeling for treatment delivery that enables clinicians to preemptively think about potential outcomes or complications that may arise from a decision and to modify a plan before the decision is made or a complication arises [4], and (4) providing continual monitoring during and after treatment using AI to analyze imagery, sensor data, or reports from patients to verify that healing is occurring and to include patients as participants in their own care [5]. These functions enable AI to deliver more tailored, safer, and potentially more effective care than standard delivery methods alone.

In the following sections, we evaluate how AI is changing various aspects of dental treatment and planning. In Sect. 6.2, we examine how AI assists in creating personalized treatment plans by assessing patients' individual data, including an integrated medical history, habits, and clinical records—and using predictive and decision-analytic modeling to provide patient-specific treatment planning, outcomes, and risk estimates. Section 6.3 reviews the integration of AI in restorative and prosthetic dentistry, with a particular emphasis on the increasing precision, aesthetics, and efficiency of the design and fabrication of restorations (fillings, crowns, bridges, and dentures) aided by AI. Section 6.4 explores AI applications in orthodontic treatment planning and management of tooth movement using braces or clear aligners, predicting treatment time and final alignment. Section 6.5 examines how AI supports endodontic execution by highlighting root canal anatomy on radiographs, estimating working lengths, and providing complex treatment decision-making. In Sect. 6.6, we consider AI in the management of implantology and surgical prosthodontics, from pre-planned, computer-assisted implant placement and robotic surgery to improved accuracy, and the unique role of AI in verifying treatment outcomes. In Sect. 6.7, we examine some of the ways that AI plays an important role in periodontal care and the management of soft tissues. Section 6.8 discusses AI-assisted oral and maxillofacial surgery with applications related to orthognathic (jaw) surgery planning, facial reconstruction, and the incorporation of robotic assistance when performing surgery, thereby helping to improve outcomes. Section 6.9 covers AI applications for post-care monitoring of treatment results and coordination of communication with patients. This section discusses the use of smart algorithms to manage healing and assess the effectiveness of orthodontic treatment outcomes, as well as using tools to enhance communication with patients through teledentistry platforms, reminders, automated follow-ups, and personalized patient education. Finally, in Sect. 6.10, we provide a conclusion to summarize the transformative use of AI in dental care and the innovations shaping its future.

The above-mentioned sections demonstrate that AI is not simply an augmentation of the modern dental treatment process but is both transforming and enhancing how dental treatment is delivered. With every application shared with you, we are coming closer to better, smarter, safer, and more personalized care.

6.2 AI in Personalized Treatment Planning

All patients differ—not just in the anatomical features of the teeth and jaws, but also in biological status, medical history, behaviors, genetic predisposition, and specific treatment objectives. Treatment planning for patients has historically relied on a standardized approach, with the clinician modifying the plan for each case. Unfortunately, while modifications can aid a clinician in making each treatment unique, they may result in some specific details necessary for implementing the treatment not being fully understood. Personalized treatment planning through AI seeks to change this paradigm by using large datasets and predictive models to create personalized plans for each patient [6].

AI further demonstrates how personalized planning is achieved through data-informed risk evaluation and decision support. ML algorithms can assess patient-specific characteristics, such as periodontal measurements, caries or risk factors, bite force distribution, medical conditions, and potentially genetic markers, to forecast how a patient-specific treatment regimen might perform. For instance, AI can combine a patient's caries history, dietary habits, and salivary pH to determine their future caries risk and propose a preventive-based treatment plan rather than one that is heavily restorative, when compared with patients of different risk profiles. In periodontal care, AI models have been employed to predict the risk of tooth loss using measures of bone levels and inflammatory markers, allowing the clinician to make a more informed decision on whether to pursue aggressive periodontal surgery or to maintain a more conservative maintenance plan for a given patient [7]. Through analyzing thousands of similar data points from past cases, AI can suggest the most optimal pathways of treatment individualized to the person, rather than relying solely on broad clinical guidelines.

Another area is predictive outcome modeling. AI systems are being trained with extensive databases of treatment outcomes to determine which patient factors and treatment decisions can achieve the optimal results. With this kind of prediction of outcomes, AI will be able to help dentists and patients in their shared decisions regarding treatment strategies. A dentist may say, "In referring to this AI model that has been trained on cases like yours, there is an 85% probability that a crown on your cracked tooth will last at least 10 years, compared to a probability of just 60% if we place a large filling." These investigations support a discussion of treatment alternatives that are informed and personalized.

In areas such as implant dentistry, as the field continues to gain popularity, even minor complications must be carefully considered, and AI is providing new opportunities to predict treatment outcomes more accurately. For instance, AI models have already been successfully implemented to predict osteointegration or implant success. Systematic reviews have reported predictive accuracy rates typically ranging from 62.4 to 80.5%, depending on the study design [8]. Huang et al. [9] created a Deep Learning (DL) model utilizing preoperative Cone-Beam Computed Tomography (CBCT) scans to identify the risk of implant loss, suggesting that the model could be helpful in evaluating preoperative risks by accurately predicting implant failure within five years. Zhang et al. [10] developed a Convolutional Neural Network (CNN) that predicted implant outcomes based on periapical and panoramic radiographs, finding an 87% accuracy rate when identifying cases likely to result in failure. The development of these tools informs practitioner choices for complex cases and allows for the selection of interventions that are both clinically appropriate and economically sensible for the patient.

AI can also support the planning of multidisciplinary treatments. Complex cases, such as those involving patients requiring extensive treatment to remedy trauma from caries damage and/or severely compromised teeth, usually involve multiple specialties or a multidisciplinary plan that may even include emergency endodontics or periodontal pretreatment in order to execute morphological, functional, and aesthetic rehabilitation of the broken-down teeth and remaining periodontal and dentoalveolar structures. It is often highly challenging to develop an appropriate treatment plan and determine the best sequence for several related procedures [11, 12]. AI can assist with the myriads of connections across all specialties and suggest the optimal sequencing of different activities to achieve the best overall treatment result (e.g., deciding whether to perform orthodontic alignment before implant placement or vice versa for a patient missing several teeth). AI can support clinicians in developing comprehensive treatment plans with their patients by simulating various clinical scenarios or sequences of procedures while also determining the optimal functional and aesthetic outcomes that lead to greater efficiency, such as saving time, reducing complexity, or lowering treatment costs [13].

Additionally, AI makes possible the notion of a "digital twin" in dentistry [14, 15]. A digital twin is a virtual model of a patient which can be employed to trial treatment approaches. Utilizing intraoral scans, CBCT images, and health records, AI could create a virtually detailed model of the patient. The clinician could then carry out a procedure virtually (for example, orthodontically moving teeth or placing an implant) on the model, and AI would predict outcomes—tooth movements, changes in bite, stresses on restorations—based on its learned physics and biological response models. While still in its infancy, it could offer truly predictive planning by allowing clinicians to trial treatments in silico and determine which personalized approach is most likely to yield the highest probability of success with the actual patient.

As previously described, it is important to note that although AI in treatment planning serves as a decision support tool for the clinician, it is not intended to replace the judgment of the clinician. The dentist's knowledge and understanding of their individual patient's context are equally important. What AI can offer is a powerful integration of all the available data with evidence-based likelihood, potentially bringing to the dentist's attention possibilities they may not be aware of or substantiating an exposure with some quantitative evidence.

In conclusion, AI will usher in the era of precision dentistry. Treatment plans can be individualized and predicted to an extent that has never been conceivable. The earliest experiments suggest that AI systems will suggest treatment plans that are both in agreement with the expert panel and, in some instances, identify omissions (e.g., suggesting the need for an interdisciplinary approach for the patient that a clinician specializing in one area may not consider). As these systems continue to mature and gain confidence, we can anticipate a shift towards more data-driven procedures and processes in dental treatment planning. Patients will receive treatment planning that is appropriate to their needs, resulting in better data on outcomes and satisfaction with care. In the upcoming sections, we will see how individualized treatment planning happens in the specialty area of general practice with and through the assistance of AI—from restoring a single tooth to fully rehabilitating a mouth.

6.3 AI in Restorative and Prosthetic Dentistry

Restorative and prosthetic dentistry encompasses a variety of treatments, including fillings, inlays, crowns, bridges, dentures, and full-mouth restorations. All of these procedures require careful detail, design, and fabrication to ensure that the artificial restoration integrates with the remaining natural structure and functions properly. Time-honored approaches to making prosthetic components typically include a fair amount of manual labor and artistry (for example, a dental technician waxing up a crown or setting denture teeth). AI is changing restorative dentistry by automating protocols for design, increasing the precision of fabrication, and unlocking personalized prosthetic devices like never before [16].

One prominent use is for Computer-Aided Design and Manufacturing (CAD/CAM) of restorations, as modern CAD software in dentistry can integrate computerized algorithms and AI algorithms to modify and improve the design of crowns, bridges, and dentures. For example, AI can automatically detect the edges of a crown preparation on a digital scan that would take a technician time to analyze and quantify accurately. In fact, researchers have developed AI models that are capable of identifying and delineating the finish line of a prepared tooth at an accuracy comparable to expert technicians and can do so even when the margin is subgingival (below the gum) [17]. AI not only saves time by delineating the finish line but also achieves reliability by producing the same finish line on a prepared tooth every time (thereby reducing variability among technicians labeling different margins). By automatically detecting margins, the accuracy of crowns is improved at the margins, and better fitting restorations reduce the overall risk of gaps or overhangs, which can facilitate leakage of cement or accumulation of plaque.

Beyond detecting margins, AI-enabled CAD software can also create the overall shape and morphology of restorations. Relying on databases of tooth structure and principles of occlusion, AI can intelligently design crowns that are anatomically correct and harmonious with adjacent and opposing teeth. For example, if an upper first molar crown is needed, the AI will inspect the patient's digital impression to see how the opposing lower molar occludes with it and propose a crown shape that not only fits the space but also provides proper contact points and cuspal guidance in movements. Often these AI-proposed designs will be a reasonable first use for the final design, requiring only minimal adjustments by the human technician if necessary. Recent studies have shown that AI-proposed crown designs are not only time-effective but also clinically relevant. Liu et al. [18] documented that AI-designed crowns had similar marginal adaptation levels to crowns made by expert designers and were able to produce crowns in a greatly reduced time (up to 900% less time compared to a wax-up). Wu et al. [19] found that AI design tools were four times faster than novice human users and produced adequate crown morphology, but experienced CAD users still produced better morphology compared to the AI. Another study by Liu et al. [20] confirmed that AI-generated zirconia crowns were comparable in shape, realism, and contact to the digitally designed crowns, with successful results in vitro and in vivo—even though there were some spatial differences on occlusal surfaces and a color difference noted on the buccal and lingual surfaces. Taking together, these studies indicate that AI-developed crown designs can equal or even outperform human designs in terms of efficiency and continue to get better in morphological accuracy.

AI is fundamentally changing the way removable prostheses are designed. A Removable Partial Denture (RPD) or complete denture has multiple elements to consider when designing, such as which teeth should be replaced, designing the metal framework or base, and arranging the artificial teeth. Various researchers have used different learning methods (e.g., using ML or computer algorithms) to classify the arch shape or type of edentulous ridge anatomy, and this information can be used to construct the denture. In one study, a CNN was trained to classify dental arch forms to help provide a better-fitting denture [21]. Along these same lines, Mahrous et al. [22] reviewed the impact of a recently developed AI-based software program, AiDental, which affected students' scores in RPD design. AiDental is a computer-based platform that helps doctors plan an RPD with the assistance of AI to create a framework based on user information [23]. This system has a comparison aspect that evaluates students' designs against an AI-generated ideal design to give immediate feedback on performance. The use of this system showed improvement in students' design performance and highlighted the potential for robotic/AI-based software to improve the quality of RPD design. AI could possibly help evaluate the fit and function of RPDs [24].

In fixed prosthodontics, AI is emerging as an advantageous adjunct to augment precision, efficiency, and standardized treatment workflows. An especially important area for AI benefits is in the assessment of tooth preparation, a variable shown to be important in the long-term success of prosthodontic treatments. Advanced AI models, particularly CNNs, have been used to automate complex tasks like margin line detection, a well-known, technique-sensitive procedure that requires expert execution. For example, Zhang et al. [25] utilized a Sparse Octree-based CNN to accurately extract the tooth preparation margin line with a reported accuracy ranging from 90.6 to 97.4%, thus demonstrating the reliability of AI at approximating high-level expert performance. The 3D-CNN framework created by Farook et al. [26] could produce a Partial Dental Crown (PDC) design from intraoral scan data and their model showed high sensitivity (1.00) and fair validation accuracy (60%). Revilla-León et al. [27] published a systematic review of AI applications for prosthodontics, including fixed prosthodontics. They identified many studies supporting AI's potential to develop automated designs of tooth anatomy, reliably detect preparation margins with high accuracies, and generally optimize the casting process, but emphasized the potential for improved clinical validation and representation of broader datasets.

Another new area is AI in shade matching and esthetics. Picking the right color for a filling or a crown is notoriously difficult despite having many available color guides. AI tools can analyze images of the patient's teeth and, with computerized shade matching, automatically determine the shade and translucency of the needed restoration while obtaining data on extrinsic variables such as the environment and neighboring structures [28, 29]. Neural Networks (NNs) can ingest large datasets of tooth images, all labeled with shade labels, and learn to provide the recommended shade, thus obtaining recommendations that are better than any experienced clinician can provide in visual shade matching. Furthermore, AI can assist in creating the characterization of prosthetics—where to stain, texture, and glaze a ceramic crown—to more accurately match the features of the patient's natural enamel. The AI will have been trained using images from large databases of aesthetically successful case presentations with implant-assisted prosthetics. In summary, AI can assist the technician's knowledge and experience in formulating their customization of a prosthesis to blend well into the overall dental architecture.

The use of AI is also changing the laboratory workflow in prosthetic dentistry. Automated milling and 3D printing are already established, but AI could further enhance workflows by nesting multiple prosthetic shapes on the same print tray or block, saving material and reducing time. An example of this could be nesting the shapes of the maxillary denture and the mandibular denture, optimizing material usage to provide a more cost-effective product for the patient [30]. Additionally, AI has the potential to predict and account for shrinkage and distortion that may occur in the manufacturing process [31]. For example, an AI model could enlarge areas of a 3D-printed denture base using previous data to allow for shrinkage that has been seen in the same resin, ensuring that when the denture base is printed and processed, the denture ultimately fits the patient. While these changes are not dramatic, they bring greater accuracy and improved fit in prosthetic appliances.

At last, AI has found its position in maxillofacial prosthetics, a subdiscipline dealing with prostheses for facial defects (e.g., artificial eye, ear, and nose) or for larger intraoral defects. Maxillofacial prosthetics can benefit from the use of AI for designing prostheses that restore not only function but also appearance. AI systems could use mirror imaging of the unaffected side of the face for symmetrical reconstruction to produce individualized, visually harmonious prosthetic options; these could be achieved through the predictive capability of the original facial features of missing tissues. Liang et al. [32] developed a Generative Adversarial Network (GAN)-based model, called CTGAN, that was able to reconstruct complete 3D mandibular structures in patients with bone defects resulting from tumors or radical oral cancer surgery. The model was trained on CT data and tested on six mandibular tumor cases to perform 3D mandibular completion. CTGAN successfully generated anatomically realistic mandibles with smooth transitions between reconstructed and healthy regions (as shown in Fig. 6.1). The AI showed promise and provided a new approach for pre-surgical planning and virtual prosthetic modeling. Hidaka et al. [33] used an AI that relied on facial recognition to objectively assess the aesthetic outcomes of different methods for medical treatment of mandibular defects. Measurements based on AI-derived symmetry help quantify cosmetic differences across treatment methods, leading to greater consistency in evaluating differences and allowing for more informed clinical decisions. AI applications are being developed for assistive technologies beyond structured reconstructions [16]. Advanced prosthetic technologies, including voice-activated reading glasses and AI-enabled artificial eyes, are creating devices and components that surpass traditional care—improving quality of life through functional innovation. While some of these are still at the cutting edge of the clinic, they represent the vast potential of AI to restore not only appearance but also independence and confidence to patients with facial disfigurement. All in all, AI significantly contributes to maxillofacial prosthetics through the ways it can facilitate how we design, fabricate, and evaluate prosthetic outcomes. Whether it is a more efficient way of modeling anatomy or a standardized approach to evaluating cosmetic quality, AI will allow clinicians to pursue a more personalized and effective rehabilitative care approach.

To summarize, AI in restorative and prosthetic dentistry provides better-fitting, longer-lasting, and more esthetic restorations and prostheses that meet the needs of the patient and clinician in a more efficient manner. The ability for AI to work in

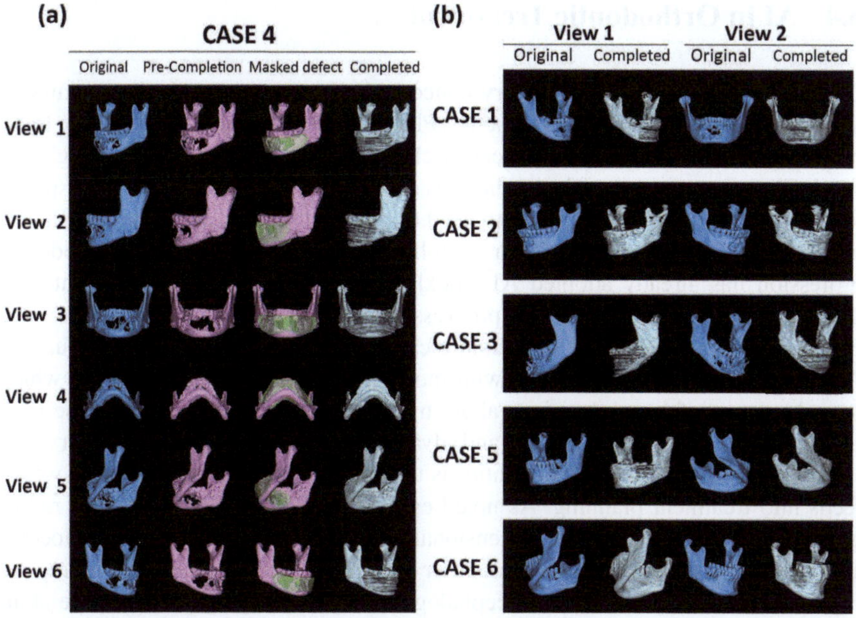

Fig. 6.1 AI-based 3D mandibular completion in six clinical cases. **a** Detailed reconstruction steps for a complex mandibular defect, showing CBCT-derived original morphology, pre-completion model, masked defect area, and final reconstruction. **b** Five additional cases illustrating the same completion workflow, each with original and reconstructed mandibles. Reproduced from Liang et al. [32], published in Scientific Reports 10 (2020) 16,431, under the Creative Commons Attribution 4.0 International License (CC BY), (https://creativecommons.org/licenses/by/4.0/). Font style and text size were adjusted for improved readability; the figure content is unchanged

tandem with dental professionals will allow routine design procedures to be automated, enabling humans to focus on subtle adjustments and decisions that require complex personal judgment. This equals better care—crowns seat with little adjustment, dentures fit right away, and smiles look appropriate and natural. Lastly, as AI continues to monitor and learn from its increasing caseload, we can expect even more incredible advancements, such as AI-designed smiles tailored to individual facial proportions or AI systems that will handle the entire workflow, from scan through to fabrication with little to no human influence. It is certain that soon, dentists' and technicians' roles will not be going away but rather taking on a new function of overseeing and supervising computer systems, confirming the output of AI to ensure it meets the subtle needs of every patient case.

6.4 AI in Orthodontic Treatment

Orthodontics is an area of dentistry concerned with correcting teeth and jaws as needed to improve function and esthetics. Planning and completing orthodontic treatment, either with conventional braces or clear aligners, is anything but straightforward. Clinicians need to make predictions about the movement of teeth in response to different forces, whether any teeth need to be extracted in order to provide space, and whether the patient's growth or compliance may cause issues. The orthodontic profession has already adopted AI quickly to enhance diagnosis, treatment plan development, and even treatment progress monitoring [34, 35]. AI systems have processed large numbers of orthodontic cases and their outcomes. Consequently, AI systems provide orthodontists with more background information from which to make more informed decisions about treatment options while at the same time improving efficiency in patient care and advancing personalized orthodontic services.

One basic use of AI in orthodontics is the analysis of diagnostic images, which feeds into treatment planning. As noted earlier in Chap. 5, AI can analyze radiographs, photographs, and three-dimensional scans to determine the type of malocclusion or classify anatomical landmarks. For example, AI can automatically complete cephalometric analysis of lateral cephalograms by identifying points of the skull and jaw, as well as measuring angles and distances used by orthodontists in diagnosis. This analysis saves considerable time and provides a consistent tool with intra-operator variability removed. Commercially available programs and packages exist, such as WebCeph, CephX, Dolphin Imaging, and AudaxCeph, that use AI to perform cephalometric tracing instantly and give a preliminary diagnosis based on those measurements [36].

In addition to static diagnostic analysis, AI is increasingly being applied to the ability to predict orthodontic treatment outcomes, which is particularly important in cases involving irreversible treatment interventions like extractions or interproximal enamel reduction [37]. Forecasting the outcome allows orthodontic treatment decisions to be made more strategically, leading to reduced chances of unproductive outcomes and enhanced patient satisfaction. The prominent use of AI in these circumstances is in automated virtual tooth setups that allow orthodontists to simulate treatment and visualize the final expected occlusion. Previously, creating these setups required extensive manual oversight to ensure accurate segmentation and setup of each individual tooth. However, AI-assisted systems have been developed to automate this process, most notably in clear aligner therapy. Woo et al. [38] compared three automated digital setup systems against manual setups, and while the automated option was effective in all cases and improved efficiency, there were instances when clinical cases required manual editing.

Not only can AI be used to evaluate dental alignment, but it may also be utilized to characterize skeletal and facial changes during orthodontic therapy. For instance, Park et al. [39] utilized a CNN model to estimate the cephalometric changes of Class II patients after they underwent treatment with modified C-palatal plates, and they achieved an overall mean difference of 1.79 ± 1.77 mm between ground truth and prediction. Furthermore, Tanikawa et al. [40] developed AI models capable of predicting 3D facial morphology following orthognathic surgery and orthodontic treatment based on previous treatment outcomes. They designed two AI systems employing landmark-based geometric morphometric methods combined with DL techniques, achieving prediction errors of less than 1 mm in both groups. Park et al. [41] developed a conditional GAN (cGAN) to estimate the 3D facial changes following orthodontic treatment. The model was trained to predict the patients' facial changes based on individual characteristics and treatment conditions. The mean prediction error was 1.2 ± 1.01 mm, with an accuracy of 80.8%. Notably, more than 50% of experienced orthodontists were unable to distinguish between the real and AI-predicted images.

Improving aligner therapy (clear aligners) is certainly one of the most evident areas of AI contribution in orthodontics [37, 42, 43]. The clinical efficacy of these systems is highly dependent on the accuracy of the aligner design. AI systems can play a major role in designing custom aligners for the distinct dental anatomy of each individual patient. By analyzing 3D intraoral scans, AI algorithms are able to create a complete digital model of the patient's teeth and jaw structures and produce aligners with precisely matched forces to control tooth movement. Unlike traditional management of this treatment, where forces are standardized or based on norms in a manual treatment plan, an AI-based aligner treatment planning approach allows for full individualization, automatic and immediate customization, and treatment with adaptive algorithms that optimize force distribution across the teeth with ongoing and gentle pressure for more predictable tooth movement. This will improve not only treatment outcomes but also patient comfort.

An additional benefit of the AI-promoted improvement in design accuracy is the faster aligner production [42]. Traditional manufacturing can take weeks and includes many manual steps. Conversely, AI-driven design and production systems can perform the majority of the design and manufacturing process automatically, significantly shortening the wait time. As a result, patients can receive sequential aligners sooner, reducing downtime between aligner placements and keeping treatment on track. AI-assisted treatment planning has been shown in clinical studies to reduce the total number of aligners needed per case by around 20%, mostly due to decreased mid-course corrections. Patients also reported less discomfort with aligners that had adaptive contours and fit better [42]. The ability of AI to cut down delivery time, lower the total number of aligners needed, and decrease discomfort are just a few examples of how AI is changing clear aligner therapy in terms of accuracy, speed, and patient satisfaction.

Orthodontic treatment is not a standalone event; rather, it is a continuum that usually spans 1–3 years, during which patients undergo adjustments and monitoring. As the field of orthodontics grows, patients undergoing clear aligner therapy experience a radical transformation in monitoring. Smartphone applications are also increasingly utilizing DL to analyze patients' photographs. They are also assessing whether the aligner fits properly and whether the patient may advance to the next aligner [44]. In these situations, AI-driven systems provide a level of automated oversight that allows for quick flagging of teeth that are "off-track" and timely intervention (for example, AI may suggest to the user that they need to adjust the next aligner if the tooth is not moving as desired) [42]. New research has also shown that AI systems can facilitate remote monitoring systems (e.g., Dental Monitoring), which significantly reduce the number of in-clinic checkups without sacrificing treatment quality [45]. AI monitoring systems allow patients to actively engage with their treatment by providing real-time feedback and minimizing clinic visits. Beyond the engagement benefits, AI monitoring systems ensure that practitioners are remotely monitoring whether clear aligner therapy is proceeding according to the treatment plan while also enabling the practitioner to make mid-course corrections when needed. In summary, not only does AI play an integral role in the planning process of clear aligner therapy, but it also interfaces with patients during treatment to save time, enhance the patient experience, and promote outcomes.

It should be stated that while AI provides strong recommendations and automation, orthodontic care is still based on the orthodontists' clinical judgment. AI, for instance, may predict non-extraction; however, the orthodontist knows from clinical experience that the treatment's success ultimately depends on the patient's profile and patient-specific preferences, which may warrant extractions. The goal is a combined approach between the orthodontist and AI, where together they may achieve outcomes that neither could be achieved separately. AI can do heavy calculation and pattern detection and supply the options ranked according to the probability of success, and the orthodontist needs to weigh that against other considerations the AI algorithm may not fully understand, such as the potential for patient compliance, oral hygiene, as well as psychosocial factors.

In conclusion, AI's emergence in orthodontics is already starting to change the way treatments are planned, managed, and monitored [36]. Patients experience more individualized plans (i.e., fewer unnecessary extractions and shorter treatment times where possible), while practitioners benefit from decision-support systems and efficient workload. As data from orthodontic practices around the world continues to be collected, we expect that AI will be able to provide more accurate and complete models. Orthodontics produces a significant amount of quantitative data, making it an ideal, fertile area for AI innovation, and ongoing developments will continue to improve patient smiles for many years to come.

6.5 AI in Endodontic Procedures

Endodontics, as a discipline of dentistry dealing with dental pulp and root canal therapy, has historically been a field that requires careful decision-making and accuracy. Consider procedures such as root canal therapy, which require understanding complex root canal anatomy, removing all of the infection, and filling the canals in three dimensions—often outside the clinician's direct sight. Perhaps the most challenging aspect of endodontic treatment involves deciding whether treatment is even possible or likely to succeed (as opposed to extracting the tooth), which is a nuanced clinical decision based on several factors. AI is making important contributions to

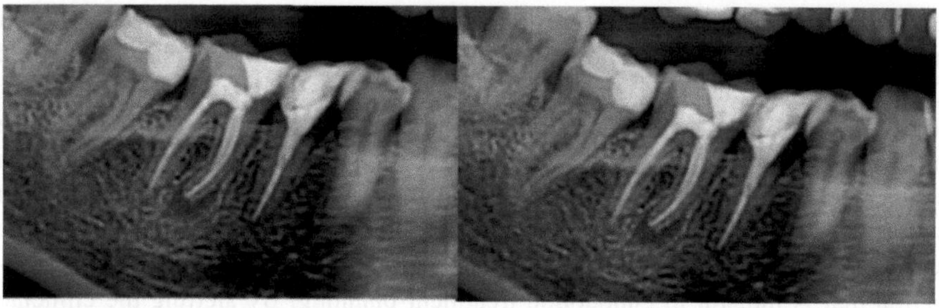

Fig. 6.2 AI segmentation of a periapical lesion on a dental radiograph. The image on the left shows the ground truth, and the image on the right is the segmentation from the AI's model. Reproduced from Boztuna et al. [48], published in BMC Oral Health 24 (2024) 1332, © 2024, with permission from Springer Nature

endodontics through enhanced root canal system detection and mapping, aiding in clinical decision-making, and potentially directing instruments with enhanced accuracy [46, 47].

AI is already having an immediate effect on endodontics in the area of diagnostic imaging related to root canal therapy, as diagnosis and mapping of the root canal system are critical to a successful treatment plan. AI-enabled image analysis of periapical radiographs and CBCT scans, compared to simply analyzing images with the human eye, allows clinicians to visualize and reliably assess periapical lesions (infected bone areas at the tips of the roots of a tooth). For example, studies have shown the potential for performance comparable to that of expert endodontists using DL models (such as variants of U-Net) to automatically segment periapical radiolucencies on radiographs [48]. This type of segmentation can improve treatment plan decisions; for instance, if the AI algorithm highlights a subtle periapical lesion on a tooth that the clinician was only going to restore, the clinician may now opt for a dental root canal first to treat that periapical infection. Figure 6.2 depicts how an AI system splits apart an apical lesion in an X-ray image using the above procedures.

Not only does AI detect lesions, but it is also helpful for classifying root canal anatomy. Each tooth has varying numbers of canals, and those canals have twists and turns as well. Understanding the number and morphology of canals before and during the procedure is fundamental since missed canals are among the most common reasons for root canal failure. In this respect, Lahoud et al. [49] developed and validated an AI-based tool for fully automated tooth segmentation on CBCT images using a feature pyramid network. The system was trained and tested on 433 images of single- and double-rooted teeth with varying anatomical characteristics. In addition to demonstrating excellent performance and strong agreement with clinical reference segmentations, the AI-based approach significantly outperformed manual segmentation in speed, reducing the average processing time from 6.6 min to only 0.5 min. This is a substantial leap in segmentation technology, allowing rapid and accurate identification of individual tooth structures and enabling downstream applications such as root canal mapping and anatomical classification. Hiraiwa et al. [50] evaluated the diagnostic capacity of a DL system for recognizing differences in root morphology of mandibular first molars on panoramic radiographs. Their research considered dental CBCT images as the gold standard and used images of 760 teeth from 400 patients to distinguish between single roots and additional roots in the distal portion of the molars. The DL model for diagnosing differences in root morphology was trained on segmented image patches from panoramic radiographs. In distinguishing between single and extra distal roots, the DL model yielded an accuracy of 86.9%. These studies demonstrate how AI-assisted investigations are advancing anatomical evaluation that is integral to endodontic treatment planning. By alerting the clinician to potential extra canals or complicated anatomy, AI ensures that the clinician can prepare correctly to address these complications—whether with a modified access cavity or specialty instruments—and contribute to the thoroughness and success rate of subsequent treatment.

AI is being used for treatment planning in a way that predicts outcomes and supports decision-making based on how an experienced endodontist would think. For example, in the case of a heavily decayed tooth, a clinician may wonder whether to attempt a root canal or whether the case is so poor that extraction and implant placement may be the better treatment option. AI systems are trained to estimate the outcomes (probability of success or failure) of root canal therapy on tens of thousands of cases of various types [51–53]. It can factor in the size of a lesion, a crack in the tooth, and the periodontal loss of support of the tooth, etc., which can be plugged into the model, and the model will output a recommendation or prediction. Sudeep et al. [47] discussed the various applications of AI in endodontics and included case-based reasoning systems that can provide treatment recommendations based on the outcomes of cases that had previously been treated. One case-based reasoning system may suggest treating a previous root canal if it finds a pattern similar to many of its previous successful retreatment cases, whereas another example may suggest extraction if the combination of factors indicates similar cases that had poor outcomes. In a nutshell, AI can be used as an expert second opinion to help not only general dentists but also endodontists make difficult decisions in complex cases.

AI has also been helpful in considering case complexity, and thus the decision-making surrounding a referral. There are established endodontic difficulty assessment forms (notably the American Association of Endodontists (AAE) Case Difficulty Assessment), but AI could automate this. AI systems may analyze radiographs and other patient data to assess the difficulty of managing a case. If AI predicts a case will be very complex, the general dentist may decide to refer the case to a specialist earlier. This will ensure the patient has their case treated by someone with the proper case management expertise, potentially improving the outcome. For example, Mallishery et al. [54] used 500 AAE Endodontic Case Difficulty Assessment forms to develop an ML model, and they demonstrated a high sensitivity (94.96%) in predicting case complexity and the need to refer. Their method offers a relatively rapid and reliable tool to assist general dentists in making referral decisions, especially in circumstances where a specialist is not available. In a more radiograph-centric approach, Karkehabadi et al. [55] trained several DL models on 1,386 periapical radiographs for the automated assessment of endodontic case difficulty. They achieved an accuracy rate of 87.62% for their best-performing model, which was higher than that of both general dentists and endodontists suggesting the value of AI as a tool to support objective, image-based triage in endodontics. In the transformation from clinical diagnosis to surgical planning, Qu et al. [56] trained and validated ML models exclusively on CBCT images—using 341 teeth from 261 patients—to predict the difficulty of cases in endodontic microsurgery. Qu et al.'s XGBoost model outperformed the other algorithms and achieved the best predictive performance across all measures (e.g., $R^2 = 0.7967$). The model ranked lesion size, distance between the apex and adjacent anatomical structures, and root canal–related features (such as filling density, curvature, and number of canals) as the most influential factors in determining surgical difficulty, providing an effective tool for preoperative risk assessment. When deciding to refer patients, the development of an efficient tool for clinicians should be of the utmost priority.

One of the most exciting potentials of AI in endodontics is real-time guidance for endodontic procedures. There is research being done to develop "smart" endodontic systems, where AI-enabled algorithms assist clinicians during root canal instrumentation. Take electronic apex locators, which assist clinicians in detecting the canal terminus through electrical impedance, as an example; if the apex locator were AI-enabled, it could take readings of electrical resistance and provide clinicians with an even more precise working length by filtering out noise and recognizing patterns associated with typical readings at the true apex. To illustrate this concept, Saghiri et al. [57] assessed an Artificial Neural Network (ANN) for determining working length through the use of a cadaver model. Their ANN was able to accurately identify the location of the minor apical foramen in 96% of trials and significantly outperformed endodontists with various levels of experience, who were able to accurately identify the location of the minor apical foramen only 76% of the time when both groups were assessed based on measurements regarding the true working length recorded by a stereomicroscope as the gold standard following tooth extraction. While research clearly continues to evolve in this setting, the results of the study demonstrate that ANNs can improve accuracy related to the precise location of the apical foramen, thereby enhancing the ability of AI to assist clinicians in determining optimal working lengths in the future. Accurate working length is essential, as under-preparation or over-preparation will jeopardize the success of the procedure. As such, AI certainly has the potential to enhance successful treatment outcomes by improving accuracy related to such important steps in the endodontic process.

It is also essential to understand that using AI in actual treatment is just beginning, as most uses of AI in endodontics have been diagnostic (primarily through radiographic interpretation). Even in diagnosis, it is impacting treatment. If AI identifies a vertical root fracture in a tooth that you intended to treat with a root canal, then this changes your treatment plan, potentially to extraction in most cases [58, 59]. AI can identify these fractures on 3D scans and even in 2D images at a level and with a sensitivity that is beyond human sight. This level of detection can prevent patients from undergoing unnecessary procedures, which can have real-world consequences—accurate diagnosis ultimately leads to more appropriate treatment.

As an example, let's look at a complex retreatment scenario. The patient has a previously root-filled molar that is failing. The decision is to either redo the root canal, perform endodontic surgery (apicoectomy), or extract the tooth. An AI model might analyze the radiograph and identify, for example, two separate untreated canals in one root (often overlooked). It would then generate a prediction for the likelihood of success for proper retreatment, as addressing these missing canals would fix the clinical problem. Conversely, if the AI finds a fracture line or extremely poor remaining tooth structure, it would report a low chance of success for retreatment, and the recommendation would then lean toward extraction. With this information, the endodontist can make a more confident recommendation directly to the patient. The patient can agree or disagree while understanding the reasoning through AI visualizations, such as heatmaps on the image, which indicate problem areas.

In conclusion, AI is likely to become an integral part of endodontic practice by enhancing diagnostic accuracy, treatment-planning quality, and maybe even the execution of endodontic procedures [47]. Early studies and applications indicate that AI has already demonstrated the ability to detect conditions (e.g., periapical lesions, extra canals, and apical foramen location) that significantly relate to treatment success. The predictions made by AI can assist clinicians in determining which treatment modality is applicable for the outcomes of each individual case and help us evolve into an era where the practice of endodontics is determined more by the uniqueness of patient needs than by generic standardization. It's likely not that far down the road when we will be using endodontic microscopes in which AI will be able to outline a tiny canal or crack while the dentist is looking into the microscope, or be able to hear an AI voice connected to the earpiece double-checking or proclaiming during a root canal, "You have 1 mm remaining to working length in this canal." With intelligent assistive technology and the dexterity of the endodontist, there is little doubt that we will achieve better success rates and increase the odds of maintaining natural teeth, which remains our singular goal in endodontics.

6.6 AI in Implantology and Surgical Prosthodontics

Implantology, which often coincides with surgical prosthodontics, usually includes the surgical placement of implants into the jawbone and the restoration of those implants with prosthetic teeth. This specialty encompasses thoughtful surgical planning to avoid vital structures and provide implant stability, the surgical placement of the implants, and the planning of the prosthetics that are going to be placed on the implants. The use of AI technology is rapidly growing in the field of implant dentistry, from imaging for planning to intraoperative guidance, and even designing the final implant-supported restoration [16, 60].

Predictive analytics is a key application of AI in the field of implantology, enabling clinicians to accurately predict desired treatment outcomes. By analyzing different types of patient data (e.g., X-ray images, medical histories), ML algorithms can indicate the probability of either a successful implant outcome or a poor prognosis, prior to or during the treatment. Clinically, this helps clinicians identify those patients at high risk for complications, personalize the treatment plan, and be more proactive in the treatment process to improve prognosis. There are several recent studies that demonstrate the possibility of these predictive models. For example, Mameno et al. [61] studied whether ML could be used to predict peri-implantitis (a common inflammatory consequence of implant surgery), and the authors found that a Random Forest (RF) model achieved approximately 70% accuracy (Area Under a Curve, AUC ~ 0.71) for predicting disease onsets. Zhang et al. [62] used ML on a series of trabecular bone scans to identify quantities of marginal bone loss around implants and demonstrated that a Support Vector Machine (SVM) model could, with good accuracy (AUC ~ 0.967, with 91.67% sensitivity, and 100% specificity), estimate clinically significant levels of severe bone loss around implants. In order to look at healing outcomes, Oh et al. [63] used DL to analyze postoperative radiographs and developed a model to predict whether the implant had osseointegrated with the jawbone (i.e., fused as part of the healing process), achieving approximately 80–84% mean accuracy for this task. These predictive models enable clinicians to estimate expected healing times and determine if additional interventions (or additional healing time) may be beneficial for a given patient.

In implantology, treatment planning is another area that will be forever changed by AI. Part of planning dental implants is the analysis of imaging (primarily with CBCT) to find areas of sufficient bone volume and density, and the best angle and depth of implant insertion. On a typical evaluation, a clinician will evaluate the CBCT scans manually. However, many AI algorithms are able to make things easier by segmenting anatomical structures (e.g., the mandibular nerve canal or maxillary sinus) and can also assist in determining bone quality. For instance, an AI system could be trained to take a scan of the jawbone and then classify areas according to density [64, 65]. One example of an AI system indicated that it could evaluate panoramic and periapical images in order to pull attention to areas of potential bone loss or low density that could negatively affect implant stability [10]. An AI has the ability to map or highlight areas of interest and allow the clinician to choose sites that have the best amount of bone or otherwise indicate the need for bone grafting if the preferred site of interest is lacking.

Once implant planning has been completed, it is ultimately possible to have AI tools assist in converting this plan into surgical guides. In fact, several recent studies have investigated the automatic design of surgical guides. For example, Wei et al. [66] created a DL workflow to design surgical guides for tooth transplants and found that it was able to recreate the design of an expert guide with comparable accuracy and reduce the amount of time it takes an expert to design a guide. In implantology, and with an AI approach, these processes could be similarly automated to lessen manual input in the planning process and improve consistency. Mangano et al. [67] presented a planning process that uses AI to automatically segment and align CBCT and intraoral scan data, and once processed, it exported for guide design and manufacturing. In their case, they found that their combined AI and mixed-reality approach was efficient and achieved small differences, although their proposed method did require calibration and allowed for minor yet predictable deviations between the planned and actual implant positions. Their methods show how such systems can simplify and possibly remove steps that previously required significant manual effort in planning and managing implant surgery and significantly improve guide fabrication accuracy.

In the surgical procedure itself, AI-assisted navigation and robotic systems act as intelligent co-pilots for the implant surgeon, supporting precise execution through real-time monitoring and guidance. These systems continuously track the position of the surgical drill relative to the planned implant site and provide immediate feedback to the operator, allowing fine adjustments during the procedure. Engagement with such AI-assisted systems goes beyond accuracy; it introduces adaptive control and real-time response mechanisms that enhance operational safety. Integrated with advanced sensors and algorithms, these systems can detect excessive forces or unintended proximity to vital anatomical structures and take immediate corrective actions, such as stopping the drill, thereby minimizing the risk of complications like nerve injury or sinus perforation. Saeed et al. [68] reviewed the emerging role of robotics and AI in implant dentistry; they noted not only the benefits of accuracy but also the real-time feedback offered during surgery. Their review showed that robotic systems using sensors and AI algorithms were able to precisely place the implant while reducing human error, thus improving the overall treatment outcome. Another advantage is consistency; these systems are able to consistently achieve highly accurate placement even under adverse situations (e.g., posterior sites, angled implants), therefore improving surgeon confidence to exploit the opportunity for advanced procedures such as immediate loading. Once a surgeon is confident that the implant is properly positioned and optimally oriented (and often with excellent primary stability due to the accurate osteotomy), the clinician should feel more comfortable placing a provisional crown the same day, providing immediate function and aesthetic benefit to the patient.

The result of optimal planning with robotic execution is implants placed in ideal positions; this provides multiple advantages. First, prosthetic outcomes benefit—an implant that is precisely angled and centered in a tooth position makes it easier to produce a crown that has ideal occlusion and aesthetics. For example, in full-arch cases (like an All-on-4 denture), robotic precision can place multiple implants such that a prefabricated interim prosthesis will fit right away. Indeed, a striking observation made from clinical trials was that in some robot-assisted full-arch implant placements, certain temporary prostheses made before surgery seated with minimal or no adjustment immediately after implant placement because the implant was positioned exactly where the digital plan intended [3]. Not only does this save time (no extensive chairside adjustments), but it also means a patient leaves that day with a well-fitting new set of teeth after treatment, a huge satisfier for patients. Second, correct placement of the implants means better force distribution, which leads to more predictable longevity. If an implant is tilted or placed off-center, forces may apply uneven stress to the implant, which could lead to bone loss or mechanical failure over time. In AI planning, principles of prosthetic-driven and biomechanical loading have to be integrated; the quality of bone and the expected loading direction are taken into account in AI planning to propose the best implant position. Together with robotic surgery, this means that the implants are placed not only where bone is available but also at the correct orientation that provides ideal force support and surface area, thereby increasing the longevity of the implant and its prosthetic.

The other primary benefit of AI in implantology is that it can optimize crown geometry for natural function. AI generative models, such as the 3D-Deep Convolutional GAN (3D-DCGAN), have already been trained on hundreds of tooth scans to design crowns that imitate natural anatomy. Ding et al. [69] performed a recent study comparing a crown designed by 3D-DCGAN with the natural tooth, as well as crowns generated by CEREC Biogeneric, and by an experienced dental technician using conventional CAD software. The authors reported that, in terms of general morphology, the 3D-DCGAN crown was closest to that of a natural tooth (as shown in Fig. 6.3). Finite element analysis confirmed that the 3D-DCGAN crown distributed bite forces nearly the same as a real tooth (~26.73 MPa stress at the crown's center for the 3D-DCGAN crown, ~23.97 MPa for a natural tooth). The authors also found that the 3D-DCGAN crown and natural tooth had very similar fatigue lifespans under cyclic loading, while a conventional CAD design showed greater deviation in the cusp angle and more adverse fatigue behavior. The authors concluded that this AI method can "mimic both the morphology and biomechanics of natural teeth," in addition to possibly improving the biomechanical performance and longevity of the crown.

In conclusion, AI's value in both implantology and surgical prosthodontics is as a facilitator for the clinician to think in an all-encompassing manner and then execute flawlessly. AI offers the benefit of digital precision combined with the expertise of the clinician, resulting in longer-lasting implants that function more naturally. With technological advances, we may be looking at some simple cases of implant placement being done autonomously (under human supervision) or ultra-minimally invasive implant techniques performed entirely by a machine guided by AI (i.e., an implant placed with a tiny keyhole incision accurately at the target). What certainly lies ahead is the continued integration of AI in surgical procedures to optimize implant rehabilitation so that it is safer, faster, and more individualized to the patient's anatomy and requirements.

6.7 AI in Periodontal and Soft Tissue Therapies

Periodontal therapy consists of procedures on the supporting structures of the teeth—the gums (gingiva) and bone, in particular, in the presence of diseases such as gingivitis and periodontitis. Soft tissue therapy may include periodontal plastic surgeries (i.e., gum grafts), laser treatments, or the management of conditions related to oral mucosal tissue. The pretreatment process consists primarily of assessing disease severity and documentation in the form of diagnostic radiographs, specific measurements (pocket depth), and monitoring of tissues over time. AI's clinical applications are newly emerging in periodontal therapy, primarily in diagnosis and risk prediction (which drives a more individualized and proactive approach based on risk) [70].

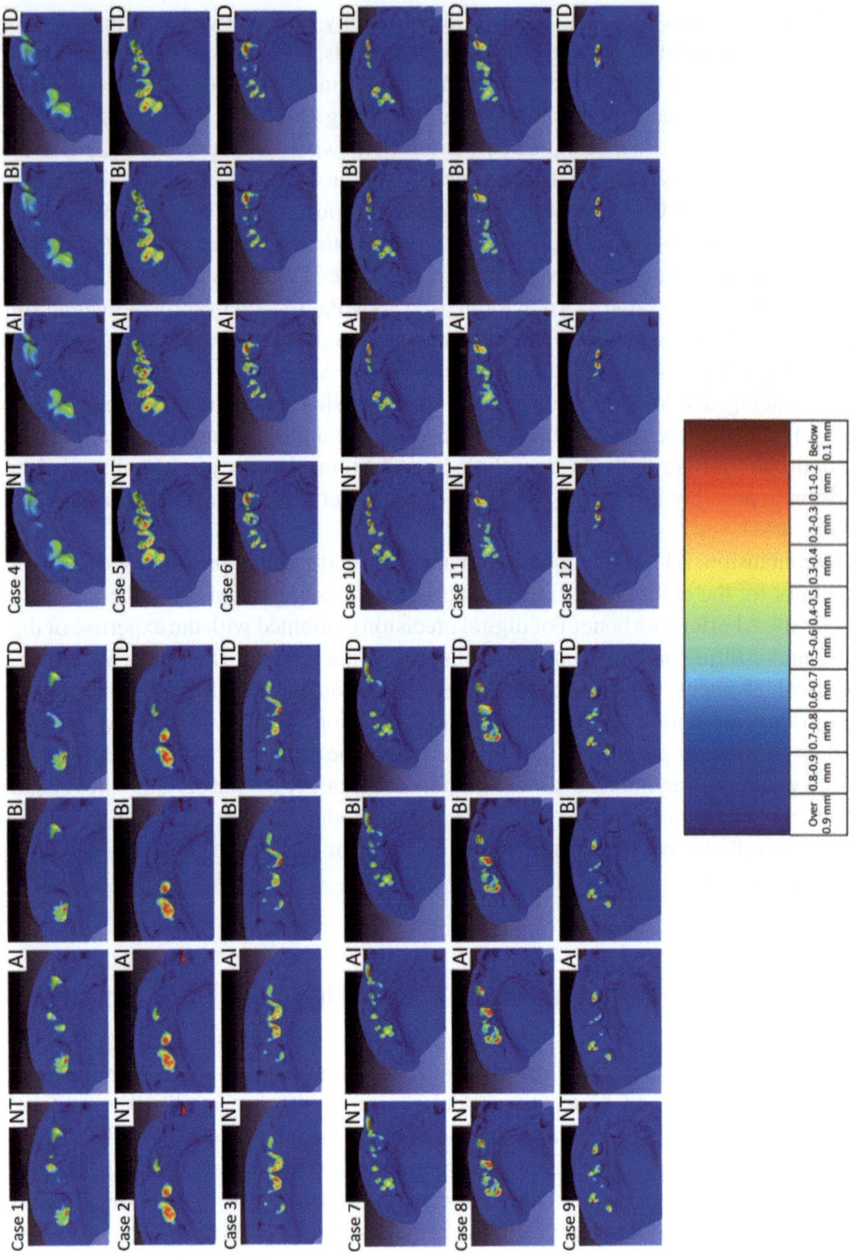

Fig. 6.3 Comparison between the occlusal contact number and the area of a natural tooth (NT), and the crowns generated by AI, CEREC Biogeneric (BI), and by an experienced dental technician using conventional CAD software (TD) for 12 cases. Reproduced from Ding et al. [69], published in Dental Materials 39

Once again, AI's role in the execution of periodontal treatment has yet to be charted, yet it is contributing significantly to the planning and maintenance of periodontal health.

In periodontics, one of the core applications of AI is periodontal disease risk assessment and personalized treatment. The rate of periodontitis progression and the response to treatment for any given individual may vary significantly. These algorithms allow AI to analyze combinations of patient data, such as plaque level, periodontal pocket depth, bleeding on probing, and medical history (which often includes information about diabetes status), in order to assign levels of risk and predict disease progression [70, 71]. For example, the ML model could make an assessment of a patient being at high risk of rapid periodontal breakdown because of certain combinations of risk factors. This can trigger a more aggressive treatment and maintenance plan for that patient (e.g., more frequent cleanings, adjunctive antibiotic therapy), whereas the low-risk patient may be kept on a more standard recall cycle. These personalized periodontal strategies ensure that resources are directed toward those who need them most while preventing overtreatment of others.

AI technology will increasingly be used to optimize periodontal surgical planning, especially for regenerative procedures. Advanced imaging and ML can combine to identify bony defects and may even recommend treatment rationales based on prior learning from previously treated cases [72, 73]. For example, DL algorithms have been developed to classify intrabony defect morphologies (i.e., one-wall, two-wall, and three-wall defects) from radiographs. However, the morphology of the defect is key to determining outcomes, as it correlates with predictable regenerative results. Piroonsan et al. [74] showed that a CNN could successfully classify three-walled intrabony defects on intraoral X-rays with clinically acceptable accuracy (AUC ~ 0.75) and thus utilize AI to recommend the easiest defects most accessible to regeneration, as well as aid in clinical decision-making during treatment planning. AI allows data-driven estimates of defect geometry, providing indications for the type of material and method to be utilized in regenerating bony defects. Abu et al. [72] developed a DL system to determine the radiographic defect angle of intrabony lesions, a crucial prognostic factor, which achieved up to 95% accuracy after image enhancement. They emphasized that narrow defect angles (<25°) were associated with significantly improved clinical attachment gains following regenerative therapy compared with wider defect angles (>37°), indicating that AI can assist in choosing the appropriate therapy based on defect type. If an AI system could classify a defect quickly and compare it to a database of successful treatment options and inform the periodontist of an evidence-based probability of success, the incorporation of clinical outcomes into the surgical decision-making process would happen quickly and easily, allowing the most effective regenerative strategy for the case.

Higher-level prototypes of decision-support systems are being developed. Allahverdi and Akcan's expert system using fuzzy logic is one AI-based approach intended to assist in the decision-making process [75]. In the future, incorporating AI classification and recommendation tools into surgical planning software could lend real-time assistance to clinicians during periodontal surgery planning. Specifically, a clinician might receive data-driven recommendations on which sites to graft, as well as recommendations on which biomaterials to use based on the patient's defect morphology and risk profile.

In conclusion, AI aids in periodontal and soft-tissue therapy through personalized care, shared decision-making, treatment planning, and delivering better patient outcomes. It is able to stratify patients based upon their risk, allowing the clinician to take action sooner or more aggressively if needed. It can predict treatment outcomes, thus improving the chances for successful therapeutic interventions. In the future, AI may provide surgeons with real-time guidance (for example, dynamically adjusting laser settings to an individual pocket's needs), or recommend adjunctive therapies such as probiotics or antibiotics based on genetic or microbial profiles and the bacterial signatures identified in subgingival plaque samples. Overall, technological innovations like AI exist to help us preserve oral health through disease prevention and limit the recurrence of disease, which is the underlying aim of periodontal therapy.

6.8 AI in Oral and Maxillofacial Surgery

Oral and Maxillofacial Surgery (OMFS) includes all surgical procedures in the oral cavity, jaws, and face, from the extraction of impacted molars to jaw fracture repair to more complex surgeries, including orthognathic (corrective jaw) surgery, cleft palate surgery, and removal of oral tumors. Regardless of complexity, the best surgical results often depend on careful planning and execution. The use of AI in OMFS continues to grow in a variety of areas, including planning and preoperative processes through advanced AI (e.g., predictive analytics, imaging analysis), assisting in navigation (potentially including robotic assistance), and training residents and surgeons through simulation [3, 76].

A novel application of AI that has emerged in OMFS is in surgical treatment planning and simulation, specifically for orthognathic surgery (surgery to correct dentofacial deformities such as underbites or asymmetries). Moving forward with treatment in orthognathic surgery involves predicting postoperative skeletal and soft tissue changes, or essentially how a patient will look and feel post-surgery once the jaws are repositioned. Traditionally, such surgeries were planned using cephalometric analysis and model surgery, which are limited in their ability to provide precise outcome predictions. Now, AI models, including ML and DL models, can be employed to more readily and reliably predict surgical changes. An example is an AI system called GPOSC-Net that was developed as a generative model to synthesize postoperative lateral cephalograms from preoperative data in orthognathic cases [76]. The model has elements that can predict how skeletal landmarks will move with surgery and then can generate a plausible post-surgery X-ray image. The model, which was validated using patient datasets, was able to predict postoperative jaw landmark positions with greater accuracy than cephalometric predictions and generated high-fidelity images that the surgeon would trust and feel confident in for postoperative treatment decisions. In practice, this means that surgeons can provide their patients with a visual prediction of their profile after surgery and adjust the surgical plan (i.e., how many millimeters to move the jaw) to achieve suitable functional and facial aesthetic outcomes. This use of AI to enliven clinical decision-making and patient engagement allows the surgeon to immediately iterate on the surgical plan and immediately see the simulated outcome.

In addition to lateral cephalograms, AI is also being utilized to predict 3D facial changes. Using techniques such as GANs, researchers have also made predictions of 3D facial surface changes from photos or 3D scans. For example, one method uses a Cycle-GAN to predict how a face would appear after a certain set of surgical jaw movements [77]. As shown in Fig. 6.4, the AI is able to generate quite realistic "post-op" photographs from "pre-op" photographs, which potentially have utility in planning the cosmetic aspects of OMFS procedures. It is crucial to accurately predict how soft tissue changes, as a movement of the bony jaw isn't always a 1:1 movement of the overlying skin. AI can learn those nuances from large datasets of pre- and post-op 3D images, improving the accuracy of surgical planning in terms of the aesthetic changes predicted.

Another important application of AI in OMFS is in pathology and development, specifically to assist in planning resection surgeries (like tumor resection) and reconstruction. As an example, when a surgeon removes an oral cancer, they have to determine margins—how much healthy tissue to take around the tumor. AI algorithms can learn from imaging (MRI/CT or even intraoperative fluorescent images) to outline where tumors are much better than human judgment [78]. This can help the surgeon locate clearer margins (while still ensuring preserved healthy tissue) if the AI-based segmentation is integrated into surgical navigation. Some systems use Augmented Reality (AR) to display the AI-identified tumor boundary along with the surgeon's field of vision (using either AR glasses or a regular screen), literally showing the surgeon where to cut. This could lead to the surgeon completing more complete tumor resections (reducing recurrence) while preserving important tissues so that function is maintained [79]. This is exemplified in Fig. 6.5, which illustrates how AI-enhanced fluorescence-guided surgery can assist with surgical decision-making by delineating a tumor in a near real-time fashion and facilitating better resections. In Fig. 6.6, we see an example of this integration, where a sophisticated intraoperative navigation system represents the cutting trajectories in real time with respect to tumor location; through this system, surgical accuracy and safety can be enhanced. Supporting this notion, Bollen et al. [80] implemented an automated method for gross tumor volume delineation of head and neck cancers using CNN and multimodality imaging. The AI model developed by Bollen et al. [80] largely enhanced the consistency and efficiency of tumor contouring in comparison to human manual delineation. The study indicated that multimodality AI segmentation reduces interobserver variability while decreasing planning time, demonstrating that AI could delineate tumor margins with accuracy comparable to human experts, if not better. In Fig. 6.7, the representative results of their model's performance are shown, where we can see automated tumor delineations compared to human expert contours across multiple imaging modalities.

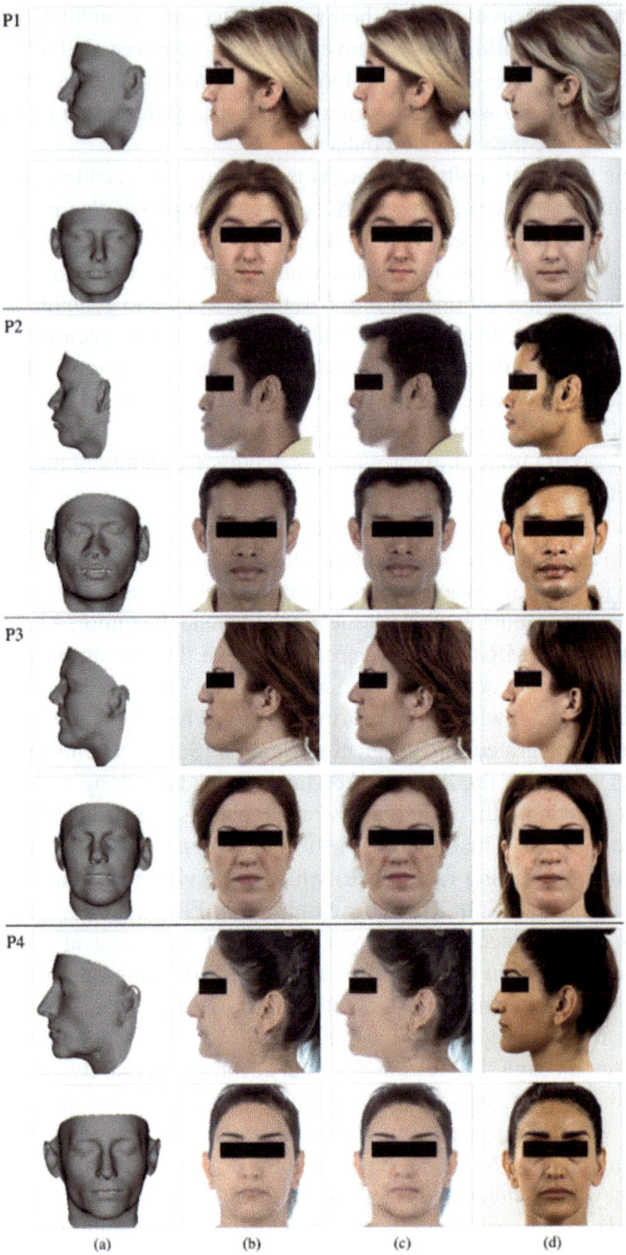

Fig. 6.4 AI-based simulation of post-operative facial appearance in orthognathic surgery for four patients. Each case includes lateral and frontal views comparing **a** simulated 3D face templates derived from surgical planning tools, **b** pre-operative facial images, **c** AI-generated predictions of post-operative appearance, and **d** actual facial images taken eight weeks after surgery. Reproduced from Andlauer et al. [77], published in IEEE Transactions on Image Processing 30 (2021) 7349–7363, under the Creative Commons Attribution 4.0 International License (CC BY), (https://creativecommons.org/licenses/by/4.0/)

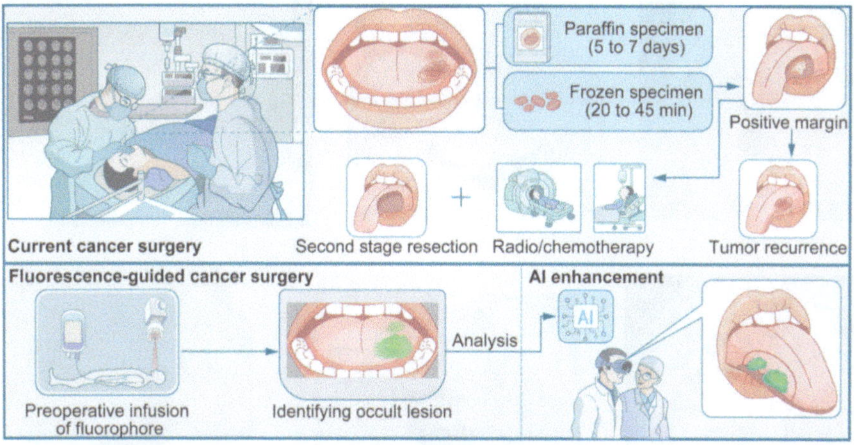

Fig. 6.5 Workflow of AI-enhanced fluorescence-guided surgery. While conventional methods lack real-time guidance, AI can improve intraoperative imaging, aiding precise tumor margin identification and supporting surgical decision-making. Reproduced from Cheng et al. [78], published in NPJ Precision Oncology 8 (2024) 196, © 2024, with permission from Springer Nature

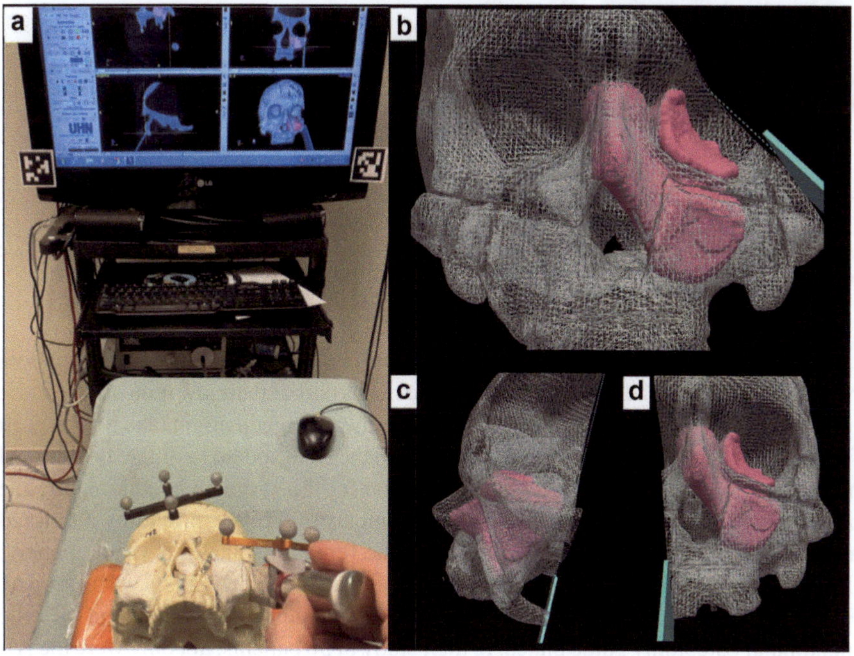

Fig. 6.6 Advanced intraoperative navigation system used during maxillofacial tumor resection. The system provides real-time visualization of surgical instruments and cutting paths in relation to the tumor in 3D space. Reproduced from Sahovaler et al. [79], published in Frontiers in Oncology 11 (2021) 723,509, under the Creative Commons Attribution 4.0 International License (CC BY), (https://creativecommons.org/licenses/by/4.0/)

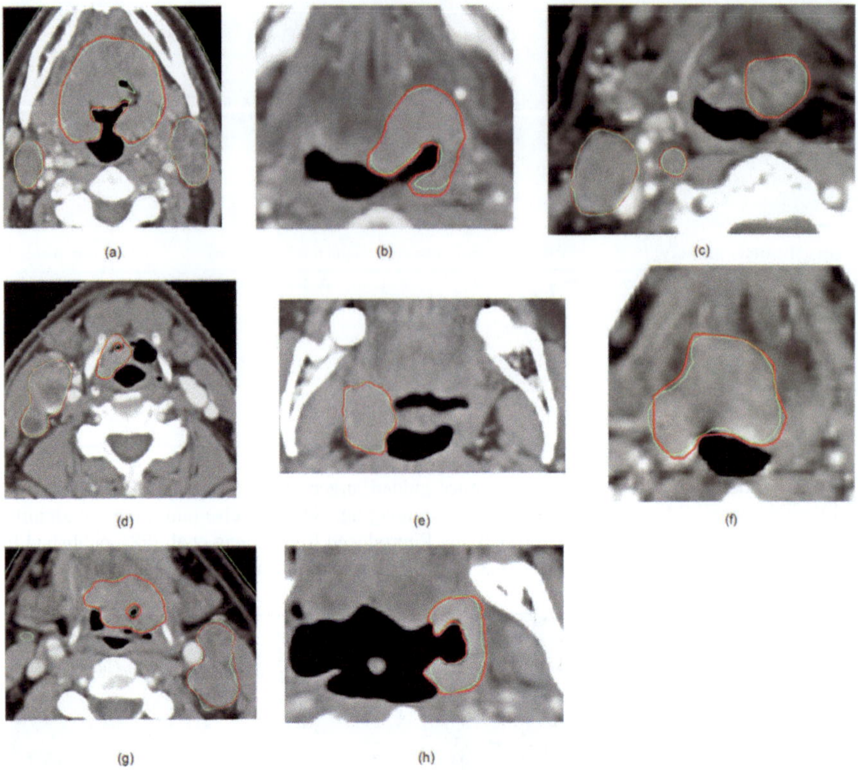

Fig. 6.7 Examples of automated gross tumor volume delineation using a Late Fusion CNN (LF-CNN) for CT + PET (**a–d**) and CT + MRI (**e–h**). Manual expert contours are shown in red, and automated AI-generated delineations are shown in green. Reproduced from Bollen et al. [80], published in Radiotherapy and Oncology 182 (2023) 109,574, © 2023, with permission from Elsevier

In the context of reconstructive surgery, AI can assist in the design of custom prosthetics and plates. Imagine a patient who needs part of their jaw removed because of a tumor. To reconstruct that segment of their jaw, a surgeon might take a bone graft from their hip and use custom plates to hold it in the right spot to facilitate healing. AI has also recently proven to be a helpful solution for this problem by automating the design process for a custom plate or even segments of the jaw, providing a tailored approach for each patient. It first examines the remaining anatomy of the patient; then it may use the anatomy of the contralateral side of the patient's jaw as a mirror. For example, Yan et al. [81] developed an AI algorithm to design patient-specific mandibular osteotomy guide plates. In their study of 50 patients, not only were the AI-generated guides made in a matter of seconds (~25 vs. ~1685 s if derived manually), but the AI-designed guides had better safety scores, while they had the same surgical accuracy (conditions were symmetry for bone cuts, proper shape/location) as the plates designed by experienced clinicians. Similarly, Mazzocchetti et al. [82] showed that a DL-based shape completion approach can automatically reconstruct missing jaw/facial segments for implant design. Overall, these investigations demonstrate how AI-based design is reshaping maxillofacial reconstruction by automating the creation of plates and implants without reducing surgical outcomes.

Robotic surgery in the OMFS field is a progressive area where AI is poised to have a significant impact. We currently possess surgical robots such as the da Vinci system for certain head and neck surgical procedures (such as transoral robotic surgery for cancers of the throat). These robots use intelligent software to reduce tremors and scale motion. However, as noted in [3], da Vinci's use in the oral cavity is limited by physical constraints. Newer, specialized robotic systems are beginning to emerge (for example, flexible robotics). Researchers are currently utilizing robots for dental extractions to enhance precision in the surgical procedure and lessen surgical trauma. Han et al. [83] described a robotic platform that performs minimally invasive extraction of impacted teeth using a pre-planned "window" osteotomy process—it drills away just enough bone to expose the tooth, removing the tooth without complication. In another example, Miadili et al. [84] performed the extraction of a median impacted mandibular tooth, also by a dental robotics method. In this example, there was no incident of nerve injury or any related events, and the patient healed excellently. In both examples, the robotic arm drilled a known, pre-calculated window of bone to expose and extract the tooth while ensuring ample protection of adjacent teeth and avoidance of nerve injury. Compared to conventional methods, surgical trauma was less, and accuracy was higher with robotics. Yet these systems remain semi-autonomous, as the surgeon remains in the loop during the procedure and because the robot demonstrates limited degrees of freedom (i.e., limited motions). Full-fledged real-time AI capabilities, with recognition of tissue and adaptive decision-making AI during surgery, are not yet available. AI-assisted robotics will enhance the consistency and precision of OMFS surgical procedures, but more research and clinical validation are required before the routine clinical application of robotics [85].

There are, of course, limitations to this approach. Head and neck anatomy is complex, and every patient has a unique pathology, so the data needed for AI models must be of very high fidelity and require a significant amount of training data to be useful. Reinforcing the ethical nature of AI recommendations and ensuring that AI considers functional outcomes as equally important as aesthetic outcomes are both essential (i.e., in the modern orthognathic surgery era, a great visual result is valuable, but not if a reduction in airway space or jaw function is among the outcomes, which means the AI models/data must consider multifactorial success criteria).

Ultimately, in conclusion, AI in OMFS plays a strong role as a supplementary and collaborative tool throughout the surgical process, through improved pre-surgical planning, the ability to predict outcomes and perform surgical simulations, and during surgery through precision navigation and robotics. Patients are benefiting from more predictability in their surgical interventions and often less invasive surgery. An example is that of a patient with facial deformities who now has improved assurances of their postoperative outcomes and an intervention that is less invasive and more consistent in achieving the predetermined surgical plan. A patient with a jaw tumor may now have it removed with increased safety margins and, for example, subsequently reconstructed with a custom plate that maintains their appearance and functional features. As the technology continues to be developed, we can envision further autonomy and intelligence in proposed surgical systems—for example, fully robotic dental-based surgical procedures for standard operations, or AI that designs an entire surgical case plan specific to each patient (including creating custom surgical instruments based on a CT, for example), the night before the surgeon operates the following day. The cooperation between the surgeon and AI in OMFS paves the future toward safer surgeries, faster recoveries, and improved outcomes for patients in an already difficult field of dentistry.

6.9 AI in Post-Treatment Monitoring and Patient Engagement

Successful dental care does not end when the patient gets out of the chair. The post-treatment stage is a very important part of the treatment, as it helps determine long-term results and ensures patient satisfaction. Post-treatment involves checking the patient's healing progress or recurrence of disease, encouraging and enabling adherence to the patient's home care requirements, and encouraging patient participation in their oral health care to reduce the possibility of future oral or systemic issues. The use of AI in the post-treatment phase is evolving, particularly by leveraging smart analysis of patient data and interactive means of communicating with patients. When AI is used to give patients continuous, personalized monitoring and support, it turns the gaps between clinic visits into opportunities for continuous care and creates opportunities for patients to be more engaged in their suite of care [5].

One of the most successful applications is remote observation using AI-enabled apps and devices. To demonstrate how this works, we can reference orthodontic treatment. For most of orthodontics' history, an orthodontist would see a patient to check their braces or aligners every 4 to 6 weeks to assess progress. With systems like Dental Monitoring (DM; Paris, France), patients are able to take periodic scans or photos of their teeth with their smartphones, which the AI algorithms analyze for tooth movement, aligner fit, and appliance concerns. The AI is able to determine if the patient can proceed to the next aligner or if a bracket is loose or a rubber band is not being used properly by generating a match for discrepancies in tooth positions or for tethered attachments [36, 86]. A report is provided to the orthodontist, and feedback is provided to the patient. The benefit of this approach is that any minor issues can be addressed early on; if, for instance, an aligner is not fully seated on a tooth, the AI raises an alert, and the orthodontist can have the patient use chewies or go in for a check, rather than discovering weeks later that progress had not occurred. This also means less need for office visits when progress is happening, because the AI will show that everything is on track.

The testing of such AI systems in an in vivo context has now established some level of clinical validity. Homsi et al. [87] tracked 24 orthodontic patients for an average of 13.4 months to test DM's tooth-tracking precision. The patients were scanned at regular intervals, and the DM app was used in conjunction with the iTero Element 5D intraoral scanner (Align Technologies, San Jose, CA). The 3D models provided by the two systems were compared, with no clinically significant difference found, which helped to show that DM's AI modeling algorithms can provide tracking of tooth movement and appliance fit within clinically acceptable limits. Morris et al. [88] tested the accuracy of DM's smartphone-based 3D dental models by comparing them to intraoral scanner models on orthodontic typodonts. They recorded no clinically significant difference when comparing DM-generated models (either photo or video mode) with iTero scans. The authors concluded that DM's remote models had sufficient accuracy for clinical use. Marks et al. [89] carried out a comparative trial of clear aligner therapy with DM remote monitoring versus in-office traditional monitoring. Both groups showed a significant level of success in occlusal improvements using the Peer Assessment Rating (PAR) index to assess treatment outcomes, with no statistical differences in terms of final alignment quality between patients monitored using DM and those monitored conventionally. This shows that AI-driven remote monitoring can be just as effective as standard care while also providing the potential to limit in-person visits.

The capability of AI-driven remote monitoring was greatly demonstrated during the COVID-19 pandemic. Caruso et al. [90] described two case reports that were effectively managed during a complete lockdown, utilizing the DM platform. The first involved a child's impacted canine and eruption guidance, while the second concerned an adult incisor crossbite correction. For each treatment, the AI application utilized the patient's smartphone scans to assess both the fit of the aligner and dental tooth movement, allowing each treatment plan to continue without the need for in-office visits. Patients found the system effective and well accepted when they complied with the protocol. AI functions as the orthodontist's virtual "eyes" between appointments, offering ongoing treatment oversight and enhancing the efficiency of orthodontic management and responsiveness for patients.

The same principles hold true in a post-surgical follow-up context. Patients may utilize apps to photograph their surgical sites (for example, after periodontal surgery or implant placement). These systems can proactively recognize potential issues such as inflammation, infection, or gingival recession by examining visual clues, such as redness, swelling, or exudate. If there are early signs indicative of problems, clinical teams can be alerted and initiate timely interventions, such as requesting that the patient visit the clinic or discussing the need to alter the care plan. This approach offers another level of oversight during the early and most vital healing stages, which may enhance outcomes and patient comfort.

Patient engagement and education are other fields that have already been transformed through AI. Now, various chatbots and virtual health assistants can communicate with patients about their dental health questions or offer coaching. These AI-based tools differ from static FAQ pages or pamphlets because they often employ Natural Language Processing (NLP) to provide personalized, on-demand advice. Santonocito et al. [91] found that, after a randomized trial, orthodontic patients who engaged with an AI-driven chatbot for assistance had better oral hygiene outcomes compared to a group that received typical leaflets. Additionally, the chatbot patient group had significantly lower increases in gingival inflammation and plaque, demonstrating better compliance with oral hygiene instructions. The authors of the study concluded that validated AI chatbots are effective in improving patient education and satisfaction throughout orthodontic treatment. Similarly, Helvacioglu-Yigit et al. [92] analyzed three publicly available AI chatbots (OpenAI's ChatGPT-3.5, Google's Gemini 1.5 Pro, and Microsoft's Copilot) for their responses to common patient questions in oral and maxillofacial radiology. Their analysis indicated that all the models provided scientifically correct and accurate answers, but the responses also tended to have notably high readability levels, with an average Flesch–Kincaid Grade Level (FKGL) score of 12.97. The score indicates that the responses were at a reading level appropriate for someone at least in the 13th grade (college freshman) level. The authors concluded that while AI chatbots can potentially answer frequently asked questions, the involvement of dental professionals is still required to ensure that the information is clear, understandable, and patient-focused. Pithpornchaiyakul et al. [93] demonstrated the applicability of AI to enhance engagement between tutor coordinators and caregivers in pediatric dentistry during the COVID-19 pandemic. Based on their findings, a 21–30-day period of using AI-powered chatbot significantly increased parental oral health knowledge and enhanced communication regarding their children's brushing habits, particularly in encouraging twice-daily brushing. Caregivers reported high satisfaction and described the chatbot as caring, engaging, and supportive of improved oral hygiene routines.

Another area of development is AI-based appointment and recall management. Many dental offices already have pre-programmed automated reminders, but AI can personalize the recall intervals based on individual patient risk. For instance, an AI system can review a patient's historical record—analyzing incidents of caries, periodontal status, and compliance history—and adaptively set the recall frequency over time as a function of the patient's individual issues or changes in those issues [94]. This individualized approach allows more regular visits for at-risk patients, while low-risk patients are not put on a recall schedule too soon, as there is better alignment between the timing of recall and patient need, improving preventive care outcomes.

AI is more than just recall optimization and is changing the larger task of scheduling appointments. Scheduling has generally been, and can still be, a manual and error-prone task, but with intelligent algorithms, scheduling is now moving toward an automated process [95]. In these situations, AI scheduling systems take into account clinician availability, patient preferences, and treatment duration in order to generate schedules automatically that are efficient and free of conflict. In these systems, automatic scheduling reduces waiting times and decreases the likelihood of errors such as double booking. These systems are expected to lead not only to greater patient satisfaction but also to a more productive clinic. In addition, predictive models powered by AI are being developed to solve the no-show problem. Alabdulkarim et al. [96] used an ML model to predict no-shows to dental appointments, achieving an AUC of 0.718 and an F1 score of 66.5%. By estimating which patients are most likely not to show for their appointments, clinics can adjust scheduling by making changes to previous schedule plans, reallocating patients, shortening time slots, reducing missed appointments, and more effectively utilizing chair time.

Overall, AI-based post-treatment monitoring and patient engagement are changing dental care from something that happens only during appointments to something that continues every day, helping patients stay connected to their oral health. Patients will feel better cared for and directed, even if they are not physically at the dental office. Dentists now benefit by being able to catch problems early (when fixes are less complicated) and have greater insight into their patients' day-to-day oral health behaviors and status. Lastly, better outcomes will occur, restorations will last longer due to patients caring for them appropriately, there will be fewer emergency visits when early warning signs are caught, and patient satisfaction will be higher as patients feel looked after by their dentist throughout their health journey rather than only when they visit the chair for their 6-month recare cleaning. One can envision a future where every dental patient has an AI dental assistant on their phone or smart home device. If they eat something hard and notice a crack, they could ask, "AI, I think I cracked my tooth, what should I do?" and it could triage and advise ("If there is no pain and no piece missing, schedule a check within a week; if you see a sharp edge or pain, see your dentist in 1–2 days."). It may even schedule the appointment or set up an e-consult automatically. The integration of AI into day-to-day life will enable oral health care to be seamless and effective, ensuring that the work of the dentist and patient during treatment is not only protected but also leveraged long after the treatment itself is concluded. In other words, AI extends the dental continuum into the patient's home and day-to-day activities, facilitating improved prevention and personalized care.

6.10 Conclusion

Dentistry is rapidly undergoing transformation due to AI across the full continuum of treatment—from when a treatment plan is developed, to when the treatment itself is performed, and even into the subsequent long-term maintenance. As described in this chapter, AI tools and systems are driving a clinically precise treatment planning process, producing more precise treatment outcomes, and enabling a more proactive and responsible follow-up than has ever been imaginable in dentistry. Collectively, these advances represent a true paradigm shift toward data-driven, patient-centered care that promises to enhance clinical outcomes and improve the patient's experience in a significant way.

A main advantage of AI in dental treatment is improved accuracy and predictability. AI in treatment planning uses algorithms that analyze large amounts of clinical data to create a tailored plan for each patient's anatomy and risk profile. Each patient's situation is personalized at a level previously unattainable. This could mean using AI to identify the best implant location with the least risk, to create a crown designed to fit a specific patient's occlusion, or to predict the visual outcome of jaw surgery on the patient's face. Algorithms rely on patterns derived from large amounts of data and provide the practitioner with a recommendation that is based on clinical evidence. Thus, the treatment plan generated by analyzing big data is smarter and more likely to work on the first attempt, negating the need for trial and error or adjustment.

AI is changing accuracy and efficiency on the procedural side of practice during clinical procedures. AI, robotics, and computer-assisted systems can execute treatment steps consistently in ways that human hands alone could often not achieve [3]. We have witnessed, in implantology as well as endodontics, how AI-assisted robots and navigation systems have eliminated the potential for human error—for example, placing an implant in the exact target site in bone to avoid and preserve critical nerves, or preparing a root canal to the exact length specified without overextending past the apex. These procedures allow for more conservative, minimally invasive treatments, retaining healthy tissues and reducing recovery times. From a safety perspective, using AI systems helps reduce risk, as the systems assess and evaluate critical matters (e.g., drill trajectory or force) and can stop just before the point of no return. Executing procedures with consistent AI performance means patients should expect excellent outcomes regardless of human variability from day to day, a significant step toward quality assurance.

One key theme that has emerged throughout the chapter is improved patient engagement and empowerment. AI not only assists the dentist, but it also engages patients directly—empowering them and keeping them informed and engaged in their care [5, 36]. Intelligent apps and virtual assistants can help educate patients with personalized tips and information at the time of need, answer their questions 24/7, and motivate healthy behaviors and well-being in a customized, interactive way. In this way, AI is demystifying treatments and home care so that patients can truly become partners in their oral health. An informed, engaged patient is much more likely to follow through with instructions (wear that retainer, use that fluoride, keep those recall visits), leading to dramatically higher treatment outcomes in the long term. In this way, AI is helping shift the paradigm of dentistry from reactive care (one-time appointments every six months) to preventive, continuous care (identifying issues early and positively reinforcing good behaviors continuously).

Looking into the future, the ability of AI to assist in dental treatment is extremely broad and still evolving. We can expect even more AI systems to be integrated into the clinical work environment—imagine a comprehensive AI software hub that listens and observes throughout a procedure to provide on-the-spot advice or even alert the dentist to subtle signs. A dual-purpose AI system could operate as a second expert set of eyes and ears in the dental operatory.

Another future aspect of AI is adaptive learning. AI systems will always be learning with each case; the more they observe or assist in a process, the better their recommendations will become. This will create a situation where the more AI is used, the smarter and more effective its recommendations become, thus creating a virtuous cycle that leads to continuous improvements in the quality of care received.

In addition, as data from different disciplines merge (i.e., dental records combined with medical and genomic records), AI will assist in the development of truly holistic, personalized medicine in dentistry. For example, AI could take into account a patient's diabetes status or genetic markers when providing recommendations for a periodontal maintenance plan, taking systemic factors into consideration that may influence aspects of their oral health. This could lead to predictive models for very long-term outcomes. For example, AI could predict a patient's tooth loss over the next 20 years if no interventions take place, allowing the dentist to prepare—with the ultimate goal of preserving teeth or planning for substitutes.

Certainly, there are challenges with the incorporation of AI into practice. Most notably, accuracy, data privacy, and the human element of patient care are important factors to consider. However, AI is meant to be a supportive resource, not a replacement for the dentist's clinical skills and the dentist–patient relationship. When properly implemented, AI can help give clinicians more time to think and perform those human activities that require empathy, creativity, or judgment while allowing AI to manage repetitive or data-centric tasks. Not only will that produce better clinical outcomes but also a more humanistic practice—a dentist who doesn't do all the repetitive work can focus more on listening to and advising their patients, and patients will feel they are provided with the resources and support to undertake their journey.

In closing, AI has proven to be a disruptive technology in the areas of dental treatment planning, delivery, and aftercare. In all aspects of dental treatment and patient care, AI systems are providing very real value by improving the precision, efficiency, and personalization of care, ultimately leading to improved oral health outcomes for patients. The examples and studies presented in this chapter suggest that AI is now a reality in dental care. AI is advancing the clinical practice of dentistry every day, whether through the automated detection of a small canal on a radiograph or the smartphone application that guides the healing of a surgical patient. With the advancement of technologies and the growing familiarity and confidence of practitioners, we can expect to see even greater impact from AI in the not-too-distant future. The future of dental treatment will be one of greater capability for dentists as they work alongside intelligent systems, with care that is ultimately more effective and more patient-centered—and, as a result, more successful. Exciting and meaningful progress will be achieved through these advances when the well-being of patients and ethical conduct remain central, and the promise of AI is realized in full in the practice of dentistry—leading to a future where dental diseases can be managed with unmatched precision and preventive care is maximized and optimized, making the maintenance of oral health easier for both patients and practitioners alike.

References

1. S. Sharma, P. Kumari, K. Sabira, A.S. Parihar, P.D. Rani, A. Roy, P. Surana, Revolutionizing dentistry: the applications of artificial intelligence in dental health care. J. Pharm. Bioallied. Sci. **16**, S1910–S1912 (2024)
2. M. Ghaffari, Y. Zhu, A. Shrestha, A review of advancements of artificial intelligence in dentistry. Dent. Rev. 100081 (2024)

3. C. Liu, Y. Liu, R. Xie, Z. Li, S. Bai, Y. Zhao, The evolution of robotics: research and application progress of dental implant robotic systems. Int. J. Oral Sci. **16**, 28 (2024)
4. Y. Chen, K. Stanley, W. Att, Artificial intelligence in dentistry: current applications and future perspectives. Quintessence Int. **51**, 248–257 (2020)
5. R. Kaushik, R. Rapaka, A patient-centered perspectives and future directions in AI-powered teledentistry. Discoveries **12**, e199 (2024)
6. A.M. Batra, A. Reche, A new era of dental care: harnessing artificial intelligence for better diagnosis and treatment. Cureus **15** (2023)
7. T. Rebeiz, G. Lawand, W. Martin, L. Gonzaga, M.-R. León, S. Khalaf, J.-M. Megarbané, Development of an artificial intelligence model for optimizing periodontal therapy decision-making: a retrospective longitudinal cohort study. J. Dent. 105780 (2025)
8. M. Revilla-León, M. Gómez-Polo, S. Vyas, B.A. Barmak, G.O. Galluci, W. Att, V.R. Krishnamurthy, Artificial intelligence applications in implant dentistry: a systematic review. J. Prosthet. Dent. **129**, 293–300 (2023)
9. N. Huang, P. Liu, Y. Yan, L. Xu, Y. Huang, G. Fu, Y. Lan, S. Yang, J. Song, Y. Li, Predicting the risk of dental implant loss using deep learning. J. Clin. Periodontol. **49**, 872–883 (2022)
10. C. Zhang, L. Fan, S. Zhang, J. Zhao, Y. Gu, Deep learning based dental implant failure prediction from periapical and panoramic films. Quant. Imaging Med. Surg. **13**, 935 (2023)
11. M. Palazzo, L. Massai, The importance of the operating sequence: a multidisciplinary treatment approach. Pract. Proced. Aesthet. Dent. **19**, 483–489 (2007)
12. K.-W. Tu, C.-H. Kuo, C.-C. Hung, D.-Y. Yan, J.L.P. Mau, Strategic sequencing of orthodontic treatment and periodontal regenerative surgery: a literature review. J. Dent. Sci. (2025)
13. H. Chen, P. Liu, Z. Chen, Q. Chen, Z. Wen, Z. Xie, Predicting sequenced dental treatment plans from electronic dental records using deep learning. Artif. Intell. Med. **147**, 102734 (2024)
14. S. Ahn, J. Kim, S. Baek, C. Kim, H. Jang, S. Lee, Toward digital twin development for implant placement planning using a parametric reduced-order model. Bioengineering **11**, 84 (2024)
15. Y. Maddahi, S. Chen, Applications of digital twins in the healthcare industry: case review of an IoT-enabled remote technology in dentistry, in: Virtual Worlds, MDPI, pp. 20–41 (2022)
16. A.P. Karnik, H. Chhajer, S.B. Venkatesh, Transforming prosthodontics and oral implantology using robotics and artificial intelligence. Front. Oral Health **5**, 1442100 (2024)
17. H. Lerner, J. Mouhyi, O. Admakin, F. Mangano, Artificial intelligence in fixed implant prosthodontics: a retrospective study of 106 implant-supported monolithic zirconia crowns inserted in the posterior jaws of 90 patients. BMC Oral Health **20**, 80 (2020)
18. C.-M. Liu, W.-C. Lin, S.-Y. Lee, Evaluation of the efficiency, trueness, and clinical application of novel artificial intelligence design for dental crown prostheses. Dent. Mater. **40**, 19–27 (2024)
19. Z. Wu, C. Zhang, X. Ye, Y. Dai, J. Zhao, W. Zhao, Y. Zheng, Comparison of the efficacy of artificial intelligence-powered software in crown design: an in vitro study. Int. Dent. J. **75**, 127–134 (2025)
20. C.-M. Liu, T.-Y. Lu, C.-S. Wang, S.-W. Feng, Y.-C. Lin, S.-Y. Lee, W.-C. Lin, Evaluation of the accuracy, occlusal contact and clinical applications of zirconia crowns using artificial intelligence design versus human design. J. Dent. Sci. (2025)
21. T. Takahashi, K. Nozaki, T. Gonda, K. Ikebe, A system for designing removable partial dentures using artificial intelligence. Part 1. Classification of partially edentulous arches using a convolutional neural network. J. Prosthodont Res. **65**, 115–118 (2021)
22. A. Mahrous, D.L. Botsko, A. Elgreatly, A. Tsujimoto, F. Qian, G.B. Schneider, The use of artificial intelligence and game-based learning in removable partial denture design: a comparative study. J. Dent. Educ. **87**, 1188–1199 (2023)
23. AiDENTAL, (n.d.). https://www.aidental.app/design/. Accessed 31 May 2025
24. A. Sikri, J. Sikri, R. Gupta, Artificial intelligence in prosthodontics and oral implantology—a narrative review. Glob. Acad. J. Dent. Oral Health **5**, 13–19 (2023)
25. B. Zhang, N. Dai, S. Tian, F. Yuan, Q. Yu, The extraction method of tooth preparation margin line based on S-Octree CNN. Int. J. Numer. Method Biomed. Eng. **35**, e3241 (2019)
26. T.H. Farook, S. Ahmed, N. Bin Jamayet, F. Rashid, A. Barman, P. Sidhu, P. Patil, A.M. Lisan, S.Z. Eusufzai, J. Dudley, Computer-aided design and 3-dimensional artificial/convolutional

neural network for digital partial dental crown synthesis and validation. Sci. Rep. **13,** 1561 (2023)
27. M. Revilla-León, M. Gómez-Polo, S. Vyas, A.B. Barmak, G.O. Gallucci, W. Att, M. Özcan, V.R. Krishnamurthy, Artificial intelligence models for tooth-supported fixed and removable prosthodontics: a systematic review. J. Prosthet. Dent. **129**, 276–292 (2023)
28. F. Rashid, T.H. Farook, J. Dudley, Digital shade matching in dentistry: a systematic review. Dent. J. (Basel) **11,** 250 (2023)
29. S. Shetty, S. Gali, D. Augustine, S. Sv, Artificial intelligence systems in dental shade-matching: a systematic review. J. Prosthodont. **33**, 519–532 (2024)
30. Evident Launches EviSmart Nest Automates Dental Nesting, (n.d.). https://www.evidentdigital.com/blog/evismart-nest? Accessed 17 Sept 2025
31. A. Omairi, Z.H. Ismail, Towards machine learning for error compensation in additive manufacturing. Appl. Sci. **11**, 2375 (2021)
32. Y. Liang, J. Huan, J.-D. Li, C. Jiang, C. Fang, Y. Liu, Use of artificial intelligence to recover mandibular morphology after disease. Sci. Rep. **10**, 16431 (2020)
33. T. Hidaka, S. Miyamoto, K. Furuse, Y. Fukunaga, A. Oshima, K. Matsuura, T. Higashino, Evaluation of aesthetic outcomes of mandibular reconstruction using artificial intelligence. Head Neck **46**, 2699–2708 (2024)
34. F. Albalawi, K.A. Alamoud, Trends and application of artificial intelligence technology in orthodontic diagnosis and treatment planning—a review. Appl. Sci. **12**, 11864 (2022)
35. A. Monill-González, L. Rovira-Calatayud, N.G. d'Oliveira, J.M. Ustrell-Torrent, Artificial intelligence in orthodontics: where are we now? A Scoping Rev. Orthod Craniofac Res. **24**, 6–15 (2021)
36. P. Fawaz, P. El Sayegh, B. Vande Vannet, Artificial intelligence in revolutionizing orthodontic practice. World J. Methodol. **15** (2025)
37. J. Liu, C. Zhang, Z. Shan, Application of artificial intelligence in orthodontics: current state and future perspectives, in: Healthcare, MDPI, 2023: p. 2760.
38. H. Woo, N. Jha, Y.-J. Kim, S.-J. Sung, Evaluating the accuracy of automated orthodontic digital setup models, in: Semin Orthod (Elsevier, 2023), pp. 60–67
39. J.H. Park, Y.-J. Kim, J. Kim, J. Kim, I.-H. Kim, N. Kim, N.R. Vaid, Y.-A. Kook, Use of artificial intelligence to predict outcomes of nonextraction treatment of Class II malocclusions, in: Semin Orthod (Elsevier, 2021), pp. 87–95
40. C. Tanikawa, T. Yamashiro, Development of novel artificial intelligence systems to predict facial morphology after orthognathic surgery and orthodontic treatment in Japanese patients. Sci. Rep. **11**, 15853 (2021)
41. Y.S. Park, J.H. Choi, Y. Kim, S.H. Choi, J.H. Lee, K.H. Kim, C.J. Chung, Deep learning–based prediction of the 3D postorthodontic facial changes. J. Dent. Res. **101**, 1372–1379 (2022)
42. D.B. Olawade, N. Leena, E. Egbon, J. Rai, A.P.E.K. Mohammed, B.I. Oladapo, S. Boussios, AI-driven advancements in orthodontics for precision and patient outcomes. Dent. J. (Basel) **13**, 198 (2025)
43. D.C. Ruiz, S. Mureşanu, X. Du, B.M. Elgarba, R.C. Fontenele, R. Jacobs, Unveiling the role of artificial intelligence applied to clear aligner therapy: a scoping review. J. Dent. 105564 (2025)
44. T. Ferlito, D. Hsiou, K. Hargett, C. Herzog, P. Bachour, N. Katebi, O. Tokede, B. Larson, M.I. Masoud, Assessment of artificial intelligence–based remote monitoring of clear aligner therapy: a prospective study. Am. J. Orthod. Dentofac. Orthop. **164**, 194–200 (2023)
45. A. Sosiawan, J. Jordana, D.E. Dhywinanda, J.F. Salim, N.F. Ramadhani, R. Nurdiansyah, I.G.A.W. Ardani, A.P. Nugraha, Artificial intelligence driven dental monitoring and surveillance of malocclusion treatment in orthodontic patients. World J. Adv. Res. Rev. **16**, 49–53 (2022)
46. A. Aminoshariae, J. Kulild, V. Nagendrababu, Artificial intelligence in endodontics: current applications and future directions. J. Endod. **47**, 1352–1357 (2021)
47. P. Sudeep, P.M. Gehlot, B. Murali, A.B. Mariswamy, Artificial intelligence in endodontics: a narrative review. J. Int. Oral Health **15**, 134–141 (2023)

48. M. Boztuna, M. Firincioglulari, N. Akkaya, K. Orhan, Segmentation of periapical lesions with automatic deep learning on panoramic radiographs: an artificial intelligence study. BMC Oral Health **24**, 1332 (2024)
49. P. Lahoud, M. EzEldeen, T. Beznik, H. Willems, A. Leite, A. Van Gerven, R. Jacobs, Artificial intelligence for fast and accurate 3-dimensional tooth segmentation on cone-beam computed tomography. J. Endod. **47**, 827–835 (2021)
50. T. Hiraiwa, Y. Ariji, M. Fukuda, Y. Kise, K. Nakata, A. Katsumata, H. Fujita, E. Ariji, A deep-learning artificial intelligence system for assessment of root morphology of the mandibular first molar on panoramic radiography. Dentomaxillofacial Radiol. **48**, 20180218 (2019)
51. D. Dennis, S. Suebnukarn, S. Vicharueang, W. Limprasert, Development and evaluation of a deep learning segmentation model for assessing non-surgical endodontic treatment outcomes on periapical radiographs: a retrospective study. PLoS ONE **19**, e0310925 (2024)
52. C. Bennasar, I. García, Y. Gonzalez-Cid, F. Pérez, J. Jiménez, Second opinion for non-surgical root canal treatment prognosis using machine learning models. Diagnostics **13**, 2742 (2023)
53. Y. Qu, Z. Lin, Z. Yang, H. Lin, X. Huang, L. Gu, Machine learning models for prognosis prediction in endodontic microsurgery. J. Dent. **118**, 103947 (2022)
54. S. Mallishery, P. Chhatpar, K.S. Banga, T. Shah, P. Gupta, The precision of case difficulty and referral decisions: an innovative automated approach. Clin. Oral Investig. **24**, 1909–1915 (2020)
55. H. Karkehabadi, E. Khoshbin, N. Ghasemi, A. Mahavi, H. Mohammad-Rahimi, S. Sadr, Deep learning for determining the difficulty of endodontic treatment: a pilot study. BMC Oral Health **24**, 574 (2024)
56. Y. Qu, Y. Wen, M. Chen, K. Guo, X. Huang, L. Gu, Predicting case difficulty in endodontic microsurgery using machine learning algorithms. J. Dent. **133**, 104522 (2023)
57. M.A. Saghiri, F. Garcia-Godoy, J.L. Gutmann, M. Lotfi, K. Asgar, The reliability of artificial neural network in locating minor apical foramen: a cadaver study. J. Endod. **38**, 1130–1134 (2012)
58. S. Ozsari, K. Kamburoğlu, A. Tamse, S.E. Yener, I. Tsesis, F. Yılmaz, E. Rosen, Automatic vertical root fracture detection on intraoral periapical radiographs with artificial intelligence-based image enhancement. Dent. Traumatol. (2025)
59. M. Fukuda, K. Inamoto, N. Shibata, Y. Ariji, Y. Yanashita, S. Kutsuna, K. Nakata, A. Katsumata, H. Fujita, E. Ariji, Evaluation of an artificial intelligence system for detecting vertical root fracture on panoramic radiography. Oral Radiol. **36**, 337–343 (2020)
60. S.F. Khan, A. Siddique, A.M. Khan, B. Shetty, I. Fazal, Artificial intelligence in periodontology and implantology—a narrative review. J. Med. Artif. Intell. **7** (2024)
61. T. Mameno, M. Wada, K. Nozaki, T. Takahashi, Y. Tsujioka, S. Akema, D. Hasegawa, K. Ikebe, Predictive modeling for peri-implantitis by using machine learning techniques. Sci. Rep. **11**, 11090 (2021)
62. H. Zhang, J. Shan, P. Zhang, X. Chen, H. Jiang, Trabeculae microstructure parameters serve as effective predictors for marginal bone loss of dental implant in the mandible. Sci. Rep. **10**, 18437 (2020)
63. S. Oh, Y.J. Kim, J. Kim, J.H. Jung, H.J. Lim, B.C. Kim, K.G. Kim, Deep learning-based prediction of osseointegration for dental implant using plain radiography. BMC Oral Health **23**, 208 (2023)
64. M. Widiasri, N. Suciati, C. Fatichah, E.R. Astuti, R.H. Putra, A.Z. Arifin, Alveolar Bone Quality Classification from Dental Cone Beam Computed Tomography Images using YOLOv4-tiny, in: 4th International Conference on Informatics, Technology and Engineering 2023 (InCITE 2023) (Atlantis Press, 2023), pp. 584–593
65. J.-H. Lee, J.-H. Yun, Y.-T. Kim, Deep learning to assess bone quality from panoramic radiographs: the feasibility of clinical application through comparison with an implant surgeon and cone-beam computed tomography. J. Periodontal Implant Sci. **54**, 349 (2024)
66. L. Wei, S. Wu, Z. Huang, Y. Chen, H. Zheng, L. Wang, Autologous transplantation tooth guide design based on deep learning. J. Oral Maxillofac. Surg. **82**, 314–324 (2024)

67. F.G. Mangano, K.R. Yang, H. Lerner, O. Admakin, C. Mangano, Artificial intelligence and mixed reality for dental implant planning: a technical note. Clin. Implant Dent. Relat. Res. **26**, 942–953 (2024)
68. A. Saeed, M. Alkhurays, M. AlMutlaqah, M. AlAzbah, S.A. Alajlan, M. Alkhurays Sr, Future of using robotic and artificial intelligence in implant dentistry. Cureus **15** (2023)
69. H. Ding, Z. Cui, E. Maghami, Y. Chen, J.P. Matinlinna, E.H.N. Pow, A.S.L. Fok, M.F. Burrow, W. Wang, J.K.H. Tsoi, Morphology and mechanical performance of dental crown designed by 3D-DCGAN. Dent. Mater. **39**, 320–332 (2023)
70. R.M. Sarakbi, S.R. Varma, L. Muthiah Annamma, V. Sivaswamy, Implications of artificial intelligence in periodontal treatment maintenance: a scoping review. Front. Oral Health **6**, 1561128 (2025)
71. A.S. Parihar, S. Narang, S. Tyagi, A. Narang, S. Dwivedi, V. Katoch, R. Laddha, Artificial intelligence in periodontics: a comprehensive review. J. Pharm. Bioallied. Sci. **16**, S1956–S1958 (2024)
72. P.A.R. Abu, Y.-C. Mao, Y.-J. Lin, C.-K. Chao, Y.-H. Lin, B.-S. Wang, C.-A. Chen, S.-L. Chen, T.-Y. Chen, K.-C. Li, Precision medicine assessment of the radiographic defect angle of the Intrabony defect in periodontal lesions by deep learning of bitewing radiographs. Bioengineering **12**, 43 (2025)
73. S. Kurt-Bayrakdar, İŞ Bayrakdar, A. Kuran, Ö. Çelik, K. Orhan, R. Jagtap, Advancing periodontal diagnosis: harnessing advanced artificial intelligence for patterns of periodontal bone loss in cone-beam computed tomography. Dentomaxillofacial Radiol. **54**, 268–278 (2025)
74. K. Piroonsan, K. Pimolbutr, K. Tansriratanawong, Classifying three-wall intrabony defects from intraoral radiographs using deep learning-based convolutional neural network models. Eur. J. Dent. **19**, 721–728 (2025)
75. N. Allahverdi, T. Akcan, A Fuzzy Expert System design for diagnosis of periodontal dental disease, in: 2011 5th International Conference on Application of Information and Communication Technologies (AICT) (IEEE, 2011), pp. 1–5
76. I.-H. Kim, J. Jeong, J.-S. Kim, J. Lim, J.-H. Cho, M. Hong, K.-H. Kang, M. Kim, S.-J. Kim, Y.-J. Kim, Predicting orthognathic surgery results as postoperative lateral cephalograms using graph neural networks and diffusion models. Nat. Commun. **16**, 2586 (2025)
77. R. Andlauer, A. Wachter, M. Schaufelberger, F. Weichel, R. Kühle, C. Freudlsperger, W. Nahm, 3D-guided face manipulation of 2D images for the prediction of post-operative outcome after cranio-maxillofacial surgery. IEEE Trans. Image Process. **30**, 7349–7363 (2021)
78. H. Cheng, H. Xu, B. Peng, X. Huang, Y. Hu, C. Zheng, Z. Zhang, Illuminating the future of precision cancer surgery with fluorescence imaging and artificial intelligence convergence. NPJ Precis. Oncol. **8**, 196 (2024)
79. A. Sahovaler, H.H.L. Chan, T. Gualtieri, M. Daly, M. Ferrari, C. Vannelli, D. Eu, M. Manojlovic-Kolarski, S. Orzell, S. Taboni, Augmented reality and intraoperative navigation in sinonasal malignancies: a preclinical study. Front. Oncol. **11**, 723509 (2021)
80. H. Bollen, S. Willems, M. Wegge, F. Maes, S. Nuyts, Benefits of automated gross tumor volume segmentation in head and neck cancer using multi-modality information. Radiother. Oncol. **182**, 109574 (2023)
81. Y. Yan, C. Lv, B. Wang, X. Wang, W. Han, M. Sun, B.S. Kim, Y. Zhang, J. Bao, L. Lin, Applying artificial intelligence algorithm in the design of a guide plate for mandibular angle ostectomy. J. Plast. Reconstr. Aesthet. Surg. **84**, 595–604 (2023)
82. S. Mazzocchetti, R. Spezialetti, M. Bevini, G. Badiali, G. Lisanti, S. Salti, L. Di Stefano, Neural shape completion for personalized Maxillofacial surgery. Sci. Rep. **14**, 19810 (2024)
83. L. Han, H. Wang, Q. Guan, Y. Yang, X. Li, Y. Yu, Y. Wang, Digital robot-assisted minimally invasive impacted tooth extraction: a case report. Heliyon **10** (2024)
84. M. Miadili, W. Zhang, Y. Zhang, Y. Gao, H. Mutalifu, X. Li, J. Zhang, Robot-assisted extraction of impacted mandibular tooth: a clinical report. BMC Oral Health **25**, 1–8 (2025)
85. R. Bahrami, M. Pourhajibagher, N. Nikparto, A. Bahador, Robot-assisted dental implant surgery procedure: a literature review. J. Dent. Sci. (2024)

86. J.H. Park, L. Rogowski, J.H. Kim, S. Al Shami, S.E.I. Howell, Teledentistry platforms for orthodontics. J. Clin. Pediatr. Dent. **45**, 48–53 (2021)
87. K. Homsi, V. Snider, B. Kusnoto, P. Atsawasuwan, G. Viana, V. Allareddy, P. Gajendrareddy, M.H. Elnagar, In-vivo evaluation of artificial intelligence driven remote monitoring technology for tracking tooth movement and reconstruction of 3-dimensional digital models during orthodontic treatment. Am. J. Orthod. Dentofac. Orthop. **164**, 690–699 (2023)
88. R.S. Morris, L.N. Hoye, M.H. Elnagar, P. Atsawasuwan, M.T. Galang-Boquiren, J. Caplin, G.C. Viana, A. Obrez, B. Kusnoto, Accuracy of dental monitoring 3D digital dental models using photograph and video mode. Am. J. Orthod. Dentofac. Orthop. **156**, 420–428 (2019)
89. J. Marks, E. Freer, D. Ong, J. Lam, P. Miles, Evaluating dental monitoring effectiveness compared with conventional monitoring of clear aligner therapy using the peer assessment rating index. Am. J. Orthod. Dentofac. Orthop. **166**, 350–355 (2024)
90. S. Caruso, S. Caruso, M. Pellegrino, R. Skafi, A. Nota, S. Tecco, A knowledge-based algorithm for automatic monitoring of orthodontic treatment: the dental monitoring system. Two cases, Sens. **21**, 1856 (2021)
91. S. Santonocito, M. Cicciù, V. Ronsivalle, Evaluation of the impact of AI-based chatbot on orthodontic patient education: a preliminary randomised controlled trial. Clin. Oral Investig. **29**, 1–13 (2025)
92. D. Helvacioglu-Yigit, H. Demirturk, K. Ali, D. Tamimi, L. Koenig, A. Almashraqi, Evaluating artificial intelligence chatbots for patient education in oral and maxillofacial radiology. Oral. Surg. Oral. Med. Oral. Pathol. Oral. Radiol. (2025)
93. S. Pithpornchaiyakul, S. Naorungroj, K. Pupong, J. Hunsrisakhun, Using a chatbot as an alternative approach for in-person toothbrushing training during the COVID-19 pandemic: comparative study. J. Med. Internet Res. **24**, e39218 (2022)
94. M. Mathew, R. Reji, AI in streamlining NHS dentistry. Br. Dent. J. **236**, 734 (2024)
95. Samera | How AI will Change Running a Dental Practice - Samera, (n.d.). https://samera.co.uk/learning-center/how-ai-will-change-running-a-dental-practice/#Streamlining_appointment_scheduling_and_patient_management_with_AI. Accessed 20 June 2025
96. Y. Alabdulkarim, M. Almukaynizi, A. Alameer, B. Makanati, R. Althumairy, A. Almaslukh, Predicting no-shows for dental appointments. Peer J. Comput. Sci. **8**, e1147 (2022)

Chapter 7
AI in Dental Education and Practice Management

This chapter examines the impact of Artificial Intelligence (AI) on dental education and practice management, two areas of tremendous importance that typically lag behind the clinical applications of AI in diagnosis and treatment. In dental education, AI is changing the way learners learn through high-fidelity simulators, virtual patients, and intelligent tutoring systems that provide personalized feedback, performance analytics, and adaptive learning experiences. These technologies have a stronger effect on psychomotor skill development and clinical reasoning, while also being used for data-informed curriculum development and the monitoring of at-risk students through learning analytics and predictive modeling.

The chapter also focuses on the potential for AI to impact the operational side of dental practices and academic clinics. From intelligent patient scheduling and patient communication systems to intelligent tools for managing Electronic Dental Records (EDRs), AI has the potential to streamline workflows and enhance both patient and staff engagement. The chapter discusses the potential for new methods like Federated Learning (FL) to sustainably manage data across institutions while preserving security and patient confidentiality. In addition to examining opportunities brought about by AI, the chapter explores challenges related to data privacy and the need for training faculty and staff.

This chapter provides evidence of AI not only as a clinical intervention but as a strategic and adaptive facilitator of better educational practices and practice management, focusing on an important and non-clinical aspect of dentistry. AI can improve education and empower health professionals at all levels, including students, instructors, administrators, and clinicians through thoughtful implementation and ethical oversight.

L. Tayebi et al., *Artificial Intelligence in Medicine and Dentistry*,
https://doi.org/10.1007/978-3-032-15977-9_7

7.1 Introduction

AI is increasingly infiltrating every facet of dental practice beyond clinical diagnoses and management of treatment. Chapter 7 addresses two important but frequently under-discussed areas, namely education and the management of schools or practices, while intentionally excluding clinical diagnostic and treatment management, as discussed in earlier chapters. In educational institutions, AI is creating opportunities to change how students learn, and instructors teach. Similarly, within the processes and management of dental schools and clinics, AI tools are enhancing efficiency and improving practices from patient scheduling to record-keeping. In a nutshell, this coverage ranges from the dental classroom and simulation lab to the clinic's front desk and back office. While neither of these tasks involves the actual drilling of teeth or radiograph interpretation, they do influence the efficiency and effectiveness associated with providing dental care.

AI has now become an important disruptive force in several industries, including dentistry, not only in clinical care but also in operational workflows [1]. To grasp the significance of AI in contemporary dental schools and clinics, it is essential to highlight that dentistry is an increasingly technology-oriented profession. Future dentists will have to use AI tools, and it is important that they are trained in their use during dental education. The integration of AI into dental education will ensure that new dentists are familiar with working in health centers that rely on high technology. On the side of clinic management, AI is helping to solve productivity issues that have plagued administration for many years. AI will improve appointment systems, lower clerical errors, and streamline communication with patients. AI is reducing time spent on tedious tasks and fostering data-informed practices to allow educators and staff time to devote to student learning and working with patients.

In order to present an organized and coherent discussion, this chapter will be divided into two sections: AI in dental education and AI in managing dental practice. The first section will evaluate how AI-based tools improve education at the preclinical and clinical stages of training and how those tools can be used in developing and implementing curricula and assessments. The section will include information related to AI-based simulators during preclinical training, virtual patients and AI-based tools during clinical training, and AI-assisted curriculum analysis and planning. The second section will describe AI applications that assist in and enhance the operation of dental schools and practice management, with details related to smart patient scheduling and communication and AI tools for patient data management and security. In discussing these topics throughout the chapter, challenges will be raised regarding matters such as data privacy, ethical considerations, and the need for a human touch. Upon completion of the chapter, readers will understand how the impact of AI in dentistry goes beyond smart diagnostics, redefining education for future providers and potentially changing the way care is delivered at the organizational level.

7.2 AI in Dental Education

Innovations in AI are impacting dental education in ways that enhance the effectiveness, personalization, and scalability of teaching tools. From high-fidelity simulators that utilize AI to provide coaching on hand skills to intelligent tutoring systems that personalize content and support a student's individual learning pace, AI systems help to bridge gaps between theoretical and clinical learning contexts. This section will examine how AI is enhancing preclinical dental education (with simulators and adaptive learning), training in clinical practice (with virtual patients and AI decision support), and even the analysis of curriculum and academic analytics. The goal is to support the formation of dentists who are not just clinically competent but also comfortable working with AI systems in their future practice.

7.2.1 AI in Preclinical Dental Education

Traditionally, preclinical dental education involves students executing procedures such as crown preparations or cavity preparations on plastic teeth or manikins, observed by instructors. Over the past few years, this core aspect of dental education has been greatly enhanced, employing complex technologies including intelligent tutors, haptic feedback devices, adaptive e-learning, and Virtual Reality (VR). High-fidelity VR simulators, providing visual and haptic feedback and a 3D display for procedures like drilling simulations, have begun to reshape the learning of psychomotor skills [2]. Such systems allow learners to perform dental procedures on virtual teeth while receiving lifelike force feedback and feedback on the performance of their skills.

Evidence suggests that simulator training can enhance student performance and bolster self-confidence. For instance, in a study led by Farag and Hashem [3], novice students were asked to perform Class I cavity preparations. These students were then trained by a haptic VR simulator and had them repeat the cavity preparation procedure. The results were remarkable, showing that post-simulator training, student preparation times were significantly shorter and cavity quality scores improved. These results suggest that VR simulators may better aid skill acquisition than traditional methods.

Beyond educational value, these technologies have practical benefits such as decreasing costs and reducing the waste associated with plastic teeth and disposable typodont materials. From the learner's perspective, the use of a simulator is often linked to higher student engagement. For example, in one survey, approximately 90% of students stated that a mixed reality and haptic-based dental simulator would raise their interest in learning, and 82% of students indicated that they would use the simulator again for future skills training [4]. Fig. 7.1 illustrates a student using a mixed reality simulator while wearing Augmented Reality (AR) glasses. The student uses a haptic device while operating within a realistic virtual operative field. This immersive setup aids in bridging the abstraction of simulation and clinical practice by replicating the real world.

In spite of these developments, the vast majority of existing simulators are predicated on established instructional rules and static scoring features, such as total tissue resected or deviations from an ideal preparation path, and do not offer adaptive or context-sensitive feedback. To help overcome these issues, there is growing interest

(a)

(b)

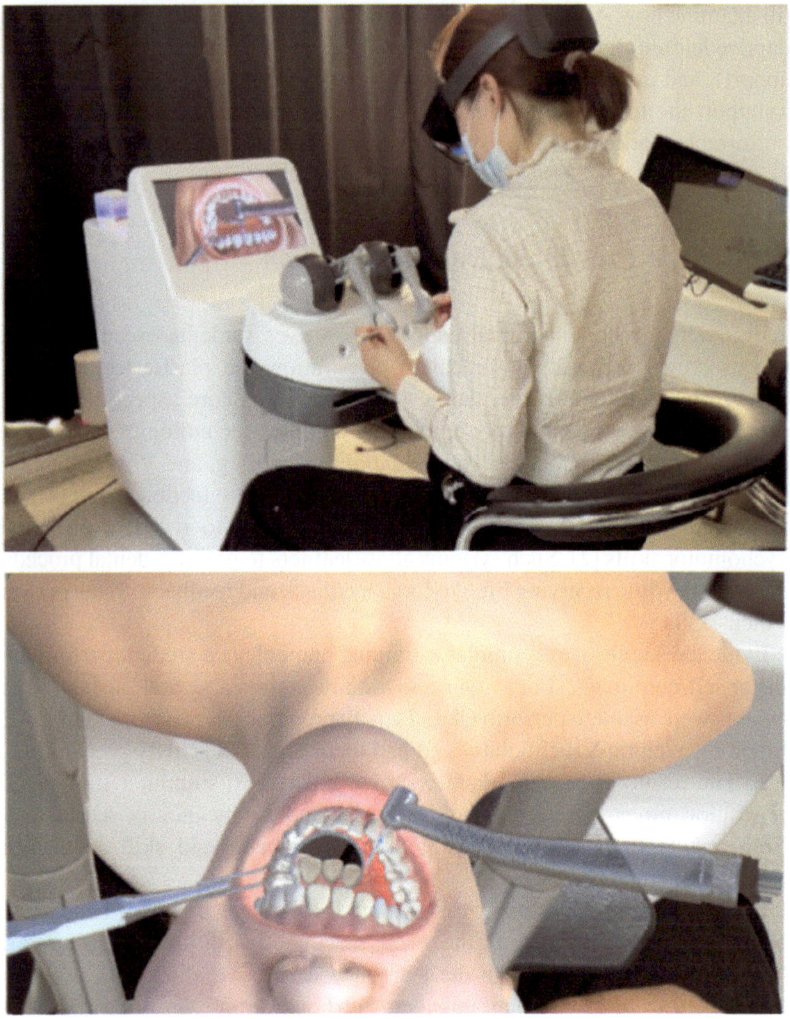

Fig. 7.1 **a** Exterior training scene of the Unidental Mixed Reality (MR) Simulator, and **b** view from the head-mounted display (HMD) of the virtual training environment. Reproduced from Li et al. [4], published in JMIR Serious Games 10 (2022) e30653, under the Creative Commons Attribution 4.0 International License (CC BY), (https://creativecommons.org/licenses/by/4.0/)

in AI-enabled simulation platforms. AI-enabled systems can provide individualized, data-driven skill assessments and real-time procedural instruction, advancing preclinical training to even higher levels of effectiveness.

An intelligent dental simulator developed by Rhienmora et al. [5] was one of the first systems to utilize AI in this application, assessing student performance while simulating virtual crown preparations using Hidden Markov Models (HMMs). A screenshot of this simulator design appears in Fig. 7.2 and includes a virtual dental mirror to practice using indirect vision. The simulator's ability to analyze the movement characteristics of dental instruments allowed the system to classify novice and expert users with high accuracy. Unlike traditional simulators, which simply replicate haptic sensations, this AI-enabled platform analyzed the recorded data and provided analytics with individualized scoring. The simulator was able to recognize 13 sequences of a crown preparation and give real-time feedback to students based on their performance while performing each sequence. Students would receive stage-specific feedback such as "try to lower the degree of rotation around the X axis" and "force in minus Z direction should be 2 times higher" whenever a student engaged in the task and diverged from expected performance. This level of feedback provides students with granular insights that facilitate early adjustments to establish new competence without continuous monitoring because it is delivered in stages. These accounts of the feedback discussed herein demonstrate that practicing intentionally in a virtual environment removes risks to patients and conserves physical resources.

Collaborating on these innovations, Collaço et al. [6] created an immersive VR platform that utilizes haptic feedback alongside Machine Learning (ML) to train and assess students in administering anesthesia to the inferior alveolar nerve, one of the most stressful parts of dental training. A total of 163 dental students tested the system, which utilized an HMD along with a real syringe mounted on a haptic device to simulate the injection in a highly realistic fashion. The system captured the students' movements through kinematic data and implemented a ML model to analyze technical performance. The machine learning method was validated, with an accuracy of 84%, as a good classifier to assess a student's needle insertion point performance. Fig. 7.3 shows the simulator in use—here you can see a student engaging with the system in full immersion, a design that mimics the physical and cognitive workload of real-world clinical training experiences. A comparative study was conducted by Sallaberry et al. [7], which compared ML algorithms for assessing user performance in the context of a VR-based dental anesthesia simulator. The authors studied classifiers including Naive Bayes, Random Forests (RFs), Multilayer Perceptrons, and Support Vector Machines (SVMs). Their findings showed that when an SVM was integrated with ReliefF feature selection, it achieved the highest accuracy (76%). Their investigation highlights the potential of ML integrated with VR systems to efficiently assess performance at scale in dental education. Collectively, these advances suggest a shift from fixed simulation models to intelligent, adaptive learning environments. The combination of AI and haptics with immersive VR allows new dental simulators to provide objective assessment and real-time, individualized feedback. These systems lessen faculty workloads and offer equitable access

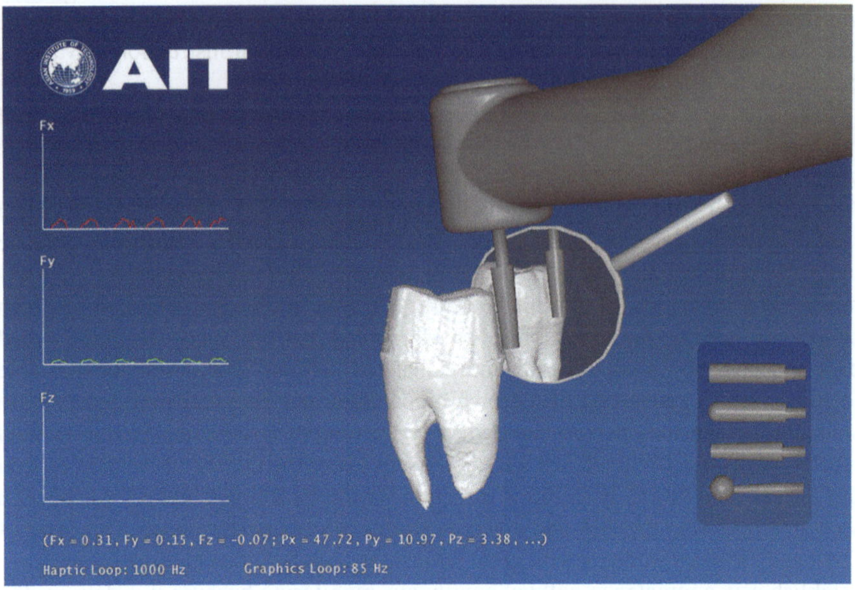

Fig. 7.2 Screenshot of an intelligent dental simulator prototype, featuring a virtual dental mirror to support indirect vision training. Reproduced from Rhienmora et al. [5], published in Artificial Intelligence in Medicine 52 (2011) 115–121, © 2011, with permission from Elsevier

to high-quality training while providing standardized competency assessments. As technology advances, AI-powered simulation platforms are expected to be pivotal in shaping the future of preclinical dental education.

In addition to procedural simulators, AI-based tutoring systems are also being used for educational purposes in dental education. These systems can assess students on content knowledge in foundational subjects (anatomy, theory), evaluate and analyze their responses, and adapt the content's level of difficulty or focus accordingly [8]. By modeling each student's knowledge with ML, an AI tutor has the potential to identify a student's weak performance areas and provide targeted practice to improve those weaknesses. For instance, an AI tutor can recommend more practice exercises in pharmacology or radiology if it detects that the student is not performing well in those areas. This method moves the teaching experience away from a singular "one-size-fits-all" approach; instead, the system continually adjusts lessons in real time to maximize each student's understanding and progress. A recent meta-analysis compared AI-based learning interventions with non-AI-based learning interventions and found that AI instruction greatly enhances students' knowledge acquisition (on average, approximately a 46% increase over non-AI instruction) and increases learner satisfaction [9], indicating the potential for personalized tutoring in dental education.

An example of an intelligent tutoring system in a dental context is one that was developed to support students in navigating virtual patient cases in a problem-based learning format [10]. This tutor applied a Bayesian network that enabled the modeling

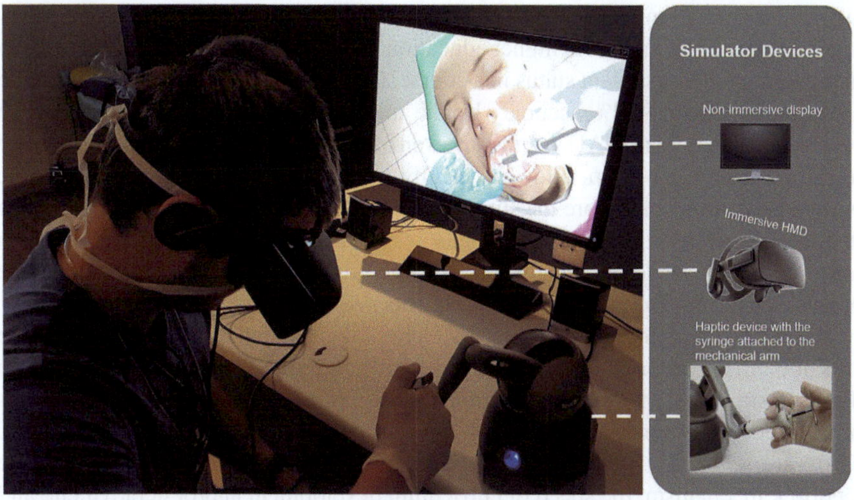

Fig. 7.3 Setup of the immersive VR dental simulator: a student wears the HMD and holds a physical syringe connected to a haptic device while training on the inferior alveolar nerve block procedure. The monitor simultaneously displays the virtual environment rendered in the HMD, illustrating the system's immersive and interactive design. Reproduced from Collaço et al. [6], published in Journal of Dental Education 85 (2021) 589–598, © 2020, with permission from John Wiley and Sons

of the evolving student knowledge state and subsequently generated hints or remedial feedback when the student struggled. Dental students who worked with this intelligent tutoring system achieved clinical reasoning gains equivalent to those obtained from human-tutored sessions. These results indicate that well-designed intelligent tutors can model expert guidance and be effective in providing feedback-rich learning in preclinical education.

In addition to more structured tutoring programs, conversational AI chatbots are also being studied as virtual dental educators. AI chatbots can offer answers to students' questions in straightforward language at any hour (with no anticipated response time for feedback), providing on-demand clarification and coaching beyond regular class hours. In a study conducted in a clinical education setting, a custom-developed chatbot was integrated to support students' clinical inquiries. Students reported significantly higher engagement and satisfaction, along with reduced anxiety, when using the chatbot compared with the traditional platform. The immediate responses to their questions enhanced interactivity and helped reduce faculty workload [11]. This 24/7 AI tutor availability is beneficial if a student chooses to study late at night and wants guided help with a more challenging concept or topic, allowing them to reinforce or deepen their understanding when an experienced human instructor might be unavailable.

Another benefit that AI-based tutoring systems can provide is the ability to identify which students are at risk of falling behind. The data collected through these systems, including quiz scores, response times, and hint usage, can be used in predictive algorithms to inform instructors of learners in need of additional assistance. Early applications of ML models in higher education have shown a high degree of accuracy in predicting at-risk student status in a course, for example, identifying students who are struggling with ~90% accuracy by the mid-point of the course [12]. Through performance patterns, an AI system may even be able to predict that a student is likely to fail an upcoming exam, allowing faculty members an opportunity to intervene with remediation well before the student reaches a crisis. It is through this approach that intelligent tutoring systems not only respond to student performance but also reformulate the academic mentoring and coaching dynamic to include a proactive process, ensuring that no student is left unsupervised to fail.

It is essential to note that AI tutoring technologies in dental health education are still in their infancy and have not spread to all programs [8]. The data we have to date is positive, but many dental programs are still utilizing AI as part of pilot studies or as a secondary format to in-person learning, not as a main format of education. There are still many issues related to the ability of AI to provide an appropriate feedback mechanism, the speed of curriculum development and/or deployment, and whether faculty will take on the student-educator role—and to what degree faculty roles may change with AI-enhanced learning experiences and educational delivery models in dental education. Regardless, there is no doubt that intelligent tutoring systems and AI-assisted technologies will be present in more dental programs in the future, as they can provide an individualized, adaptive learning experience at any time of day or night—as an ongoing tutor or assistant—and will ultimately advance dental education in preclinical environments while better preparing future dental professionals.

7.2.2 AI in Clinical Dental Education

Once students reach the clinical stage of their education (where they begin treating patients under supervision), AI technologies can potentially remain a supportive educational tool. The focus at this stage changes from isolated psychomotor skill development to clinical decision-making, patient management, and the evaluation of student performance. AI can be utilized to enhance clinical education through tools including virtual patient simulation, chairside decision support while treating patients in educational clinics, and AI-enhanced student evaluation tools.

To prepare students for interacting with real patients, educators are increasingly using virtual patient simulators and case-based learning platforms [13–17]. Virtual patient simulators provide another avenue for education and an opportunity for dental students to continue working toward building their clinical competencies in a safe environment and to use feedback to help them improve. The purpose of virtual patients is to provide workplace exposure to case-based learning for early-stage learners while avoiding the potential negative outcomes of early exposure to patients. These platforms are designed to facilitate relatable patient interactions so students can practice patient interviewing, risk assessment, and treatment planning before seeing patients in clinical settings. In short, virtual patient platforms help bridge the gap between preclinical experience and patient care responsibilities.

One of their most important benefits is the flexibility they provide, allowing students to engage repeatedly and reflectively with different clinical encounters at any time during their training. In one study, Mardani et al. [18] found that the application of virtual patient-based training can improve learning and clinical decision-making ability of dental students. In another study, Wu et al. [19] developed a Virtual Dental Clinic (VDC) and found that students using VDC demonstrated improved performance compared to a control group. VDC users demonstrated higher scores on qualification tests and also reported that using VDC was beneficial for their clinical reasoning process. Fig. 7.4 shows a sample conversation from one of the VDC cases. Students view virtual cases as a valued addition to their clinical training. Students who are exposed to a broader array of virtual cases will encounter a range of experiences beyond the limits of clinical rotations. They will also serve as a bridge in training from preclinical learning to experiences with real patients. Emerging virtual patient platforms can adapt to student input—for example, an AI-driven chatbot can use learner responses to role-play patient interactions—thus following, to some degree, the nature of real interactions with patients [20]. Overall, the incorporation of AI-driven virtual patient simulations into dental curricula is a novel approach that has a potential to enhance students' treatment planning capabilities and confidence before they treat real patients.

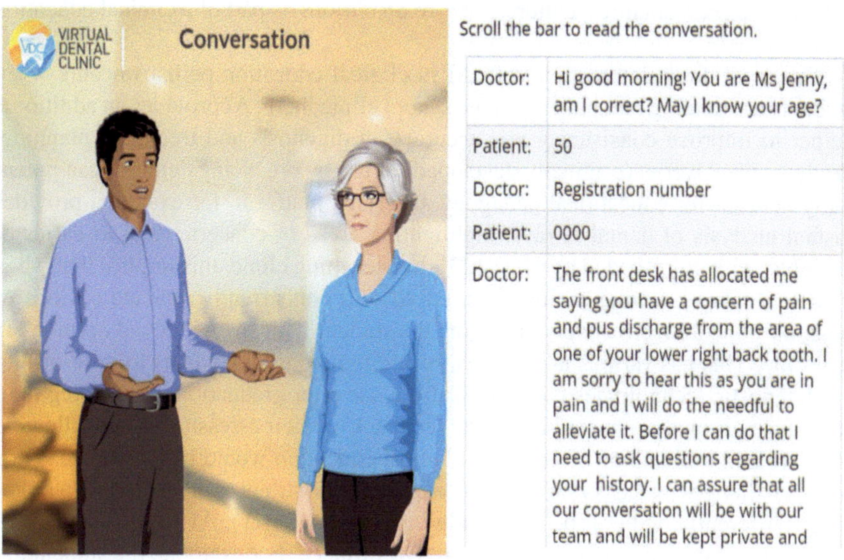
VIRTUAL DENTAL CLINIC
Conversation
Scroll the bar to read the conversation.
Doctor: Hi good morning! You are Ms Jenny, am I correct? May I know your age?
Patient: 50
Doctor: Registration number
Patient: 0000
Doctor: The front desk has allocated me saying you have a concern of pain and pus discharge from the area of one of your lower right back tooth. I am sorry to hear this as you are in pain and I will do the needful to alleviate it. Before I can do that I need to ask questions regarding your history. I can assure that all our conversation will be with our team and will be kept private and

Fig. 7.4 A sample conversation from one VDC. Reproduced from Rehman et al. [21], published in BMC Medical Education 25 (2025) 585, under the Creative Commons Attribution 4.0 International License (CC BY), (https://creativecommons.org/licenses/by/4.0/)

Utilization of AI chatbots as either patient-simulators or supervisor-simulators represents a new avenue for clinical training. For example, an AI chatbot can be assigned a persona (e.g., a patient with a toothache) through which the student must take the history through either text or voice conversation. The AI can then respond in real time with either the necessary information or appropriate emotional reactions potentially associated with that scenario. Jones et al. [22] created an AI chatbot based on Generative Pre-trained Transformer (GPT) technology to simulate a patient consultation followed by a discussion with a clinical instructor. The students connected with two AI chatbots: the first simulated a patient, and the second simulated a clinical supervisor engaging with the student. The findings were positive—educators observing the exercise offered feedback indicating the AI role-play "facilitated peer discussion, highlighted gaps in history taking, and promoted peer learning." In a post-exercise survey, students indicated that the AI-simulated patient encounter was authentic and relevant to the clinical practice context, and 86% of students reported strong agreement that their simulation felt real. This suggests that, with thoughtful design, AI chatbots can create effective simulations of patient interactions to enhance students' communication and diagnostic questioning skills in a controlled environment. They offer unique opportunities to repeat interviews, as a student could interview the patient again and try something different or new, which may not be feasible with an actual patient at will. With AI models continuing to improve in sophistication, it is feasible to create even better virtual patients or even AI "standardized patients" for examinations and training, including the ability to have various personalities, cultures, or rare conditions as part of a clinical education experience.

The most direct interaction with AI in clinical education perhaps occurs when students are treating real patients in the school clinic; here, AI provides an additional helper to improve consistency and accuracy in diagnosis and treatment planning. Products like Overjet (originally developed for use by practicing dentists) can potentially be used for educational pedagogy. Overjet's platform, for example, provides instant analysis of dental X-rays, highlighting areas of concern, such as caries or calculus, with color-coded overlays [23]. In a teaching clinic, this implies that when a student takes bitewing radiographs, an AI will concurrently indicate cavities or quantify bone loss, effectively providing the student with an "AI second opinion" in real time. This has various advantages, including exposing students to state-of-the-art diagnostic technologies they are likely to use after graduation, reinforcing their learning by providing immediate visual feedback on their assessments, and allowing standardized evaluations of findings. Clinical education would benefit because one of the challenges it faces is variability (i.e., different instructors may interpret a radiograph differently, with all being equally valid perspectives). AI would standardize the baseline evaluation to reduce interpretive variance. For example, if a student did not identify an incipient interproximal caries on an X-ray, the AI overlay would call attention to it (color-coded) to help facilitate that teachable moment. Early adopters have reported that AI-embedded tools in clinics have enhanced students' diagnostic accuracy. An investigation at the University of Florida determined that students who trained using Overjet's AI improved their ability to detect cavities in X-rays by more than 40% [24]. These AI platforms also provide a faculty dashboard where faculty members can track students' performance, including overall review cases, diagnostic accuracy, and clinical alignment, to determine which students need support and in what areas [23]. It adds a data-driven aspect to evaluating students' progress, complementing the observation and grading by the instructor. In this manner, AI can act like another instructor in the clinic, one who never gets tired and is always there to point out details.

A further use of AI in clinical dental training includes the utilization of performance assessment tools via AI. Currently, this could be viewed through the lens of Objective Structured Clinical Examinations (OSCEs), which are established clinical competency evaluations for students who demonstrate their clinical knowledge and skills through a series of structured stations or scenarios. While traditionally human raters score the students, AI is beginning to analyze performance on OSCEs. It is worth mentioning that most existing research and examples of AI-assisted OSCE evaluation come from the medical field, offering valuable insights that could inform future dental applications. For example, Geathers et al. [25] designed and tested a system to automatically assess OSCE scores based on the Master Interview Rating Scale (MIRS) using Large Language Models (LLMs). They compared the performance of four state-of-the-art LLMs (GPT-4o, Claude 3.5, Llama 3.1, and Gemini 1.5 Pro) in evaluating OSCE transcripts across all 28 items of the MIRS under the conditions of zero-shot, chain-of-thought, few-shot, and multi-step prompting. Tekin et al. [26] evaluated the performance of ChatGPT-4o and Gemini Flash 1.5 in scoring students' clinical skills during an OSCE and compared the results of the AI and human evaluators. Their findings showed that AI consistently rated the students' performances higher but more uniform than the human evaluators, suggesting potential for standardization in future AI-based assessment systems. They found that inter-rater consistency was higher for visually observable steps, while auditory tasks led to greater discrepancies between AI and human evaluators. They suggested that AI is promising as a supplemental tool for OSCE evaluation, especially for visually based clinical skills.

Such findings in medicine may serve as a foundation for exploring similar AI-driven assessment approaches in dental education, particularly where clinical tasks are also visually observable. AI systems in dentistry could one day evaluate a student's technique based on video analysis, observing the student's adherence to clinical protocols. While the incorporation of AI-based evaluation in medical education is still in its infancy, these AI-based assessments have the potential to bring greater rigor, objectivity, and scalability to dental evaluations as well. AI evaluation tools may assist in managing the large volume of assessment work, thereby increasing faculty time spent on remediation or instruction. Further, validating assessment systems to ensure they function equitably, remain free of bias, and provide fair assessments will be essential for their successful integration into dental education.

In conclusion, AI, as it relates to clinical dental education, serves as both a coach and a safety net. It enhances students' confidence by providing supportive analyses and guidance during the provision of care. Similarly, AI enhances students' skills for the future; as AI becomes commonplace in practice, today's students must demonstrate proficiency in using these resources. Early results of students learning in clinics involving AI are promising [24]. Students become better at interpreting AI outputs and make more consistent diagnoses. Virtual patients and chatbots also build readiness by improving decision-making and communication skills in a simulated environment. Some challenges with respect to AI in clinical education highlight the need to prevent students from relying on AI too heavily, to ensure they master the fundamental clinical skills, and for faculty to be present to address technical issues and provide oversight of inaccuracies. The future generation of dentists will use AI as a commonplace part of their decision-making process, so including AI in education isn't just helpful—it is necessary. AI, when properly integrated, can yield more competent, confident, and tech-savvy clinicians.

7.2.3 From Learning Analytics to Adaptive Curricula: The Evolving Role of AI in Dental Education Systems

AI is having an increasingly transformational impact at different levels of dental education, not just improving individual teaching tools, but also spearheading changes in curriculum design, student support systems, and programmatic planning. This section will discuss how AI, along with learning analytics based on data, is being utilized to optimize the curriculum structure, personalize student pathways in their learning, enable early identification of at-risk students, and support decision-making at the programmatic level based on evidence. From adaptive learning platforms and predictive modeling to faculty development and competency-based frameworks, AI is changing how dental schools develop, deliver, and continually optimize their education model.

One of the key applications of AI in education is learning analytics, which can be described as the utilization of student performance and engagement data to inform educational strategies. An example from dental education is the study by Alwadei et al. [27], which, while not specifically using AI algorithms, demonstrates the power of a data-informed approach to curriculum optimization. These researchers used data on student interactions in an adaptive learning platform to predict final exam performance in a blended learning course. The study did not use AI algorithms, but the way researchers have found to use behavioral and performance data derived from e-learning platforms allows scalability in educational interventions and in principles related to AI-enabled systems. An example would be dental schools using such analytics to identify "at-risk" students and to simulate the potential consequences of curricular changes (e.g., targeted remedial modules for underperforming students).

Data-driven approaches have also been used to investigate curriculum structure at the program level, enabling visualization of course relationships and identification of key patterns. Ren et al. [28] conducted a study employing data science methods—specifically network modeling and visualization analysis based on complex network theory—to examine the structure of China's undergraduate dental curriculum. These data-driven and network-based methods are widely applied in educational data mining and curriculum analysis, providing a foundation for more advanced AI applications. By applying Pearson correlation coefficients to quantify the correlation between courses using student performance data, and analyzing topological measurements such as degree, betweenness, and clustering coefficient, they constructed a dynamic course network. Their findings showed that the whole course network exhibited an obvious small-world characteristic with a large clustering coefficient and a small average path. Furthermore, highly interconnected core courses—particularly Pathology, Pathophysiology, Oral Anatomy and Physiology, and Oral Biology—form the backbone of the program. The study concluded that while the curriculum follows a progressive structure from basic professional knowledge to professional skills, efforts toward curriculum reform are needed, particularly to address that the academic performance in skills and practical courses was lower than in public and theoretical courses. Their approach, although not strictly classified as an AI method, is illustrative of an emerging field of systems-level modeling framework used to analyze curriculum structures and identify inefficiencies. As demonstrated through this study, advanced data-driven techniques can reveal areas for improvement and support evidence-based curriculum reform, moving institutions away from anecdotal or arbitrary decisions toward intentional, data-informed design.

At the institutional level, learning analytics has transitioned from retrospective to real-time, actionable insight based on the implementation of dynamic dashboards that allow students, instructors, and administrators alike to visualize levels of mastery, progress towards learning objectives, and comparisons with the performance of peers [29]. Student-facing dashboards allow students to reflect on their learning, stay motivated, and self-regulate their learning, often enhanced by personalized recommendations, prompts, or alerts. Teacher-facing dashboards typically aggregate data on student engagement and learning outcomes to portray performance trends, allowing instructors to monitor students who may be struggling and adjust their pedagogy to provide interventions and reach out to individual students needing help. Finally, compared to student- and teacher-facing dashboards, administrator-facing dashboards could provide visibility into systemic issues and outcomes of pedagogy, supporting decision-making for curriculum changes and the distribution of resources accordingly. While not strictly AI-based, these platforms form the backbone of more sophisticated AI-enabled decision-support systems that continue to evolve with advances in AI.

A highly significant application of AI in education is the ability to proactively identify students at risk of failing or dropping out. ML models can be trained on historical student data to identify early indicators, including declining test scores, low engagement in digital systems, or multiple unexcused absences. Research in educational data mining has shown that academic measures and contextual factors such as family income and absenteeism can greatly improve predictive accuracy [30]. For example, Mustofa et al. [31] constructed a hybrid AI model using Logistic Regression (LogReg) and a Neural Network (NN) to predict student dropout with high accuracy (up to 96%) based on various factors. Such predictive models can help an institution intervene in a student's academic experience through academic or counseling support before it leads to significant problems.

Several Learning Management Systems (LMS) have started to incorporate such capabilities directly into their platforms through early alert systems. These LMS can look for indicators such as frequency of access, timing of assignment submissions, and levels of participation. If disengagement is detected, alerts can be sent out to instructors or academic advisors for appropriate intervention to enable quick action. Studies have shown that these types of systems can have a positive impact on educational attainment. Han et al. [32] reported that using academic alert systems to prompt action helped reduce course withdrawal rates and increase the proportion of students earning at least a C grade. LMS platforms such as Moodle now have learning analytics engines, including ML algorithms, to analyze students' risk levels based on quizzes, forum involvement, and assignment submissions [33]. Additionally, tools such as Dropout Detective utilize AI to evaluate LMS data and analyze students' situations to determine the likelihood of retention or withdrawal. These systems can generate early-detection alerts about student engagement along with recommendations to support interventions with students before new or imminent academic difficulties arise.

The value of early warning systems in a dental education context, given its significant course load and professional obligations, is even more critical. The nature of dental education is fairly intense and demanding for students, which increases their risk of burnout and mental health problems, and affects, to varying degrees, their academic and clinical performance. Furthermore, a snapshot survey of dental trainees during the COVID-19 pandemic indicated that 12.7% had intention to leave their education; students experiencing anxiety, depression, or burnout were between ~ 8 and 11 times more likely to consider leaving their educational program [34]. Early warning signs, such as a noticeable drop in simulation lab scores, repeated underachievement on quizzes, or a reduction in attendance, can be detected by AI and trigger a summary alert to the faculty before the condition escalates or worsens. Faculty members can intervene by providing timely academic support, mentoring, or counseling, effectively reducing the risk of attrition while helping students get back on track. Predictive models act as a safety net to ensure students do not fall through the cracks in the system.

In addition to support and monitoring, there is a growing acknowledgment of the need to evolve dental education itself to better equip future dentists for integrating AI-powered technologies into clinical practice. Educators and professional organizations have increasingly articulated the value of incorporating AI knowledge and skills into the foundational curriculum. For example, Schwendicke et al. [35] provided a proposed framework for an AI curriculum in dental education that would cover fundamental concepts such as principles of ML, applications to clinical practice, evaluation of performance, and ethical considerations. Ultimately, the idea is that graduates acquire relevant knowledge to understand, evaluate, and use AI tools appropriately in delivering patient care. Other studies have uncovered similar support for AI reforms in the curriculum, calling for AI-related topics and ethical considerations to be introduced as early as possible in undergraduate education [36].

Support from faculty members is also strong; in a recent survey, 81% of dental faculty acknowledged the need for and limited opportunities available to learn AI, thereby emphasizing the urgency of developing contextually relevant AI training programs [37]. As a result, many dental schools are beginning to implement changes by including dental informatics courses and providing exposure to AI functions through AI-assisted diagnostic tools.

One area that holds tremendous promise for impacting the educational landscape is the development of personalized, adaptive curriculum pathways for students—an area where AI's potential to transform education is particularly obvious. Often, dental curricula are designed around a one-size-fits-all model. However, students learn at vastly different rates, come from different backgrounds, and have different visions for their careers. AI could provide an adaptive learning experience by adjusting the delivery, difficulty, and pacing of content based on a student's individual progress in the curriculum [38]. Furthermore, these AI-based adaptive learning systems can provide mastery-based progression, whereby a student is held back from proceeding through the curriculum until they demonstrate competence—a valuable function in a precision-based profession like dentistry. AI can supply real-time feedback and continuously adjust the student's learning path to ensure foundational gaps are addressed before they engage in advanced procedures. This is also an effective way to maintain the engagement of faster learners while supporting students who might require more time to learn.

The purpose of integrating personalized learning pathways is ultimately to ensure every student is fully competent upon graduation, with no weaknesses left unaddressed. Research indicates that adaptive e-learning platforms lead to increased levels of engagement and motivation, ultimately resulting in superior exam performance in dental training programs [39]. Adaptive e-learning platforms are designed to continuously assess student strengths and weaknesses, providing educators with feedback to modify instruction and implement focused interventions. For example, if a skill gap in diagnosis or hand techniques develops, it can be identified and remediated within the educational experience long before it becomes a potential risk in practice. Through data-driven, real-time analysis with personalized support, AI is paving the way for a new dental education model that maximizes student potential, supports greater equity, and raises the bar of overall professional competency. AI presents the opportunity to disrupt dental education in a way that optimally improves the educational experience and, subsequently, the quality of care provided by future dentists.

7.3 AI in Managing Dental Practice

Managing dental practice involves operating in a complex milieu of administrative, management, and clinical responsibilities, such as patient scheduling, billing, insurance, supply management, patient records management, and regulatory compliance. Traditionally, the management of a dental office has been process-oriented, tedious, laborious, and subject to human error. Advancements in AI are replacing or automating many facets of back-office business functions in dentistry. This section reviews how technologies enabled by AI can advance practice management with respect to patient scheduling, patient flow, and the management and security of patient data. In these examples, AI-backed technologies have the potential for both increased productivity and fewer errors. In addition, AI usage allows clinical teams to spend less time performing administrative tasks and more time focusing on patient care rather than paperwork.

7.3.1 AI's Role in Patient Scheduling, Workflow, and Communication

AI is changing the way dental clinics perform patient scheduling, workflow, and communication. In a typical dental clinic, scheduling is based on unsophisticated phone calls, a static calendar, and human judgment, all of which typically have difficulty accommodating changes in patient flow. The typical inefficiencies of scheduling may lead to a provider sitting idle due to unfilled time slots or patient no-shows. AI-based systems, in contrast, by harnessing predictive analytics, automatic booking, and communication, enhance clinic efficiency and patient experience [40]. AI systems assess historical data on patient flow and scheduling to determine demand and peak days/times for patients. This predictive optimization feature can benefit both the patient and the practitioner, as clinics reduce rigid time blocks and implement a responsive and data-driven approach based on the individual clinic's patient flow.

A powerful example of the application of AI in dental practice management is the ability to reduce no-show rates using predictive analytics and smart communications. An AI system will initially analyze a patient's demographic and past behavior data to identify and predict whether they will show up for their scheduled appointment [41]. From there, instead of just flagging their appointment, modern platforms engage patients proactively long before the appointment date with personalized and multi-channel reminders via SMS, email, or automated phone calls, all timed at an AI-optimized period [42, 43]. These systems not only confirm attendance but also offer patients an easy way to reschedule or find alternatives through conversational AI. In practices that use an AI solution, no-show rates have decreased from 12–15% to as low as 4–6%, resulting in a 60–70% reduction in lost revenue each year [43]. In one example of implementation on a larger scale, a practice's no-show rate dropped from 15.1% to 5.9%, with nearly $10 million in cost savings within a year, demonstrated by improved scheduling efficiency and appointment capacity utilization [42]. AlSerkal et al. [44] designed and tested an AI-based no-show prediction model for primary health care centers and a real-time dashboard. The system achieved a 50.7% reduction in no-show rates and reduced average wait times for patients by 5.7 min. While the study was in a clinical setting, the fundamental approaches described may be transferred to a dental setting facing similar problems.

AI systems not only facilitate workflow efficiency but also allow for real-time rescheduling or "on-the-fly" management of a waitlist. If a cancellation occurs, the system can simultaneously notify patients on a waitlist through automated chat or rapid notification and fill the cancellation in real time [40]. That means there can be no downtime for the patient and clinician, with much less overhead. Such integrated AI systems mean that dental practice can maximize the schedules of the clinician, as well as work to improve patient engagement and experience while reducing administrative human overhead and time. As algorithms and AI technology are capable of scheduling single patients (individuals), they are also capable of predicting patient demand on a daily basis, thus allowing clinics to anticipate patient demand and be ready staff-wise. For example, if the AI system predicts an influx of patients for pediatrics or hygiene in the morning, it can recommend specific staff (assistants, front-office) to be available at particular times/durations to ensure room turnover efficiency and workflow. When clinics proactively adjust staffing to match the demand forecast, they can avoid operational bottlenecks that disrupt flow in the clinic, and they can maintain a pace that is sustainable throughout the day. This also creates a more optimal and less stressful clinical environment for providers to stay on schedule and gives patients timely and well-coordinated care.

A major component of these AI-enabled improvements depends on the effective integration of the scheduling solution and communication tool into a practice's existing dental Practice Management System (PMS). When the AI-driven solution shares the same appointment database as the front desk, any booking or change made by a human or AI will sync in real time. This two-way synchronization prevents double bookings and mistakes in data entry for staff and clinicians who rely on an updated shared schedule [45]. This integration further enables robust analytics and continuous improvement. AI-enabled PMS dashboards track metrics like booking lead times, cancellation/no-show rates, confirmation response rates, and even post-visit satisfaction. The practice manager can see these indicators in real time and make changes to their practice based on the data collected.

Availability around the clock is a key feature of modern AI scheduling platforms in the field of dentistry. Conversational chatbots or voice assistants act as virtual receptionists and can process appointment scheduling, confirmations, rescheduling, and simple questions 24/7. Patients are able to interact in natural language (text or voice) at any time—even when offices are closed, to schedule or change appointments based on real-time availability. This functionality gives patients the option to not only eliminate the need to remain on hold but also the need to wait for a staff member to become available to schedule an appointment. Additionally, dental practices can expect to see increased convenience for their patients and a decrease in lost leads and opportunities. In a study, voice AI increased the number of patients willing to schedule an appointment by nearly 20% at times. Voice AI is a powerful tool in the effort to automate normal processes while also giving clinical and administrative personnel 50%–80% less work to accomplish during the day, learning inbound patient questions before they even reach the front desk [46]. AI assistants that automate normal scheduling processes as depicted above encourage staff to spend more of their valuable time on patients. Furthermore, staff are no longer needed to collect basic patient information, verify identity, or document the reason for a visit, all of which can be done without staff using the above systems that seamlessly integrate into the scheduling platform. They also manage frequently asked questions efficiently, handle appointment logistics, and even arrange post-visit follow-ups, all of which help significantly reduce administrative burden and enhance timely, consistent communication [47].

After dental treatment, for example, an AI chatbot can follow up with the patient within the last day or two to check on their recovery and ask how their pain level is, if they've been taking their medication as prescribed (if applicable), and if they have experienced any unusual symptoms [48]. The proactive follow-up provides an opportunity to detect complications early and creates other similar opportunities to intervene. Moreover, given the prevalence of dental anxiety, the system can help relieve some of the patient's worries by offering supportive communication, addressing concerns, and explaining procedures slowly and clearly, resulting in a calming experience for the patient. Over time, the AI system can learn about a patient's communication style—for example, some patients might respond better to receiving a text in the evening or an email in the morning, or even reminders based on their previous treatment, like cleanings or crowns, which allow extremely personalized and well-timed interactions.

While there is much to be gained, including efficiency and effectiveness, bringing AI into the world of dental scheduling and communication is not without its challenges. Data privacy and security are top-of-mind considerations for dentists, as AI tools will be processing information related to personal health as well as appointment booking data. Dental practices will need to have strong data protection measures, including regulatory-compliant encryption, secure hosting, and transparent consent policies. This also includes clear accountability and liability policies in case issues arise. Integration will be costly and operationally complicated, necessitating training staff, workflow redesign, and ongoing maintenance, which may limit adoption in smaller practices. Another factor is patient acceptance. In recent surveys, patients view AI as beneficial in scheduling and communication, focusing on convenience, personalization, and cost savings. Respondents are not particularly concerned with risks such as privacy and miscommunication. Acceptance increases when patients are aware of the benefits and there is transparency about data and human oversight. Adoption is not just about technology; it also involves educating our patients and staff about how it improves services and ensures information is secure.

In conclusion, AI presents a substantial paradigm shift in the manner in which dental practices schedule appointments, communicate with patients, and manage their workflow. Predictive scheduling, dynamic rescheduling, AI chatbots and systems operating 24/7, custom messaging, and PMS integration help reduce no-shows, provide smooth service, and improve patient experience while allowing staff to focus on the clinical aspect of their care. There are challenges that remain in the areas of patient privacy, integration costs, and training, but early adopters have been able to show measurable returns on investment [42, 43]. As the evidence continues to grow and the platforms mature, the use of AI to streamline patient scheduling, workflow, and communication will become necessary to support an efficient, patient-centric dental practice management system.

7.3.2 *Patient Data Management and Security with AI*

Dental practices in the modern era generate and maintain large amounts of patient data, which include EDRs, medical history, radiographs, and financial information. Managing this data is crucial for quality care and operational effectiveness, but it also presents significant security and privacy issues. For this reason, there is an increasing utilization of AI to manage, analyze, and secure patient information in dentistry. In both record-keeping and data processing, AI may help a dentist identify opportunities to improve patient care from the patient's record, streamline administrative workflows, and maintain a reliable and up-to-date database of patient records. However, there are important protections to consider when leveraging AI for data processing in dentistry, since the security and confidentiality of patient records must not be compromised in the healthcare environment [49]. This section will focus on the role of AI in the patient data management process within dental practice and highlight the steps taken to secure data and maintain patient confidentiality.

Dental clinics around the world are converting from paper charts to EDRs, which produce large repositories of digital documents where patient information is stored. AI technologies have features that facilitate the management of the digital image of patient records. For example, ML models allow the automatic extraction of clinical data from unstructured text within dental notes. In a study by Chuang et al. [50], a type of Natural Language Processing (NLP) via generative AI (GPT-4) was used to standardize dentists' free-text notes into structured data in periodontal diagnosis. The data extraction system demonstrated high accuracy, with weighted average scores of approximately 0.97 in classifying periodontal disease stage and grade, which reduces the amount of missing data in dental records and the necessity for difficult manual chart audits and reviews. The use of AI extraction will help plausibly standardize information across dental practices, allowing for a more robust analysis of patient histories and outcomes.

To effectively manage patient data using AI, it is important to have access to valid and comprehensive datasets. Dental AI systems perform well with massive amounts of data, but unfortunately, most of that data remains siloed across different clinics and organizations. Traditional data-sharing approaches are impeded by stringent privacy policies that usually preclude gathering enough data for solid model training, which results in weaker AI models. To address this issue, researchers have examined privacy-preserving collaborative learning methods, with FL being one of the most common recent approaches [51]. Using FL, clinics collaborate to develop dental AI models without sharing raw patient data. Each clinic keeps its own data, sharing only the model parameters of what they learned through training. The collaborative process thus builds a generalized model that learns from distributed data sources (e.g., radiographs or clinical notes) while preserving patient confidentiality.

In dentistry, the protection of this confidential information is of utmost importance. Even anonymous dental radiographs may contain identifiable information, such as unique anatomical features or restorative work [51]. These issues accentuate the need to advance innovative methods for leveraging data for AI, such as FL, to support ethical and scalable AI adoption into dental practice management.

Dental patient data is extremely sensitive and contains health histories, personal identifiers, insurance and payment details, and clinical notes. Breaches or improper access to this data can severely compromise patient confidentiality and trust. This may lead to identity theft or medical fraud. Therefore, any data system framework that incorporates AI in the dental profession must have strict security elements and be compliant with health privacy standards, such as Health Insurance Portability and Accountability Act (HIPAA) in the United States and General Data Protection Regulation (GDPR) in Europe. Practically, this means implementing encryption processes when storing and transmitting data, role-based access procedures, and audit logs that document who has access, backup processes, and regular audits of system security. In their commentary regarding AI cloud incorporation for dental clinics, Bedia et al. [52] suggest that data security is crucial: dental cloud platforms should utilize encryption, access control, and continuous compliance monitoring to abide by regulations while protecting patient health information. Additionally, Bedia et al. [52] caution that failing to maintain these security protocols can lead to serious business interruptions, legal issues, and loss of patient trust.

Consent and transparency are vital foundations of data security and privacy when using dental AI systems. Because these systems rely on substantial amounts of patient data, it is paramount for patients to trust that their information is being handled ethically and responsibly. This trust is grounded in explicit and easy-to-understand communication about the policy on the use of patient data, who will own the data, how the data will be used or shared, and what safeguards will be in place to protect the data. When possible, patients should have the option to opt out or have some level of control over their data use. In addition, dental providers must provide clear disclosure of the use of AI in patient data processing. Transparency not only provides accountability for ethical data management, but it also reduces potential resistance to using AI tools by giving patients the implicit idea that they will be respected and their information kept confidential.

Alongside policies and encryption solutions, there is increasing interest in how AI itself can improve cybersecurity in healthcare systems and dental practices [53, 54]. On one hand, AI software can expand the attack surface, while on the other hand, AI can assist in security by monitoring networks and systems for suspicious behavior. For example, intrusion detection systems, typically using ML, can evaluate network traffic to identify anomalous behavior in real time, such as attempts to access patient records without authorization. Identifying such anomalies before they result in harm is particularly valuable in the delivery of healthcare, where a breach may not be detected until damage has occurred.

Ultimately, AI provides tremendous capabilities to process data concerning dental patients with greater efficiency, enhancing the accuracy of records, providing data-informed decision support, and automating both standard and routine tasks—all of which can lead to an improvement in the quality of patient care and the productivity of offices. However, the above-noted efficiencies can only be achieved sustainably with data security and rigorous protection of patient privacy. Dental practices will need to balance innovation with compliance. To do this, dental practices will deploy AI systems cautiously, implementing robust security architectures, facilitating staff development, and establishing clear processes of governance to protect patient data from unauthorized access or incidental misuse. The research community is working intently on solutions like FL to balance the data appetite of AI with the ethics of privacy. By implementing the necessary security protocols and following ethical research guidelines, dentistry can leverage AI for the management of patient data while still protecting confidentiality, enhancing patient trust, and living up to the high standard of care. The future of AI in dental practice management can be smart and efficient, while also being secure and patient-centered, if we all remain diligent and innovative.

7.4 Conclusion

AI is revolutionizing dental education and the management of dental practices in significant ways. In education, AI-based solutions are improving how dentists are educated and trained, through simulators that objectively measure hand skills, virtual patients that facilitate clinical reasoning, and analytics that inform curricular revisions. These solutions are producing graduates who are better skilled, more confident, and "AI-aware." Concurrently, AI is changing how practices are operationalized by automating scheduling and safeguarding patient information, allowing practitioners to give more attention to patients. AI, in sum, covers almost every facet of dentistry, supporting educators, clinicians, and administrators.

However, there are issues associated with AI in education and practice management. First, the privacy of data and the security of patient information are of paramount importance. AI systems store sensitive material, such as student performance data and patient health data, which raises the stakes for the institutions to which the data belongs. While AI systems can improve cybersecurity, for example, through anomaly detection, institutions will still need to demonstrate sound data governance and regulatory compliance with laws like HIPAA and GDPR. Another area that needs addressing is the issue of bias and fairness in AI algorithms; anything that is used to evaluate students should be monitored closely to avoid exacerbating existing inequalities. Interoperability issues also remain, because many of the AI systems operate outside of other software systems.

Another important factor is the human-AI relationship. AI ought to be viewed as an augmentation of human judgment rather than a replacement. In the context of education, instructors must find the right balance between AI feedback and instructor-mentored feedback. In the clinical environment, dentists will need to utilize AI's comments along with their own expertise and effectively communicate results with patients. Resistance to change is also a hurdle, given that educators, learners, and practitioners may have reservations about implementing new technologies. Despite this, early adopters appear to have clearer and more salient outcomes, objectives, and confidence pertaining to AI, and the perceived value and effectiveness typically develop over time.

Looking toward the future, AI will be further integrated into dental education and dental practice. FL may provide a pathway for cross-institutional AI education research, allowing organizations to prioritize privacy while simultaneously taking larger and more significant steps toward developing large-scale AI educational systems for dentistry. In practice, AI-driven administrative workflows may one day conduct routine tasks without human engagement, from appointment booking to confirmation to insurance verification. Voice assistants may transcribe clinical notes into designated Electronic Health Records (EHRs) in real time. Robotic process automation may allow back-office tasks to be executed by a system outside of human engagement. Pursuing a "self-driving" dental office, where systems operate with little or no human engagement, similarly seems possible.

As AI becomes more woven into the educational context, AI literacy will become part of the "basic skills." Future curricula will probably focus on learning to work with decision-support systems, including evaluating AI outputs and using the tool in an ethical manner. This is already beginning to happen, with some AI curriculum guidelines suggesting that this is a skill set we should be developing for dental students. While we think about our role as instructors in teaching AI literacy, we should also think about how AI is not necessarily an endpoint but rather a dynamic tool that we will continue to evaluate. Whether it's a component of student performance or practice efficiency, dental schools or clinics will have to collect outcomes data, similar to what we do for other treatments, to demonstrate that AI systems are providing the benefits we suggest.

The fast pace of AI progress can be stimulating yet somewhat daunting. For dentists and educators, the way forward involves engaging proactively. Beginning with small introductions to AI-supported tools, such as allowing radiograph analysis by AI or reminding patients of appointments, might provide simple initial steps to incorporate AI into daily operations. Additionally, educators should adopt predictable AI-supported learning tools while sharing and collaborating with others for learning opportunities. By actively engaging in the changes that AI is propelling into our professions, we assist in the development of these technologies. The dental profession can meaningfully direct these developments toward the highest goals of the profession. In summary, AI is ushering in a new era for dental care; whether through automation, data-driven decision support, or personalized education, both patient care and education are enhanced. By engaging thoughtfully and ethically, with attention to the human aspect of dental care, AI will not replace the human element of dentistry—it will enhance it.

References

1. Transforming dental operations: The role of AI in streamlining back-office functions—CDA, (n.d.). https://www.cda.org/newsroom/newsroom-archives/transforming-dental-operations-the-role-of-ai-in-streamlining-back-office-functions/ (Accessed July 17, 2025)
2. A.L.-S. Leung, C. Yeung, S. Chu, A.W.-Y. Wong, O.Y. Yu, C.-H. Chu, Use of computer simulation in dental training with special reference to simodont. Dent J (Basel) **9**, 125 (2021)
3. A. Farag, D. Hashem, Impact of the haptic virtual reality simulator on dental students' psychomotor skills in preclinical operative dentistry. Clin Pract **12**, 17–26 (2021)
4. Y. Li, H. Ye, S. Wu, X. Zhao, Y. Liu, L. Lv, P. Zhang, X. Zhang, Y. Zhou, Mixed reality and haptic–based dental simulator for tooth preparation: research, development, and preliminary evaluation. JMIR Serious Games **10**, e30653 (2022)
5. P. Rhienmora, P. Haddawy, S. Suebnukarn, M.N. Dailey, Intelligent dental training simulator with objective skill assessment and feedback. Artif. Intell. Med. **52**, 115–121 (2011)
6. E. Collaço, E. Kira, L.H. Sallaberry, A.C.M. Queiroz, M.A.A.M. Machado, O. Crivello Jr., R. Tori, Immersion and haptic feedback impacts on dental anesthesia technical skills virtual reality training. J. Dent. Educ. **85**, 589–598 (2021)
7. L.H. Sallaberry, R. Tori, F.L.S. Nunes, Comparison of machine learning algorithms for automatic assessment of performance in a virtual reality dental simulator, in: Proceedings of the 23rd Symposium on Virtual and Augmented Reality, 2021: pp. 14–23.
8. B.J. Kukreja, P. Kukreja, Integration of Artificial Intelligence in Dentistry: A Systematic Review of Educational and Clinical Implications, Cureus **17** (2025)
9. H. Wei, Y. Dai, K. Yuan, K.Y. Li, K.F. Hung, E.M. Hu, A.H.C. Lee, J.W.W. Chang, C. Zhang, X. Li, AI-Powered problem-and case-based learning in medical and dental education: a systematic review and meta-analysis. Int. Dent. J. **75**, 100858 (2025)
10. S. Suebnukarn, Intelligent tutoring system for clinical reasoning skill acquisition in dental students. J. Dent. Educ. **73**, 1178–1186 (2009)
11. Q. Fang, R. Reynaldi, A.S. Araminta, I. Kamal, P. Saini, F.S. Afshari, S.-C. Tan, J.C.-C. Yuan, N.N. Qomariyah, C. Sukotjo, Artificial Intelligence (AI)-driven dental education: Exploring the role of chatbots in a clinical learning environment, J. Prosthet Dent. (2024).
12. E. Nimy, M. Mosia, C. Chibaya, Identifying at-risk students for early intervention—a probabilistic machine learning approach. Appl. Sci. **13**, 3869 (2023)
13. H.L. Kleinert, C. Sanders, J. Mink, D. Nash, J. Johnson, S. Boyd, S. Challman, Improving student dentist competencies and perception of difficulty in delivering care to children with developmental disabilities using a virtual patient module. J. Dent. Educ. **71**, 279–286 (2007)
14. C.K. Weiner, M. Skålén, D. Harju-Jeanty, R. Heymann, A. Rosén, U. Fors, B. Lund, Implementation of a web-based patient simulation program to teach dental students in oral surgery. J. Dent. Educ. **80**, 133–140 (2016)
15. J.R. Boynton, T.G. Green, L.A. Johnson, S.M.H. Nainar, L.H. Straffon, The virtual child: evaluation of an internet-based pediatric behavior management simulation. J. Dent. Educ. **71**, 1187–1193 (2007)
16. G.T. Clark, A. Suri, R. Enciso, Autonomous virtual patients in dentistry: system accuracy and expert versus novice comparison. J. Dent. Educ. **76**, 1365–1370 (2012)
17. F. Janesarvatan, P. Van Rosmalen, Instructional design of virtual patients in dental education through a 4C/ID lens: a narrative review. J. Comput. Educ. **11**, 523–556 (2024)
18. M. Mardani, S. Cheraghian, S.K. Naeeni, N. Zarifsanaiey, Effectiveness of virtual patients in teaching clinical decision-making skills to dental students. J. Dent. Educ. **84**, 615–623 (2020)
19. J.-H. Wu, J.-K. Du, C.-Y. Lee, Development and questionnaire-based evaluation of virtual dental clinic: a serious game for training dental students. Med. Educ. Online **26**, 1983927 (2021)
20. A. Suárez, A. Adanero, V. Díaz-Flores García, Y. Freire, J. Algar, Using a virtual patient via an artificial intelligence chatbot to develop dental students' diagnostic skills, Int. J. Environ Res. Public Health **19** (2022) 8735

21. K. Rehman, O.S. Sultan, M.G. Babar, F. Marican, S.S. Mahdi, Perceptions of virtual clinical learning in dentistry: Understanding student views on virtual dental clinics. BMC Med. Educ. **25**, 585 (2025)
22. B. Jones, A. Desu, C.D.F. Honig, artificial intelligence chatbots as virtual patients in dental education: a constructivist approach to classroom implementation, european journal of dental education (2025)
23. AI in Dental Education. How Overjet Modernizes Dental Education, (n.d.). https://www.overjet.com/blog/ai-in-dental-education-how-overjet-modernizes-dental-education (Accessed July 28, 2025)
24. Introducing Overjet for Educators: AI Built for Dental Education, (n.d.). https://www.overjet.com/blog/introducing-overjet-for-educators-ai-built-for-dental-education (Accessed July 28, 2025)
25. J. Geathers, Y. Hicke, C. Chan, N. Rajashekar, S. Young, J. Sewell, S. Cornes, R.F. Kizilcec, D. Shung, Benchmarking generative ai for scoring medical student interviews in objective structured clinical examinations (osces), in: International Conference on Artificial Intelligence in Education, Springer, (2025), pp. 231–245
26. M. Tekin, M.O. Yurdal, Ç. Toraman, G. Korkmaz, İ. Uysal, Is AI the future of evaluation in medical education?? AI vs. human evaluation in objective structured clinical examination, BMC Med. Educ. **25** (2025) 641
27. F.H. Alwadei, B.P. Brown, S.H. Alwadei, I.B. Harris, A.H. Alwadei, The utility of adaptive eLearning data in predicting dental students' learning performance in a blended learning course. Int. J. Med. Educ. **14**, 137 (2023)
28. Q. Ren, X. Peng, X. Liu, Q. Zheng, T. He, D. Hu, X. Jiang, L. Zhang, Network modelling and visualisation analysis of the undergraduate dental curriculum system in China. J. Comput. Commun. **9**, 38–51 (2021)
29. M. Saqr, U. Fors, J. Nouri, Using Learning Analytics to Understand and Support Collaborative Learning, (2018). http://urn.kb.se/resolve?urn=urn:nbn:se:su:diva-159479
30. M. Suaza-Medina, R. Peñabaena-Niebles, M. Jubiz-Diaz, A model for predicting academic performance on standardised tests for lagging regions based on machine learning and Shapley additive explanations. Sci. Rep. **14**, 25306 (2024)
31. S. Mustofa, Y.R. Emon, S. Bin Mamun, S.A. Akhy, M.T. Ahad, A novel AI-driven model for student dropout risk analysis with explainable AI insights, Computers and Education: Artificial Intelligence **8** (2025) 100352
32. K. Han, K. Meints, L. Burns, K. Loper, Instructor use of academic alerts and its impact on student outcomes: controlling for selection bias, Stud. High. Educ. (2025) 1–13
33. AI-Driven Evolution in Learning Analytics for Digital Education, (n.d.). https://www.digitallearninginstitute.com/blog/ai-driven-evolution-in-learning-analytics-for-digital-education (Accessed July 28, 2025)
34. D.L. Chi, C.L. Randall, C.M. Hill, Dental trainees' mental health and intention to leave their programs during the COVID-19 pandemic. J. Am. Dent. Assoc. **152**, 526–534 (2021)
35. F. Schwendicke, A. Chaurasia, T. Wiegand, S.E. Uribe, M. Fontana, I. Akota, O. Tryfonos, J. Krois, Artificial intelligence for oral and dental healthcare: core education curriculum. J. Dent. **128**, 104363 (2023)
36. M. Harte, B. Carey, Q.J. Feng, A. Alqarni, R. Albuquerque, Transforming undergraduate dental education: the impact of artificial intelligence. Br. Dent. J. **238**, 57–60 (2025)
37. S. Abdullah, S.R. Hasan, M.A. Asim, A. Khurshid, A.W. Qureshi, Exploring dental faculty awareness, knowledge, and attitudes toward AI integration in education and practice: a mixed-method study. BMC Med. Educ. **25**, 691 (2025)
38. Artificial Intelligence in Dental Education. CranioCatch, (n.d.). https://www.craniocatch.com/en/blogs/ai-dentistry-education (accessed July 29, 2025)
39. M. Yakin, K. Linden, Adaptive e-learning platforms can improve student performance and engagement in dental education. J. Dent. Educ. **85**, 1309–1315 (2021)
40. AI in Dentistry: Smarter Scheduling & Appointments—scanO, (n.d.). https://scanoai.com/ai-in-dentist-smarter-scheduling-system/ (Accessed August 1, 2025)

41. K. Toker, K. Ataş, A. Mayadağlı, Z. Görmezoğlu, I. Tuncay, R. Kazancıoğlu, A solution to reduce the impact of patients' no-show behavior on hospital operating costs: Artificial intelligence-based appointment system, in: Healthcare, MDPI, (2024): p. 2161
42. How AI Technology is Transforming Appointment Management and Reducing No-Show Rates in Medical Facilities. Simbo AI—Blogs, (n.d.). https://www.simbo.ai/blog/how-ai-technology-is-transforming-appointment-management-and-reducing-no-show-rates-in-medical-facilities-2598712/ (Accessed August 2, 2025)
43. The Hidden Cost of No-Shows: How DentalQuest.AI Reduces Cancellations and Protects Revenue—DynaQuest Technology Services Inc, (n.d.). https://dqtsi.com/the-hidden-cost-of-no-shows-how-dental-ai-reduces-cancellations-and-protects-revenue/ (Accessed August 2, 2025)
44. Y.M. AlSerkal, N.M. Ibrahim, A.S. Alsereidi, M. Ibrahim, S. Kurakula, S.A. Naqvi, Y. Khan, N.P. Oottumadathil, Real-Time analytics and ai for managing no-show appointments in primary health care in the United Arab Emirates: before-and-after study. JMIR Form Res. **9**, e64936 (2025)
45. The Guide to AI Patient Scheduling for Medical & Dental Offices - Sales Closer AI, (n.d.). https://salescloser.ai/ai-patient-scheduling-for-medical-dental/ (Accessed August 2, 2025)
46. Voice AI Chat for Dentists: Elevate Patient Interaction and Satisfaction, (n.d.). https://smiletactics.com/blog/voice-ai-chat-for-dentists/ (Accessed August 2, 2025)
47. H. Akpınar, Comparison of responses from different artificial intelligence-powered chatbots regarding the All-on-four dental implant concept. BMC Oral Health **25**, 922 (2025)
48. V. Thorat, P. Rao, N. Joshi, P. Talreja, A.R. Shetty, P. RAO, Role of artificial intelligence (AI) in patient education and communication in dentistry, Cureus **16** (2024)
49. C. McGrath, C.W.R. Chau, G.F. Molina, Monitoring oral health remotely: ethical considerations when using AI among vulnerable populations. Frontiers in Oral Health **6**, 1587630 (2025)
50. Y.-S. Chuang, C.-T. Lee, G.-H. Lin, R. Brandon, X. Jiang, M.F. Walji, O. Tokede, Cross-institutional dental electronic health record entity extraction via generative artificial intelligence and synthetic notes, JAMIA Open **8** (2025) ooaf061
51. R. Rischke, L. Schneider, K. Müller, W. Samek, F. Schwendicke, J. Krois, Federated learning in dentistry: chances and challenges. J. Dent. Res. **101**, 1269–1273 (2022)
52. S. V Bedia, M.A. Shapurwala, B.P. Kharge, A.S. Bedia, A. Patil, A Comprehensive Guide to Implement Artificial Intelligence Cloud Solutions in a Dental Clinic: A Review, Cureus **17** (2025)
53. The Effect of AI on Cybersecurity. Inside Dentistry, (n.d.). https://insidedentistry.net/2025/07/cybersecurity/ (Accessed August 2, 2025)
54. S.N. Qurashi, F. Sobia, W.A. Hetany, H. Sultan, Enhancing cybersecurity defenses in healthcare using AI: a pivotal role in fortifying digital health infrastructure, medinformatics (2025)

MIX
Papier aus verantwortungsvollen Quellen
Paper from responsible sources
FSC® C105338

If you have any concerns about our products,
you can contact us on
ProductSafety@springernature.com

In case Publisher is established outside the EU,
the EU authorized representative is:
Springer Nature Customer Service Center GmbH
Europaplatz 3, 69115 Heidelberg, Germany

Printed by Libri Plureos GmbH
in Hamburg, Germany